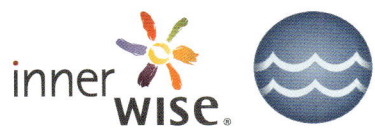

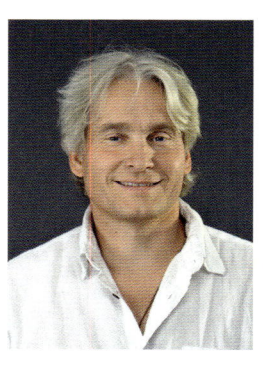

Uwe Albrecht:

I was born in 1966 and consider myself an evolutionary. Over the past 20 years, I've been developing *inner**wise***—an entirely new system for medical diagnostics and healing. More than 140,000 people are already using *inner**wise*** worldwide.

Creative lateral thinking, innovation and not accepting the status quo, coupled with practical research, make up my concept for success.

As a bestselling author, I've published more than ten books in several languages to date.

Supported by a team of mentors I've personally taught, I facilitate seminars and workshops in many countries.

For years I've been successfully applying the insights gained in my work with people to the diagnosis and therapy of systems, such as companies and organizations, projects, products, teams and crises.

This was made possible by the fact that I've been searching for the essence behind irritations, as this essence is applicable to everything. And for me, this essence is the field, which I've learned to read and transform.

"Change the field and reality follows."

UWE ALBRECHT

Intuitive Healing

THE EVOLUTIONARY METHOD

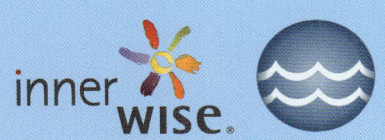

Visit our websites at:
www.innerwise.com

Important notice:
The information given in this book should not be treated as a substitute for professional
medical advice; always consult a medical practitioner. Any use of information provided in
this book is at the reader's discretion and risk. Neither the author nor the publisher can be
held responsible for any loss, claim or damage arising out of the use, misuse or suggestions
made herein, or the failure to take medical advice.

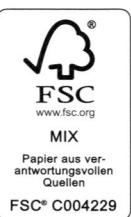

Published by Waterfront Digital Press
Cardiff California USA

English translation by Irina Pálffy-Daun-Seiler with assistance from Jill Kramer
Cover design by rootz-wingz.com
Drawings and photos by Alex Rath, Anna Badowska, Jörg Wilutzky,
Silke Kröger, Eric Frank, Katharina Kosak, Uwe Albrecht
Layout by Daniela Schulz, Puchheim
Printed and bound by Uhl, Radolfzell
Printed in Germany
ISBN 978-1-943625-64-2

2   4   5   3   1

Step out of your mind into
your intuition.
Only then will you be open to see
the world with all its miracles.
Then, your mind has meaningful things to
accomplish as well.

I am a physician; and my patients are people, animals, plants, buildings, systems,
projects, companies and organizations.
I treat all of them with the same
system: *innerwise*®.

Let your heart decide

The most important decisions in life come from the heart.
Before reading this book, ask your heart, and let it decide whether this is the
right path for you.
Take a few minutes to see how you're feeling right now:

Do you feel light or heavy inside?
Is your heart full of joy, or is there some sadness?
Do you trust in life, or are you afraid?
Do you have plenty of energy, or do you feel exhausted?
Does your breath feel open and expansive, or restricted and tight?
Can you look back at life with gratitude; or is there still guilt, anger or sadness?
Is your stance stable and do you feel grounded, or have you lost your footing?
Are you in the flow, or are you blocked?

Now, imagine that you've finished reading this book.
Do you feel lighter and fuller afterward—more joyful, trusting, open and
grounded? Do you feel like you're more in the flow and full of energy?
If you're not sure, try this once more with your eyes closed.
If you feel better when you imagine having read this book, I invite you to take
part in this exciting adventure.
If you don't feel better, or actually feel worse, it's better that you give this book
to someone else as a present and find another path for yourself.
Only do those things in life that feel good to you.
Trust your heart.

As I began to love myself, I understood that in any circumstance, I am in the right place at the right time, and everything happens at exactly the right moment. So I could be calm.
Today I know that this is "SELF-CONFIDENCE."

As I began to love myself, I found that anguish and emotional suffering are only warning signs that I was living against my own truth.
Today I know that this is "AUTHENTICITY."

As I began to love myself, I stopped craving a different life, and I could see that everything that surrounded me was inviting me to grow.
Today I know that this is "MATURITY."

As I began to love myself, I quit stealing my own time, and I stopped designing huge projects for the future. Today, I only do what brings me joy and happiness—things I love to do and that make my heart cheer—and I do them in my own way and in my own rhythm.
Today I know that this is "SIMPLICITY."

As I began to love myself, I freed myself of anything that is not good for my health—food, people, things, situations and everything that drew me down and away from myself.
At first I called this attitude a healthy egoism.
Today I know that this is "LOVE OF ONESELF."

As I began to love myself, I quit trying to always be right, and ever since I've been wrong less of the time.
Today I discovered that this is "MODESTY."

As I began to love myself, I refused to go on living in the past and worrying about the future.
Now, I only live for the moment, where EVERYTHING is happening.
Today I live each day, day by day, and I call it "FULFILLMENT."

As I began to love myself, I recognized that my mind can disturb me, and it can make me sick.
But as I connected it to my heart, my mind became a valuable ally.
Today I call this connection "WISDOM OF THE HEART."

We no longer need to fear arguments, confrontations or any kind of problems with ourselves or others. Even stars collide, and out of this collision, new worlds are born.
Today I know that THIS IS "LIFE"!

Attributed to Charlie Chaplin on his 70th birthday on April 16, 1959
(edited for clarity)

CONTENTS

Part I
Findings and Basics

The first part guides you through the basics and fundamental principles.
It serves to share experiences, deepen your consciousness and help you see more clearly.

Part II
Internal and External Tools

In the second part, you'll learn about the internal and external tools used in *intuitive healing*.

Part III
Healing All That Lives

The third part illustrates the many ways to use *inner**wise*** in the art of healing, the art of living and the art of business.

Introduction

There is only one book that is really worth reading—people themselves!
That's why I mapped out the text so that it can serve as an aid to help you read yourself.

Each chapter starts with topics and questions that you can answer intuitively, or respond to using the *arm-length test.*
Using the *arm-length test* reliably requires *spherical vision.*
We usually look at something from our personal perspective and compare what we see to our inner values. Here, we take our role as viewers very seriously. This naturally turns what we observe into a personal picture of reality. This picture, however, is of no use in our *intuitive healing* work, or with any other therapeutic system that works on such a deep level.
You need to look at something from all directions; free from intention, inner judgment, wishes or any comparison to past experiences. You need neutral *spherical vision,* an overview:

- Imagine that you see a gate in a wall in front of you. Now you're turning into an eagle and are flying high into the sky. As you look down, you now see an entire maze with an entrance.
- Or, imagine standing in the middle of a circle of people and being able to look at yourself with the eyes of all these people.

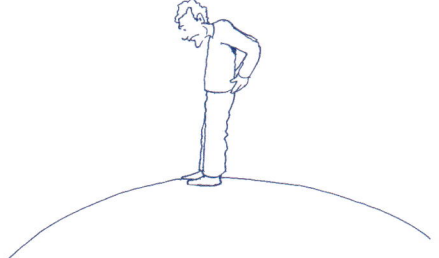

Looking at the world up close

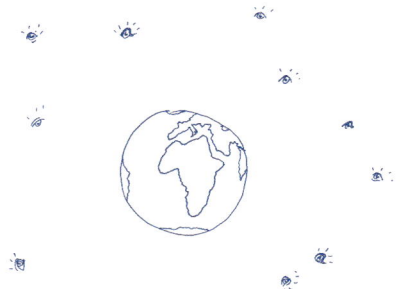

Looking at the world with the eyes of the stars

You will find the *spherical vision symbol* before each test question in this book as a reminder to apply spherical vision.

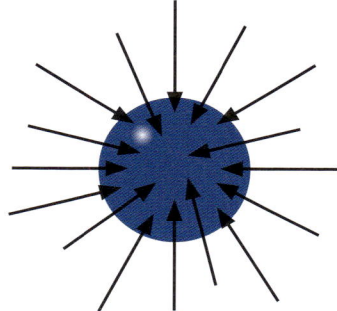

Spherical vision

The Arm-Length Test

Words are the language of the conscious mind.

The arm-length test is a way to communicate with our unconscious, with our heart. It is our body's ability to reveal fine changes on all levels.

When thinking or saying positive or negative statements, the length of our arms changes. But not only that: Our breath, stance, energy field, degree of muscle tension and much more also change when we think of something positive or negative for example; or when we simply say "yes" or "no."

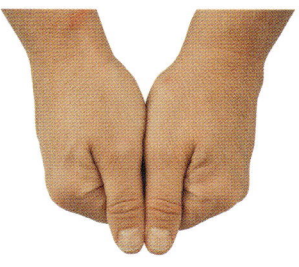

Positive statement, or "yes"

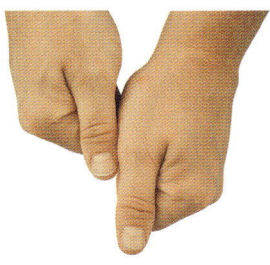

Negative statement, or "no"

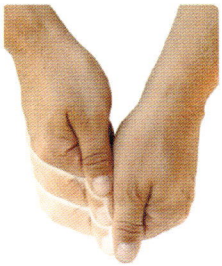

Testing position

✳ Stand up and let your arms hang loosely at your sides. Say "yes," and bring your arms together in a relaxed manner in front of your body, right at its center. When doing so, turn your thumbs to the front and compare their length. When you say "yes," your arms should be equally long.

✳ Now let them hang loosely at your sides again. Say "no," and once more bring them together in front of your body. The length of your arms, and thus, your thumbs, should differ.

In this way, your heart—your unconscious—can communicate with you through your body.

- If your arms already differ in length when saying "yes," you are out of balance; you are stressed.
- If the length of your arms doesn't change when you say "yes" or "no," you are blocked, caught in a state of rigidity.
- In both cases—stress or rigidity—the first thing to do is treat yourself.

The arm-length test: an overview

Regular test

Yes

No

Allergy/panic

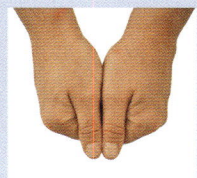 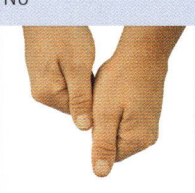 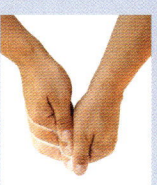

Initial stress ⟶ treat yourself

Yes

No

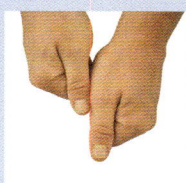 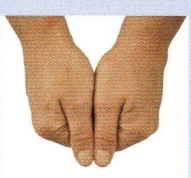

Blockage/rigidity ⟶ treat yourself

Yes

No

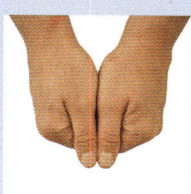 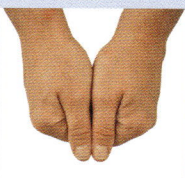

Yes

No

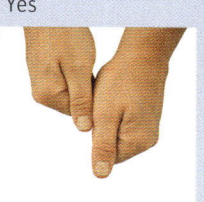 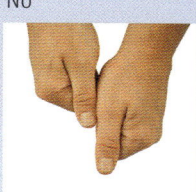

or

Stress/rigidity/blockage: treating yourself

When you think of the right remedy and imagine applying it, the stress disappears and the rigidity dissolves.

Remedies and ways to support healing:

- Drinking water
- Changing clothes
- Listening to music
- Speaking the truth
- Meditating
- Practicing yoga
- Painting
- Taking a shower
- Smelling flowers
- Drinking herbal tea
- Dancing
- Meditating with crystals
- Using homeopathy
- Going for a walk
- Treating yourself with *innerwise*

Testing

Always do the pre-tests:

- Say "yes" and test—your arms should be equally long.

- Say "no" and test—the length of your arms should differ.

- Always use spherical vision during testing.

- Am I allowed to test this? – Yes/No

- Will I receive a meaningful response? – Yes/No

Option 1 for beginners:

Make a statement or imagine something, then test.

- Your arms are equally long: **no stress.**

- The length of your arms differs: **stress.**

Option 2 for advanced practitioners:

You can now test using both statements and questions. Here, assessing the response depends entirely on how the question is phrased.

Examples:
Should I do … ? Does … harm me?

If it really harms you, your arms are equally long. Your body says "yes."

- Your arms are equally long: **yes.**

- The length of your arms differs: **no.**

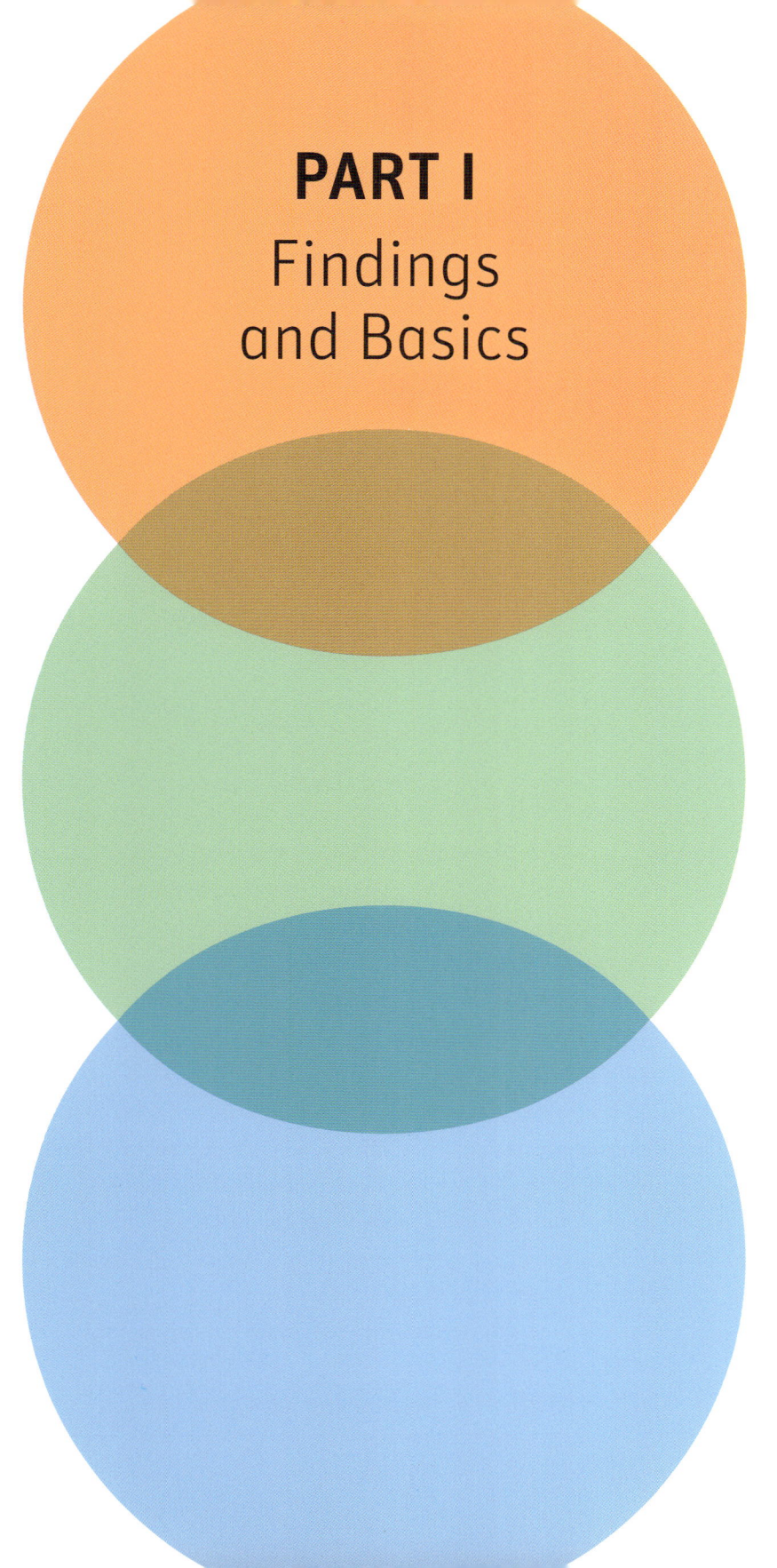

PART I
Findings and Basics

Overview

Following the tradition of the great spiritual laws, this first part sets out the basic principles and values involved in applying *intuitive healing*.

1. The Great Paradox

Our powerless mind

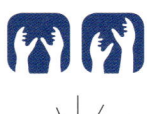
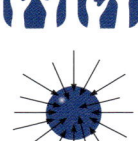

> Testing topics
>
> • I am healthy.
>
> • Imagine being happy.
>
> • I am worthy of being loved.
>
> • I am good at it.
>
> • I love myself.

The great paradox is that although everybody wants to be healthy, happy and successful, the unconscious actually wants, and thus manifests, the opposite.

Everybody wants to be healthy again. At least, that's what people claim.

Every patient who comes to see me for a treatment wants to be healthy again.

Every couple who comes to see me because they're hoping to conceive says that it's their greatest wish to have a baby.

Every entrepreneur who contacts me for coaching wants to be successful.

Every student who comes to me for coaching before an exam wants to pass that exam.

They all wish to be healthy, happy, successful, beautiful and simply good.

Then I double-check these statements using the arm-length test: I ask their unconscious how it feels about it, and in all cases, it responds without fail, "No, that's not what I want!" Consequently, there's a part in every human being that doesn't bow to the conscious mind and willpower, and has its very own ideas about life.

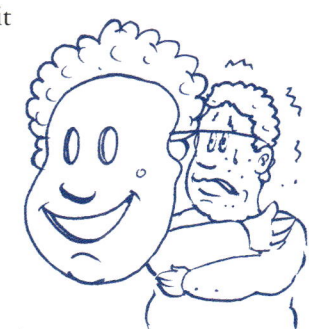

The arm-length test enables us to bypass the mind and communicate directly with the unconscious, which often yields interesting results.

The great paradox

The unconscious

- of those who are ill says, "I want to be ill; I need the illness for something!"
- of those hoping to conceive says, "A child with this partner in my current life situation with my issues won't work!"
- of unsuccessful people says, "You first need another experience; success won't do you any good right now."
- of the examinee says, "I'm not good enough ... I hate my teacher ... this reminds me of an unhealed trauma from childhood."

The big question is: How is the power of creating reality distributed across the conscious mind and the unconscious?
I tested many people and came to the following conclusion:
Usually, it was 95 to 99 percent for the unconscious, and 1 to 5 percent for the conscious mind.
I also met a few rare people whose conscious mind had reached 40 percent.

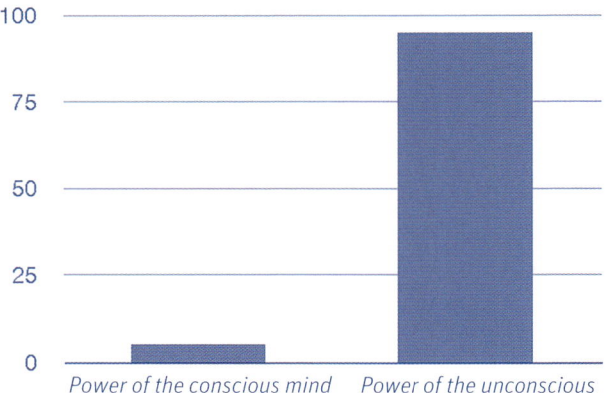

Distribution of power

This makes it crystal clear who the winner is when it comes to creating reality: the unconscious!

It explains why, for the most part, life doesn't bring us what we want.

Or, do you actually know millions of people with sexy bodies who've won the lottery, found the great loves of their lives and who own large beachfront villas?

Understanding this concept has serious consequences.

It's almost pointless to undergo therapy working solely on the level of the conscious mind and reason. We need a means of communication that reaches our unconscious, our life's main shareholder. We need remedies that can reach both the unconscious and the conscious mind and be effective in both those realms.

Let me illustrate this point once more:

When using the arm-length test, the unconscious of many people with cancer responds with a "no" when they imagine being alive, and with a "yes" when they imagine dying.

We reap what we sow … what will happen when such a message is sent out by such a powerful force?

We create our reality. It's just that we don't do it with our conscious mind, but rather, almost exclusively with our unconscious.

You can write a thousand times: "I love myself," and it won't change anything.

You can also clear the energetic charge of a deep feeling of shame from childhood and then feel more love for yourself than you did before.

2. The Principle of Integrity

Living in an unrelentingly honest way

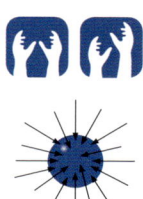

> ### Testing topics
>
> - I am honest.
>
> - I am whole and complete.
>
> - I am unbroken.
>
> - My integrity is … percent.

There's no better parameter for applying *intuitive healing* and working with *innerwise* than integrity.
Integrity means being honest, sincere, whole, sound, unbroken and unblemished. And that's exactly what *innerwise* stands for.

Since I love to make parameters more tangible and comparable, I often use a percentage scale.

If we want to measure integrity as a parameter, we first need to agree on what defines "complete integrity."
Complete integrity can only relate to a state directly between unity and duality, where the Divine and earthly life meet. I don't think that any human being can reach this state 100 percent, but I think it's possible to come very close.
Testing the mean value of the level of integrity that is actually lived out by all people on Earth shows that humanity as a whole is still very far from living with integrity.
If someone has 20 percent integrity, what is the remaining 80 percent made up of? This person may be dishonest, ill, broken … and the root cause of all of this is fear.
It is the dark part of the duality of our existence. It is the part that's always hungry for energy because it's not nourished by the divine source.

We all have it within us as long as we live in duality—that is, as long as we're alive.

Fear is the opponent of integrity.
Combined, they add up to 100 percent: integrity + fear factor = 100.

3. The Quintessence

Finding and living your soul purpose and understanding the lack of meaning and purpose

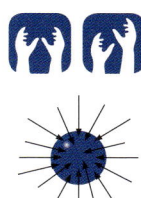

> ### Testing topics
>
> - I've found my soul purpose to an extent of ... percent.
>
> - I humbly accept my soul purpose and let it guide me.
>
> - I live my soul purpose to an extent of ... percent.

Before we go into detail, we have to ask questions about the meaning of life:
Why do we live? What is the higher purpose of life? Why did God create human beings?
Out of boredom, fun or for a specific purpose?
God—the One, the Source—is perfect; it is all that is.
But the One has a problem: just as one female human being cannot get pregnant by herself, the One needs duality to experience itself in new forms, to try itself out and to attain a new quality.
And here, humans come into play: As dual and mortal beings, they can gain experiences; and can have them either easily or with difficulty. That is, they can swim with or against the current of life.
Those who prefer the easy way start out by making an initial effort, search for and find the purpose of life, their soul purpose, and live it. In return for their trust, God offers them the gift of plenty of energy and divine providence.
Those who, in the end, prefer the difficult way, believing that they can reach their goal by using a shortcut—that is, by taking the beaten track in life instead of finding their own—don't receive the grace of plenty of energy and divine providence. As such, they will perceive life as a struggle.
Burkhard Heim was one of the greatest German researchers of the 20th century. As a young man, he lost both hands and most of his eyesight during WWII while

making a new type of explosive. Only two years later, he began to study chemistry, and after two more years, he switched to physics since he found chemistry no longer challenging enough. During his life, he underwent 36 surgeries to be able to better cope with what was left of his body. His scientific achievements are on par with those of Einstein. Some even say that they're far superior, as he was the first to create a unified field theory. Here is what he said about his fate and the purpose of his life on his 40th birthday:

> I have the impression that from the start, all that actually happens is right as it is. And that I shouldn't change much about the actual plan behind everything. From my point of view, what comes to me is right as it is and optimal for the circumstances as they are at the time.
>
> Some things may seem terrible to me, yet I think that in reality, they really aren't because everything is right as it is. Without any doubt, I have a certain purpose, since there's a point to why I even exist as a human being. Thus, it's my responsibility to embrace and live a specific purpose in life; this is the meaning and purpose of my whole existence, and fulfilling this life purpose is essential. And I will receive all I need to embrace and live my purpose, because if I didn't receive it, it would be meaningless for me to be here after all.
>
> I affirm that I have a purpose. What matters to me is finding out what this purpose is. It's imperative to work toward that. Of course, nothing falls in one's lap. I have to keep trying to drive myself eagerly and energetically so that I can succeed better in living my life purpose. This doesn't happen by itself. I can't just sit down and simply rest, saying, "It's all going to work out somehow." That's pretty obvious.

Original from "Das neue Weltbild des Physikers Burkhard Heim" (Physicist Burkhard Heim's New View of the World) by Illobrand von Ludwiger, published by Komplett Media Verlag

We will discuss Burkhard Heim again later on in this book, as his model of the 12 universal dimensions is integrated into *innerwise*.

The paths to your soul purpose

Those who have found and live their life purpose, their soul purpose or soul passion, enjoy an enriched life and inner fulfillment. They're nourished with all they need to experience abundance. Their inner glow inspires others, awakening their wish to also find, embrace and live their soul purpose.

Step 1: Finding your soul purpose

You can't search for your soul purpose. You can only find it within yourself. You can only "let it happen," as it's always there, waiting for you to finally give up your resistance to it.

This resistance is born out of our fear, which prevents you from mustering the courage to open up to, and embrace, your soul purpose.

Step 2: Embracing your soul purpose

Giving your soul purpose space in your life means surrendering to it. It means being honest with yourself and leaving behind everything in your life that keeps you from living that purpose.

It means being active, letting processes happen, trying things out and gaining new experiences.

Step 3: Living your soul purpose

You can discover the beauty in everything that your soul purpose has to offer. You can see the higher purpose of the challenges and experiences of your life, almost as if you're personally unaffected. In return, you'll have access to unlimited energy.

This past spring, I worked with a patient in the advanced stages of cancer. She spent most of her day watching TV, waiting for death. She was hoping to get more time from life. From me, she expected help and support; and from God, the grace of healing.

The following question arose in me: *What is she offering life, the Source, the Divine, in return? What is her soul purpose?*

Life doesn't work according to the principle: Once I'll be healthy again, I can do … Either we're able to do … anyway, no matter how we feel, or we'll never do it, because it's precisely doing … that gives us the strength to get healthy, to change our lives and become happier people. We're pulling ourselves up by our own bootstraps.

I suggested to this woman that she create an internet platform where she could describe how she'd given new meaning to her life by launching it; and to invite other people to also publicly share how they'd found meaning and purpose in their lives. It would be a beautiful side effect if that platform inspired others to follow her example.

The primary effect, however, was to build the platform only for herself and thereby take a step toward finding her soul passion in order to give meaning and purpose to her own healing.

Once we're able to tell life what is still ours to do as individual humans here on Earth, life will give us all we need to accomplish it.

4. Everything Is Alive!

Everything in this world has a soul

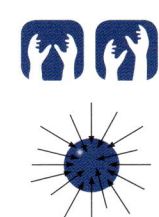

> **Testing topics**
>
> - Plants are alive and have an essence.
>
> - Buildings are alive and have an essence.
>
> - Ideas are alive and have an essence.
>
> - Projects are alive and have an essence.

"He who grasps the truth of the mental nature of the universe is well advanced on the path to mastery."

The Kybalion

If everything is alive, it all has to follow the same principles, and it must be possible to change it using the same methods.

- In an optimal state, everything is harmonious, in the flow.
- In an unhealthy state, everything is disharmonious and blocked.
- Everything has a soul, an essence; it's like a being.
- Everything is driven by fields.
- Everything can take on energetic charges.
- Everything can be perceived by different senses.
- Everything has a beginning and an end; only the time span in-between varies.

As a result, we can find ways and means of supporting everything in order to regain its flow. We can identify the essence of numerous different healing methods that can be applied to everything, so that everything can be treated.

Thus, I found that by healing the fields, the energies, the vibrations of any system by restoring harmony where there was disharmony, I could heal all that lives to the extent I'm allowed to.

Nada Brahma—the world is sound

Our world consists of sound, of rhythms. Matter is densified sound, but it remains sound, which can be harmonious or disharmonious.

> Music as we know it in our everyday language is only a miniature: that which our intelligence has grasped from that music or harmony of the whole universe which is working behind us … and which has been the source and origin of this nature. It is, therefore, that the wise of all ages have considered music to be a sacred art; for in music the seer can see the picture of the whole universe. … In the Vedas of the Hindus we read: Nada Brahma—sound, being the Creator. In the works of the wise of ancient India we read: "First song, then Vedas or wisdom." When we come to the Bible, we find: "First was the word, and the word was God," and when we come to the Qur'an, we read that the word was pronounced, and all creation was manifest. … This shows that the origin of the whole creation is sound. … When one looks at the cosmos, the movements of the stars and planets, the laws of vibration and rhythm—all perfect and unchanging—it shows that the cosmic system is working by the law of music, the law of harmony. Whenever that harmony in the cosmic system is lacking in any way, then in proportion, disasters come about in the world. …
>
> *Hazrat Inayat Khan*

What came first: matter or spirit?

I grew up as an atheist in socialist eastern Germany; by state decree, matter was the primary concern there.

Now I work equally with the spirit to transform matter.

Ever since I gave up the one-sided position of materialism and started to take spirit and matter into account, my life has become much easier. I'm also more successful as a medical doctor, and I obtain better results.

In this way, I gained access to the essence of things and grasped how they were connected; the higher principles of life revealed themselves.

It is the way in which Werner Heisenberg described it:

"The first gulp from the glass of natural sciences will turn you into an atheist, but at the bottom of the glass God is waiting for you."

Werner Heisenberg

innerwise is alive as well.

It chose its name itself, which came to me in a meditation.

innerwise—healing by reconnecting to your inner wisdom.

Discovering the intelligence inherent in *innerwise* was one of the greatest miracles I ever experienced.

Healing energies that self-adjust to the user, such as homeopathic remedies, for example, which select the optimal potency themselves and are then available in the resonance potency.

A testing system that guides the optimal way through the treatment.

innerwise—a therapeutic system with autopilot.

innerwise is a global energetic network that is perceived and sensed by all who are involved with it. This also includes the rise in the energy level of the *innerwise* system once we're able to handle higher energies based on a higher level of consciousness, without putting ourselves in danger. As soon as this rise occurs, I receive e-mails and calls from practitioners around the world who confirm that *innerwise* has evolved to a new level.

The client's safety is also taken into account: If therapists or coaches aren't balanced themselves and lack clarity, *innerwise* reduces the energies available to these practitioners to prevent damage. If therapists are completely blocked but still want to treat someone in this state, the system closes up by itself.

All of this can only work based on an inherent intelligence, and it is a privilege to be able to experience it.

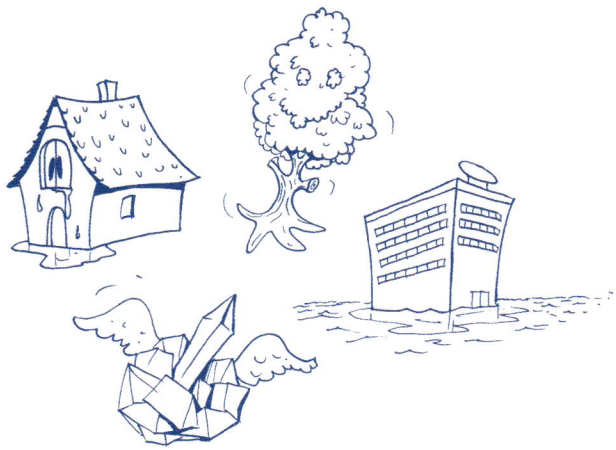

Everything is alive!

5. The Principle of the Field

Change the field and reality follows

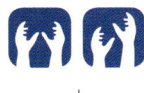

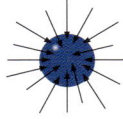

Testing topics

- I have (1, 2, 3, more than 5) energy fields.

- My energy field is homogeneous.

- My energy field is fragmented in time.

- My energy field is fragmented in identity.

"There is no place in this new kind of physics both for the field and matter, for the field is the only reality."

Albert Einstein

Fields

Fields are sound spaces, energy clouds, energetic states that contain a charge and thus a directionality, a focus.

The field always wins

Fields are the basic and all-pervasive force. Matter corresponds to densified fields, with tiny particles mixed in. Solid structures consist of minuscule particles that appear solid because they move at a nearly infinite speed. For comparison, take the image of a rotating fan presenting an impenetrable obstacle.

But a fan also depends on electricity: Increasing the power will make it oscillate faster; turning it off will bring it to a standstill.

Fields cause matter to vibrate; this is similar to how the human body follows the rhythm of music on a dance floor.

If we want to change reality, changing the fields that create reality is the easiest and most effective way.

Change the music and the body will dance in a different way.

With sharpened senses, fields of the present, past or future can be perceived and transformed energetically. This is the direct way to change reality.

The field structures reveal the interactions of different fields. This allows us to identify the causes, and understand how things are connected on a larger scale.

Reality follows the field

The world is sound—it's vibration—and reality unfolds into this sound space. Our lives' structure and experiences need a blueprint, which is contained in the sound of the fields.

Our DNA is simply an antenna for the divine sound of Creation. After mapping the human genome, scientists were so frustrated when they had to acknowledge that with some 25,000 genes, humans had only a few more genes than simple worms or fruit flies. Consequently, genes can't explain the unique characteristics of human beings. The number of genes doesn't even suffice to explain how all the different biological substances are created that we're made up of.

Imagine shredding a DVD and then trying to find the music or images with the best available microscopes.

Searching for quanta, the smallest possible entities, may lead to missing the big picture.

Exposing water to specific frequencies generates typical sound images—that is, patterns in the water. Love is one of the strongest fields; anyone who ever truly loved somebody knows that the power of love can change absolutely anything without any effort. No word, instruction or rule could ever manage to do so.

The field is a morphogenetic factor that is permanently present—like the Sun, our life-giving source of energy, whose energy enables and influences all life.

If I want to change reality, the easiest and fastest way is to change the field—to clear it of any foreign energies so that all that's foreseen in someone's life plan can occur without resistance.

Forms of energy fields

Fields are so beautiful when they're open, free, unlimited, shiny and harmonious. When living in such an environment, we can experience much joy and have a lot of fun! We can also call it a beautiful atmosphere.

And we can experience even more happiness when our field is free and beautiful. This is also evident in the way we breathe, walk, think, feel and talk.

Most people's lives look different, and so do their fields. They're blocked; energetically charged; caught in the past; burdened with patterns and imprints; deformed; loaded with guilt, fear and other junk; and linked to and intertwined with the fields of other people. In addition, there's the influence of the superordinate fields of one's respective home country, the continent, as well as the global morphogenetic field.

Altogether, they often appear to be one big noise, with infinite disharmony.

Fragmented fields

Our fields are often fragmented in different times, identities and realities.

Someone's knee was injured 20 years ago and still hurts; someone's heart broke five years ago and is still broken; someone's liver still contains the anger from 22, 18, 15, 7, 3 years ago, including the anger that arose last year.

With our right leg, we walk like our father; in our left hand, we still carry our mother's pain; the penis carries the shame from 13 years ago; in the pelvic area, there's still the soul of the child that couldn't come in to Earth 9 years ago; and our head is still buzzing with thoughts from our life thus far.

These are examples of a bunch of fragments from different times with different identities. Everything that is still within us but not yet resolved and cleared up carries an energetic charge. And this charge creates reality: pain, tension, malfunction, illness.

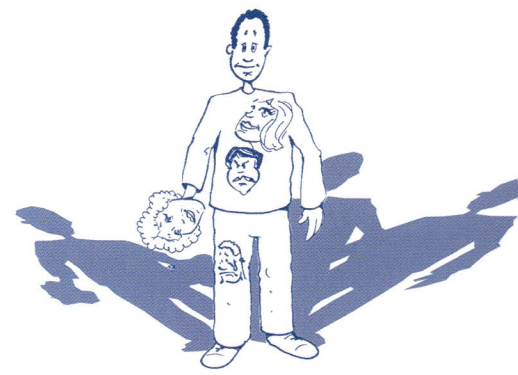

Who am I, and how many?

Fragmentation as a measured parameter

Clearing up the fragmentation of our bodies and fields is an essential step toward greater integrity.

We can test the average fragmentation value in terms of percent, but this only provides us with an overview and nothing more.

Here, we already have to take into account the fact that fragmentation and separation can occur not only in the body, but in all our fields and structures—that is, also in our energy field.

Thus, it makes more sense to test the location and level of the highest local fragmentation and to then treat that area.

For example: In one of your hands, you carry the field of your partner. In the worst case, your hand has a local fragmentation value of 100 percent, since 100 percent of this field is no longer integrated and part of your field. This value can also be 76, 34, 15, 4 (or whatever) percent.

The value isn't that important; what matters is that we treat all areas of our Being where parts are separated, and put an end to this fragmentation and separation. For only parts of our Being that are integrated are part of us and behave in this way.

Homogeneous fields

The great dream (some also call it enlightenment) is to have a homogeneous field, to be fully in the now, to be free and to be the creator of your own life. A homogeneous field is free of limitations; it's open to any development. It's simply a space where anything can happen because it's unrestricted.

This is exactly what every kind of healing modality intends to support.

The way to achieve this is by clearing up old charges: making peace with the past, being honest with ourselves, giving back the issues we carry for other people, clearing our energy field and healing our soul.

This sounds like a lot of work, but it doesn't have to take an eternity if we consistently progress along this path.

When we live with integrity, our fields are homogeneous.

The field of your soul

The original field is our individual soul field. It's modified, however, by the unresolved issues of our lives. As energetic charges, these issues re-create certain realities so that we have the opportunity to resolve the issues and learn something.

But what happens when someone doesn't have his/her own identity—that is, when the arm-length test reveals a "no" response to the statement "I am I"?

In that case, that person carries the identity of another soul, of an external field, and is subject to its influence and life plan. And in that situation, we have a big conflict: no matter what we do, we won't be happy.

For this reason, having your own identity is the most important foundation of a happy and meaningful life.

Several energy fields

It's normal to have only one field, that of our own soul. You can test this easily using the arm-length test.

- "I have one field."   *Yes/No*

- "I have two fields."   *Yes/No*

- …

- "I have more than five fields."   *Yes/No*

- …

As a therapist, I've seen patients with anywhere from 1 to 25,000 fields.

- 1 to 5 are common.

- 20 to 100 frequently occur when people are open.

- 100 to 500 can be found with therapists who take on the issues and energies of their clients until they can't take it anymore.

- Over 1,000 can be found with very spiritually open people who take on any soul and energy that's around them. Sometimes they can also see these souls/

energies and feel responsible for taking them to the Light, yet often they don't manage to do so.

Except for someone who has conceived a child, there are usually two ways to get more than one field:

1. By taking it over voluntarily —that is, if somebody has never been loved unconditionally and hopes to receive some kind of substitute love by being good or nice, by helping others or by carrying issues for other people.

2. Through manipulation. Here, a foreign energy field serves to access someone else's energy—a "hostile takeover," so to speak.

In the **first case,** the only way out is to recognize our own value and the fact that we don't help other people by shouldering their loads, as this eases the self-created pressure they need in order to change something.
We can only inspire other people through the way we lead our own lives, thereby supporting them in finding their own power and strength within, resolving their issues, putting an end to any compromises, and finding and living their soul purpose.
Building this self-worth requires resolving our lives' earliest traumas and feelings of rejection. This includes not being a wanted child at the time of our conception, our parents' doubts during pregnancy, or being loved by our parents as a substitute for the love that got lost *between* them.

In the **second case,** it's necessary to see through the manipulative games and prevent them from being used in the future.

The influence of superordinate fields

Take an evening stroll down a street of single-family homes sometime and stop in front of one of them. Close your eyes and tune in to yourself: Feel your stance, your breath, your mood, your energy field and your body structure. Once you've sensed yourself, imagine living in this house for three years and tune in to yourself again. You will feel the difference.
Go to the next house and repeat the exercise. After stopping in front of a few homes, you'll notice that with each of them, you've felt different.
Depending on the field you choose, your future can vary greatly: friends, partner, home, job …

Every time I fly back from the Americas, Asia or Africa and land in Frankfurt, I feel the heavy burden that we carry in Europe, especially here in Germany, as a consequence of a past that hasn't been dealt with. Suddenly, I feel like I have a 20-pound weight on my shoulders.

In the same way that we get used to any burden, Europeans have also gotten used to this one and don't necessarily feel it anymore. And still, it's a field that influences us constantly.

The global fear factor is even more comprehensive. I asked 20 people to test it independently of one another. They all obtained the same results: over the past 2,000 years, it rose from 10 to almost 90 percent; in 1900, it was still around 30 percent This increase to the current level has resulted from the disasters of the last century or so: two World Wars, Chernobyl, 9/11, the Fukushima nuclear incident and the global financial crisis.

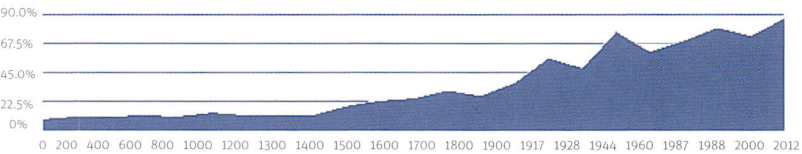

Development of the global fear factor over the last 2,000 years, in percents

When a field is ruled by fear at a 90 percent rate, it's impossible to manifest a great deal of positive things. When fear rules people's lives, joy and happiness decline.

If we want to change something on planet Earth, we first need to lower the fear factor, because if we do not, it will manifest even more chaos and destruction.

For one person alone, it's not easy to remove him- or herself from these fields and become immune to them, yet it's necessary to do so in order to be able to see clearly again and make the right decisions.

- **Choose the path that allows you to develop most freely and where you feel the happiest.**
- **Tune in to yourself first to see how your life would develop if you took a certain path or if you chose a certain field. Only then should you decide, because the field always wins.**

6. The Principle of Fear

Fear is calling

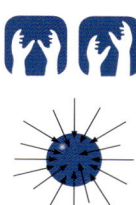

> ### Testing topics
>
> - My fear factor is … percent.
>
> - To a degree of … percent, I'm driven by my basic fears, such as the fear of pain, the fear of dying, the fear of starving to death or the fear of not being loved.

Fear is the opposite of trust.

Fear prevents flow and divine providence.

Fear manifests itself like no other force in life.

You only have to be afraid of something long enough and strongly enough and you will attain that thing or situation.

Fear kills love.

Fear likes to cling to the desire to possess—that's what's called jealousy.

Fear deprives people of freedom, including ourselves.

Fear desires safety and security.

Fear never gets enough safety—that's what's called greed.

Fear tries to cover up the wounds of the soul that aren't healing, but it can never heal them.

Most people live with a fear factor of over 70 percent. This means that their lives are ruled by fear at a rate of 70 percent. These fears are not always present at the surface; rather, they lie at a deeper level, such as the fear of:

not being loved,

suffering from pain,

starving,

not having a purpose.

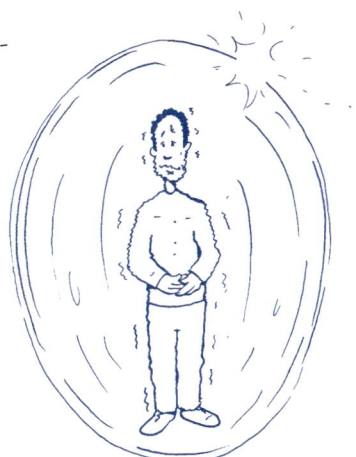

The principle of fear

A fear factor of more than 90 percent generates almost exclusively negative experiences: everybody is bad; the world is evil; it's necessary to fight against everyone and everything. In the business world, a person with this level of fear can drive one company after another into bankruptcy and then file multiple lawsuits, still trying to blame others for everything.

With a fear factor of 70 to 90 percent, there are many good ideas and approaches, but final implementation fails due to inner sabotage.

If the fear factor lies between 50 and 70 percent, life starts to be fun, and success and abundance set in. The lives of such people can be enriched by happiness and divine providence.

Very few people live with a value below 50 percent. It can be achieved for a short time in meditation, during an orgasm, or sometimes when dancing or taking drugs; but this state doesn't last, and the smallest irritation will destroy this idyllic state again.

With spherical vision and the consciousness of taking into account all fears, testing yourself can yield real and usable results.

7. From the Homo sapiens to the Homo integer—the integrated human

Nomen est omen: humans behave as they have been named

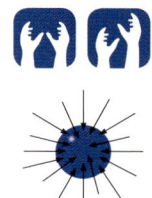

> **Testing topics**
>
> • I have integrity.
>
> • I am honest.
>
> • I am sound.
>
> • I am incorruptible.
>
> • I am whole and complete.

The meaning of "integer" in Latin is much deeper than in English. It means living with integrity. I follow the Latin roots.

Since the field always wins and creates our reality, it's crucial that we pay attention to the words and names we use, as they're a field as well. In other words, we choose certain words as an expression of their field.

With respect to *innerwise*, for instance, we changed the term "trainer" to "mentor." During the translation of our website into English, it became clear that in English, "trainer," used in the field of sports, wasn't suitable for our workshops.

The etymological dictionary explains: "trainer"—"to train": "to pull," "to draw" … so some things became clear to me. I realized that by using the term "trainer," I'd created some learning tasks myself over the past years by "training" people who matched the energy field of this word.

A **mentor** refers to someone who's experienced and can provide wise guidance, and this fits my intention.

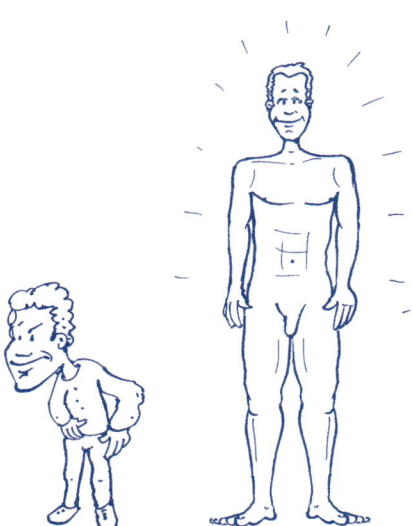

From the Homo sapiens to the Homo integer — the integrated human

Also, in organizational or product coaching, it's frequently necessary to change a name because it no longer fits the current situation. For instance, when a son takes over his father's business, often a name change needs to be made so that the son can fulfill himself, rather than managing the father's legacy.

And it's precisely the same thing with the *Homo sapiens* who is the wise, reasonable, smart, judicious, understanding, diplomatic human. But being reasonable doesn't necessarily mean being honest; being understanding isn't as broad as being circumspect, and diplomacy involves lying.

Thus, humans currently behave as they have been named.

If we want to effect global change, it will be primarily necessary to change the field. A new designation for human beings requires that we include all values needed for a new planet Earth that's worth living on.

And this designation is *Homo integer*—the integrated human—the honest, pure, decent, intact, whole, sound, unblemished, unspoiled, pristine, authentic, unbroken, complete and incorruptible human. What a world that would be!

It's time for the *Homo integer*—and for an honest, whole, sound, lovable Earth worth living in!

Nomen est omen.

8. The Principle of Now

The now is not ill

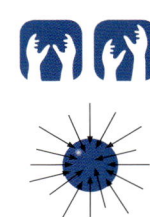

> ### Testing topics
>
> - I live in the now.
>
> - My problems stem from the past.
>
> - My problems stem from the future.
>
> - My now is free, and I can create it freely.

Illness doesn't exist in the now

In the now, there's no illness, tears, pain or failure. All this can occur only because the past is still within us, and because we don't live fully in the now with all our aspects.

When those with cancer come to see me and tell me they've had cancer for five weeks because that's when they were diagnosed, I test how long they've actually *had* cancer with the arm-length test: 5 years—yes; 10 years—yes; 15 years—yes; 20 years—no.

Often, the cancer has been in their bodies for 15 to 20 years. If I then tell them the exact year, they spontaneously remember an event: "Oh, that was when my beloved mother died; I still miss her so much." Or, "That was when we got divorced; I still hate her." Or, "That was when our child died."

Usually, cancer starts with an undigested energetic or emotional event. Over the years, it manifests itself through the different layers: the energetic, emotional, mental and biochemical levels; and at some point, it exists in the form of a cancer cell. When two to four million cancer cells have been formed, the growth is large enough to be detected in an ultrasound or x-ray exam. And for most people, that's the day they "got" cancer.

The same applies to any illness or disorder.

If we were only in the now, those issues wouldn't exist. But since we preserve old energetic charges like a museum, and often also put them on display, we give them the power to rule our lives.

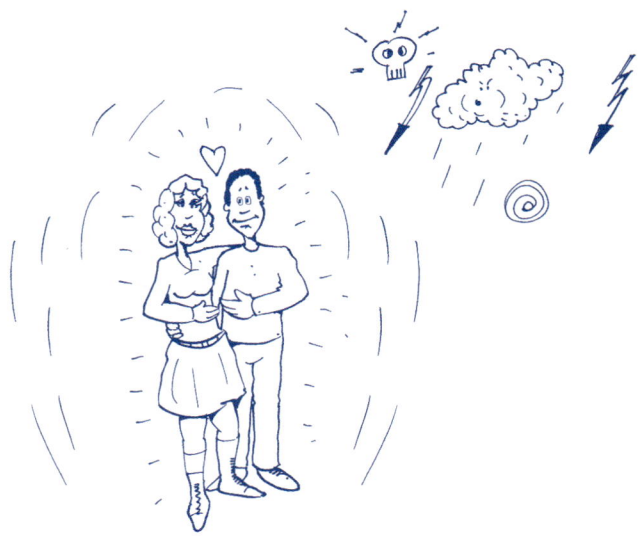

The now doesn't have a problem.

Healing in space and time

Healing is most effective at the point in time when the illness or disorder was created. In the now, healing is neither possible nor necessary.

Parts of our body that are ill or stuck in time aren't in the now. This can be determined with the arm-length test by asking in which time the specific part of the body is.

By using the arm-length test, we can identify when the primary cause of an illness or disorder occurred; with our consciousness, we can then let the healing energies unfold their effects at that point in time.

This can go back days, weeks, years or back to the time when we were in our mother's womb; it can also be related to the lives of our parents.

It can even go back several generations if the cause is there. We only have to identify the right recipient and time frame for the healing energies; then a very small impulse can have a major impact.

Reality spaces: What is time anyway?

Are their parallel worlds? Is time really as linear as it seems to us? To what extent do other people's destinies influence our lives?

I asked a 40-year-old man to imagine being 3 years old and to describe his living space at that time, with all the people who were around him. Then I worked with the healing cards, and the man described how the space changed. We worked in this way until the space he saw felt good to him, and as a result, a symptom in the now disappeared. The next day, this man's mother called and related that she'd experienced a spontaneous healing the previous day.

If you transform something in the past and heal it, this changes the now, and consequently, the future as well. Is it possible that all these times exist in parallel? When you give healing cards to clients and ask them to offer the healing frequencies as presents to the souls of long-dead ancestors, it often happens that they can see the grateful reactions of the ancestors with their inner eyes. One male patient, for example, called three weeks later saying that for the first time in his life, he'd had a really good orgasm. Previously, he'd always felt guilty about his sexual partners, although he couldn't understand why.

A small girl suddenly developed a high fever. Her parents were separated, and at the time, the girl was staying with her father for a while. The mother called and said that she wasn't surprised that her daughter had gotten ill, because she (the mother) was pregnant and had just decided to have an abortion. Despite the geographical distance, the three-year-old felt this and was shocked, which caused a state of total rigidity. With the help of the fever, she was able to "burn" herself free of this state.

This is how ingenious our bodies can be in order to help themselves. Nowadays, holistic pediatricians are actually glad when a child is still able to respond with a fever.

We have to grasp the links causing disorders or other problems systemically in space and time in order to be able to address and resolve problems at their root.

The past and the future influence the present.

We think that only past events have an effect on our now: "My life is like this because I experienced this or that in the past."

However, the future also influences the present: "Events cast their shadows before us."

The book *Theory U* by Otto Scharmer describes leading from the future as it emerges through "presencing," a process that involves precognitive sensing.

The future will only influence our reality in an energetically negative way if we aren't following our own path; we then swim against the current. Using a different image, we then move like a snow pusher: the mountain of snow in front of us gets bigger and bigger, thus requiring more and more strength to move it.

By changing the now, we can also affect the future.

If you go on an inner journey through time, moving forward through the upcoming years and sensing when and if stress arises, and you verify this with the arm-length test, you're able to perceive problems already in the now.

As everything that causes stress contains an energetic charge with the power to manifest itself, this also applies to the future.

In this way, the energetic charge of the future can already have an adverse effect on you today.

Now you can test what has to be changed in the present to freely create your future and to remove the stress.

When testing future events, it's important to understand the following:

When we test something that lies in the future, we can only perceive what will happen if people continue to follow the path they've chosen. Every decision to correct the current path in the now also changes the future.

That's why predictions about the future are so relative; in all honesty, this phrase should always be added: "If you don't change anything, this or that could happen."

Come back to the path of your soul, back in the flow, and re-create your future. So, is time real? That's an illusion.

9. The Principle of the Basic Energies

Deciphering life's energies

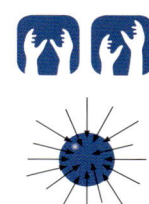

> ### Testing topics
>
> - My soul energy is …
>   (between 0 and 100) percent.
>
> - My structurizing energy is …
>   (between 0 and 100) percent.
>
> - My life energy is …
>   (between 0 and 100) percent.
>
> - My creative energy is …
>   (between 0 and 100) percent.
>
> - My love energy is …
>   (between 0 and 100) percent.

Which energies are really vital to our lives? How can we measure them and assess their impact when they change? How can we remedy deficits in these energies?

Spiritus mundi—the world ether

The world ether is the superordinate principle to human existence, the spirit of the world, or *spiritus mundi.*
It is the energy that fills the space and isn't individualized.
Out of this world ether, soul energy is created, which is the part that creates the individual, thus becoming soul energy.

The five basic energies

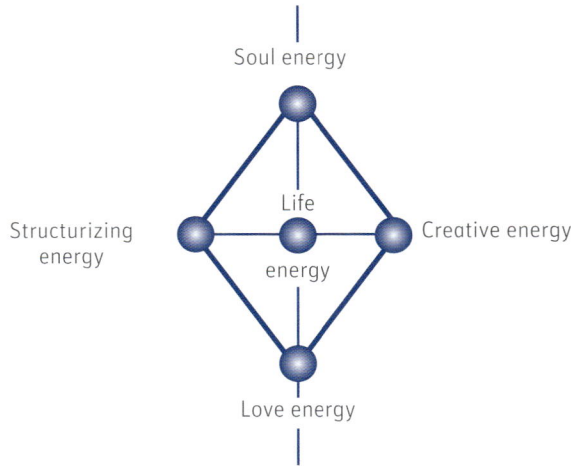

The five basic energies

All living beings have their **soul energy.** It is the individual sound that contains the basic information about this being.

When life is being created, this soul energy differentiates into three kinds of energy: structurizing energy, life energy and creative energy.

We can also see this in the yin and yang symbol: form, energy flow and evolution when considering the timeline.

Structurizing energy creates the space, the body, the temple of the soul.

Thanks to the structurizing energy, stem cells can differentiate. If this energy is strong enough, organs are created. It reflects the principle of structure.

Life energy provides the energy needed by the human system and keeps it moving. It reflects the principle of flow. It is also referred to as *qi, orgone* or *prana.* It's like the energetic charge of a battery: when the battery is full, everything works; when it's almost empty, functionality stops.

Creative energy enables a living being to be creative, in the sense of creative energy manifesting itself through the living being. The being becomes the morphogenetic canal in the process of Creation. Beethoven, for example, first saw the notes of Symphony No. 9 with his inner eye before he played them. This energy represents the creative principle.

All three kinds of energy unite to become **love energy.** By living their soul purpose, their soul passion, human beings transform their soul energy into love or heart energy, which then flows back into the *spiritus mundi,* the sounds of the worlds.

The five energies in the individual phases of our lives

1. The optimum (hardly found)

When an ovum fuses with a sperm at conception, the structurizing and life energy are each usually at a level of 100 percent.

The creative energy is still dormant; it only starts to unfold when the child is born. For this reason, we don't take it into account when the child is in the mother's womb.

During pregnancy, the structurizing energy amounts to about 80 percent, and the life energy is at 100 percent.

At birth, the structurizing energy drops below 50 percent; life energy remains at 100 percent, and the creative energy enters into play with 100 percent.

During pregnancy and one's entire life, the soul and love (or heart) energy remain at 100 percent.

It could stay like this for an entire healthy, happy and creative life. Yet that's not what happens.

2. The common scenario

During pregnancy, life, soul, love (or heart) and structurizing energy are already decreasing—sometimes only temporarily, and they recover again in part or in full.

After birth, the structurizing energy drops down to 10 to 20 percent, which disturbs the body's morphogenetic development and empowerment. The body loses form and strength; it becomes "doughy." This is typically represented in overweight children with reduced mobility. An organized body turns into a "pile of cells."

The life energy of these children already decreases to 70 or 50 percent; after they're vaccinated, it can even go down to 30 percent. These kids lose their vitality, although there's usually still enough to spend five hours watching TV, playing computer games or being on Facebook when they're a bit older. Time and again, they fall ill, catching colds, coughs or inflammations of the middle ear, and so on. These children will never climb up trees or romp around in the snow, beaming with joy all the while.

Frequently, the creative energy doesn't even reach its peak and quickly drops to minimal levels. The creative potential that's actually expressed will not lead to significant achievements.

Love energy reveals itself through inner beauty, but as it declines rapidly before the middle years of life, this beauty fades, and the corners of the mouth start to droop as a result.

As soul energy decreases, people's eyes lose their shine, and their energy field weakens.

Thus, we have the typical Homo sapiens, as we know them.

The individual energies

Soul energy

It can be tested as **"soul energy in percents."**

Usually, it's sufficient to set the soul-energy level at the time of incarnation at 100 percent and then test what has changed in comparison. It's possible that even in an unborn child, values can be as low as 20 percent, because soul fragments were lost or separated after incarnation.

One of the primary tasks of parents is to keep the soul of the unborn child whole and give birth to a child who has its full glow. As a result of profound injuries and various kinds of manipulation, soul fragments can get lost; it's not uncommon to find adults with only 2 percent soul presence left. Their eyes are dead, and their aura is often gray or dark brown to black.

Life has turned into mere survival.

In therapy, we can determine when and why this decline occurred and identify direct ways to increase these individuals' soul energy. But often, we can't treat the soul energy or presence directly; rather, we can only use it as a parameter to check where we stand in the treatment.

If we let the testing systems guide us though a treatment, the value of the soul presence increases as fundamental issues are addressed. After a treatment, this value should not be below 15 percent, with 100 percent being the optimal level.

However, the following has to be taken into account: we human beings aren't born with perfectly whole and complete souls, but only with fragments of it. As a result, there's an imperfection, a pattern of energetic charges, which is often referred to as *karma*. Finding the remaining parts and reintegrating them is the great quest of every human being.

Only individuals who've regained enlightenment have perfect souls. It's a lot of work and mostly a lifelong search, and not many people attain this state.

This means that we can test two different values of soul energy, depending on what we're referring to: the state of the soul at incarnation where only a part of the whole and complete soul was present, or the whole and complete soul when it was created out of the One, the Divine.

It's important to take all of this into account, as the comparative value has to be defined clearly for testing.

Structurizing energy

Identifying this energy took me longest to do.

Over the past few years, I kept experiencing phases of two to four weeks where I hardly ate anything anymore. There was no intention behind it, nor was I newly in love; most of my appetite simply vanished. But then life offered me great challenges so that I couldn't maintain this state and again required more food. In these phases, I always felt that I had a particularly high energy level.

I developed a scale for this energy, which was unknown to me up to that point, and correlated it with my eating habits over the course of two years.

If this energy level was low, I felt that I had to compensate for my lack of energy with food, so I gained weight.

When higher values were present, I still cleaned my plate, but I no longer went to the fridge late at night, and I was able to maintain my weight.

When these energy levels increased further, it was similar to the state of being newly in love: I felt that I was satisfied after eating just half of the usual portion of food.

Meanwhile, I was able to name this type of energy—it's "structurizing energy." It is the energy that gives shape to our body, strength to our muscles, elasticity to our tissue, dignity and pride to what we radiate from within (that is, our charisma) and straightens our spine.

When reaching a certain level, this energy serves as a fountain of youth, and it becomes possible to renew tissue and organs.

Illness and chaos arise where the internal structure and order are destroyed. Structurizing energy creates this structure and order. It ensures that the genetic program manifests itself.

As our body constantly renews itself; as each cell is replaced within hours, days, weeks or months at the latest, time and again we have the opportunity to re-create the original program, and not just the deficits. Usually, each scar, each age spot, each organic disorder, is re-created (including the disorder), since the overall and local structurizing energy is so low that it can't re-create the original—the completely healthy body.

This energy is one of the secrets of the Russian method (according to professor and academician Grigori Grabovoi), which makes it possible to re-create organs. Another secret that plays a role here is the Russian people's deep belief in the divine force.

When we measure this energy in percentages, most people's structurizing energy is below 25 percent. Regrowing organs requires lasting values of over 67 percent. Dipping briefly into very high levels doesn't suffice; it's necessary to reach a high level and maintain it on a long-term basis.

Structurizing energy scale

0–10 percent:
The body is merely a hungry mass of cells. Typical signs are lack of strength, diminished enthusiasm for exercise, pain and "food doping." Chaos and destruction run virtually freely throughout the body, which stops functioning relatively early. Money deposited into a retirement fund is basically wasted, as the person probably won't be around to claim the benefits.

10–20 percent:
By applying self-discipline with food, participating in sports regularly and sometimes putting on a mask, people manage to look fairly good and consider themselves to be performing at "normal" capacity. This is the active average human being who will reach retirement age in a more or less healthy state, and who only starts to have problems when self-discipline wanes.

20–40 percent:
Life is like being newly in love. Minor lows can be compensated for fairly quickly.

40–67 percent:
Hardly anybody can maintain this energy level on a permanent basis; however, many try to look like they do with the help of Botox and so on. We're talking about very healthy, active and radiant people who look much younger than their age.

68–100 percent:
That's the ideal level. By maintaining focus, targeted healing is possible, and we can generate vibrating energy fields in certain parts of our body that enable healing.

These lucky people have discovered the fountain of youth. It's important to take into account that frequently people's percentage levels don't remain constant and can fluctuate very strongly

It's possible to reach a level of structurizing energy of 70 percent at a therapy session or when doing qigong and then drop down to 7 percent two hours later after an argument.

The natural course of structurizing energy

When an egg is fertilized with semen, the level of structurizing energy is at 100 percent, enabling the creation of life. During pregnancy, the level goes down to 80 percent; it's still high enough for the creation of organs and structures. At birth, the value drops to 50 percent or below. This decline induces the delivery. By the age of 20, the level of structurizing energy will have gone down to merely 30 percent and continues to decrease further to 10 percent in old age. This also explains the aging process: at such low levels of structurizing energy, organs cannot regenerate, nor can natural healing occur.

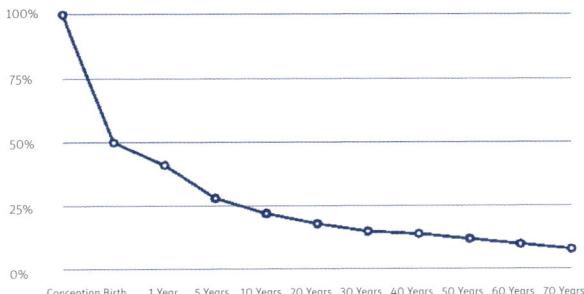

Normal decrease in the level of structurizing energy throughout life (in percents)

By working with *innerwise*, it becomes possible to change this graph.

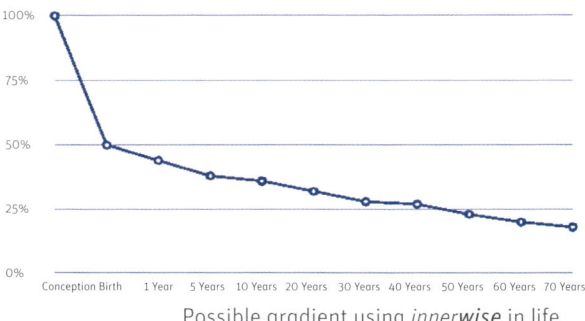

Possible gradient using *innerwise* in life

Life energy

It has many names: *orgone, qi, prana …* and it has two characteristics:

1. The energy potential, like the energetic charge of a battery.

2. Flow; flowing through the body, distributing energy. This often happens in the meridians, as described in Chinese medicine; or, when the energy rotates, like in the chakras.

Over a number of years, I energetically measured each of the 20 meridians individually (*qi* in percents) in thousands of patients and then calculated the arithmetic mean.

This mean value corresponded precisely to the level that I'd measured as life energy.

These meridian measurements also worked really well to monitor progress during treatments. With the positive effects of the treatment, the values during medical checkups also improved. But negative influences from chemotherapy also showed clearly.

When measuring life energy, surprisingly, I discovered that its level always correlated with the way people felt at that moment.

In the charts, the qi is displayed in percents from 0 to 100. A maximally round circle is the optimum; this means 100 percent qi in all meridians. Here, you can see the data of the studies:

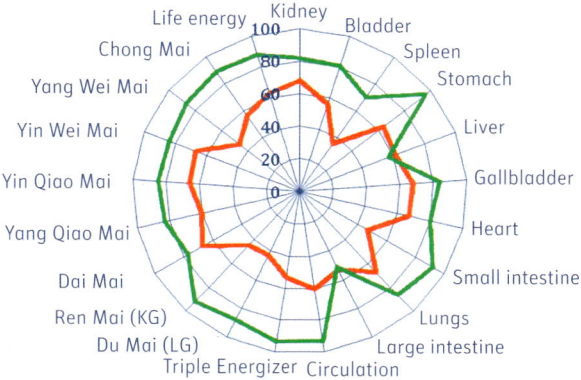

Patient has a tumor, allergies and asthma.
Meridian values, first treatment, October 6, 2002 (red line)
Second treatment, November 20, 2002 (green line)

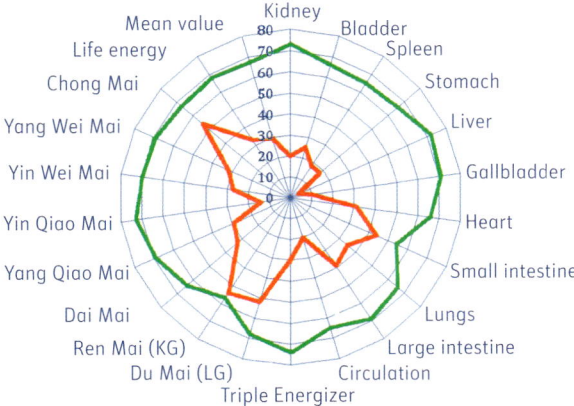

Patient has a tumor, immunodeficiency and exhaustion.
Meridian values, first treatment, June 3, 2003 (red line)
Second treatment, June 19, 2003 (green line)

This led me to develop the following scale:
We can also imagine standing in front of a wall.
At 50 percent, we're as tall as the wall. Below 50 percent, we always need to look up, and feel unable to overcome it.
At 80 percent, the wall is so low that it just takes a small step to climb over it.

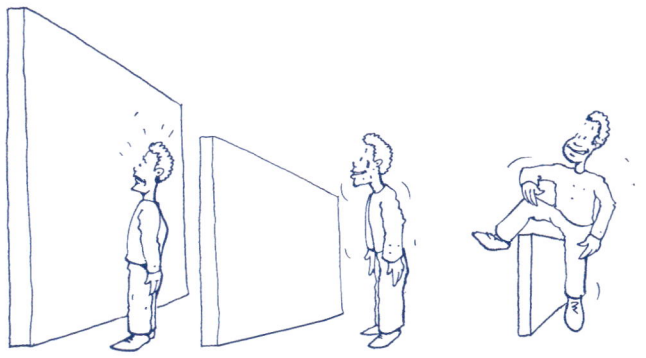

20 percent life energy, 50 percent life energy, 80 percent life energy

Life energy scale

100 percent: feels like flying, or like falling in love.
  80 percent: able to perform at full capacity, reaching your goals.
  70 percent: able to perform at normal capacity, but used to be better.
  50 percent: hanging in there, but it's no fun anymore.
  40 percent: able to perform for four to six hours.
  30 percent: exhausted after two hours of work; prone to tears.
  25 percent: severe exhaustion; nothing matters anymore.
  20 percent: the battery is empty.

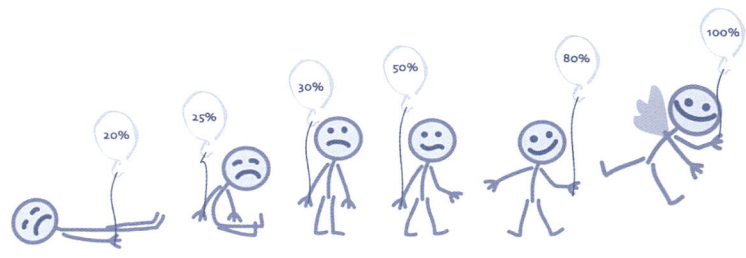

Life energy angels

What does it mean if the level of life energy is only at 30 percent? Has 70 percent been lost in this case? Disappeared into nowhere? For years, that's what I thought, thereby supporting my patients' victim behaviors perfectly. "Oh, poor you! Your life energy is only at 30 percent … do you need a tissue?"

At some point, however, I realized that none of the 100 percent of life energy could get lost; rather, life energy can exist in two forms—a nourishing and a destructive energy—whose sum total adds up to 100. If, for example, I allow for compromise in my life, I automatically allow part of my nourishing life energy to turn into destructive energy.

Now I say to such a patient: "You're *living* yourself with 30 percent, and you're *destroying* yourself with 70 percent!"

Now it's time to find out what are considered compromises in life and how these situations can be changed.

> 100 percent life energy =
>
> X percent nourishing, flowing energy
> +
> Y percent destructive, stagnating energy

This also takes into account everyone's self-responsibility for their own destiny. If we start to live against ourselves—for instance, by allowing for compromise in our lives, and for things or circumstances that harm us, such as inappropriate medications, environmental influences, adverse effects from our sleeping areas or dishonesty toward ourselves, we use our life energy against us, and it turns into destructive energy.

Creative energy

It's not *us* who are creative; rather, creativity flows *through* us.

It expresses itself through us, and we give it form.

All people who earn a living from creative pursuits, such as artists, musicians or writers, are familiar with periods where they feel blocked, where they're no longer visited by the muse. This can become an existential threat to people in these professions. At those times, often drugs and alcohol serve to compensate for these blocks.

We can talk about a "real visit" by the muse when the level of creative energy is above 50 percent.

In this respect, there's no general optimum; rather, we can test for what would be the required minimum or optimum based on profession and interests.

It's quite a challenge to reach 100 percent, and even more so to keep up this level. Raising the bar that high leads to constant frustration if the value falls through the floor once more.

Therefore, I would test for a personal value that feels good and comfortable.

Love/heart energy

Along with our soul energy, it's the most precious kind of energy we have.

It's the fire of our love, our ability to be filled with innocent amazement, the warmth of our heart or the trust that we create in others.

It is the soul energy that has been transformed through our lives and our experiences.

Usually, our heart is broken a few times in life because we're disappointed, disillusioned. Here, the word *disillusioned* can be taken literally—we are freed from an illusion.

This can only happen when we give up our self-love and project it on another person—that is, when we give someone else the responsibility for our life through expectations and claims to ownership.

"Together we're one." "When I'm with you, I always feel fine." "I can't live without you."

This is how resentment, bitterness and unfulfilled expectations create hatred; someone's heart energy transforms into the energy of hate, and the person becomes ugly.

Heart energy is also the target and point of attack of many manipulations; it is highly sought after by those stealing energy from others—also known as "energy vampires."

This type of energy stealing is often experienced as pain or a stabbing feeling in the heart.

Love/heart energy scale

0–3 percent: risk of a heart attack
4–30 percent: able to perform at a low capacity; person has a "small" heart
30–60 percent: the "normal" state
68–100 percent: a healthy, strong and loving heart; a golden heart

Experiencing abundance

When all five basic energies are strong, the *spiritus mundi,* the world ether, starts to flow through the entire human being. This is a state of ecstasy.

But watch out—it's addictive. Those who've experienced it want to do so time and again, and that requires a lot of effort.

10. The Principle of Identity

Who am I, and how many?

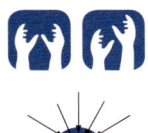

> **Testing topics**
>
> - I am I.
>
> - I am (first name).
>
> - Number of my energy fields
>
> - Whom do we work with in a treatment if there's more than one identity?
>
> - Whose life am I living if I don't live my identity?

"I am I"—I am myself

This sounds like a completely normal statement.

"Sure, who else?" replies our conscious mind without thinking.

Yet if we ask our heart and unconscious, at least 60 percent of all people respond differently: "No, this isn't me."

If we don't have our own identity, and if "I am I" shows a "no" response in the arm-length test, the key question is: "Who am I, and whose life am I living at this moment?"

In colloquial terms, we then say that we're "beside ourselves."

From time to time, it can happen that we lose our identity in life, that we try to be someone else or that strong external energy fields manage to supersede our own field.

Then, things also happen that aren't part of our soul's plan. We are beside ourselves, smaller or bigger accidents happen, we miss opportunities and many things go wrong.

It's one of the most difficult challenges in life to remain steadfast and keep living our own identity, as this requires that we don't live for other people—neither due to "helper syndrome" nor out of fear of their power. Then "I would do anything for you…" is no longer an acceptable attitude.

Ideally, we then only have one single energy field, that of our own soul.

Living our own identity is the core requirement for health, happiness and a joyous life, as our identity serves as our path through life. If we take another path, we won't reach our goals.

The number of energy fields

Usually, we have only one energy field, that of our own soul.

However, 90 percent of all people have more than one energy field.

Unless someone is pregnant, this isn't normal. There are two main reasons why this occurs:

We've shouldered someone else's load; the caretaker in us has brought this upon ourselves, so we can thank the caretaker within us.

Out of manipulation, we've taken on another, or even more, fields; or they've been "given" to us. The goal is to take control or steal energy.

When we no longer have our own identity and when more energy fields are present in us, it's totally unclear whose life plan we're living and to which energy field this plan belongs.

If we have more than one energy field, and if our own energy field is still the strongest one, it's still possible to receive a "yes" response when saying "I am I."

As of four energy fields, however, our own identity has usually disappeared.

For the most part, this is already the case when there are two energy fields (except in the case of pregnant women).

Number of energy fields: "1," "2," "10," "more than 5," "more than 10" …

To be focused, internally stable and have a homogeneous field, we need to homogenize our entire field therapeutically—that is, we have to remove all fields except our own soul field (unless we're pregnant).

Therapeutic shell game

From a therapeutic point of view, when a client has several energy fields, this is a serious situation.

In that case, albeit there's only one body in front of the therapist, he or she is still dealing with several clients and never knows with whom he or she is currently working.

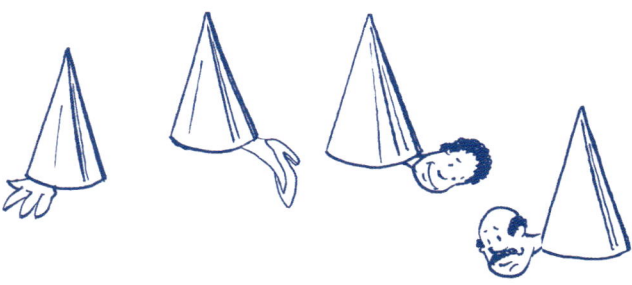

Therapeutic shell game

For days, my older daughter had the feeling that something was wrong with her. When she tested whether she should treat herself, the response was always a definitive "no."

I asked her how many energy fields she had. She tested five. Then I asked her which energy always responded to her, saying not to treat herself?

It wasn't the energy field of her own soul, but that of one of the additional fields that wanted to prevent being recognized and cleared.

Therefore—and this applies to any therapy—if there's more than one energy field, we don't know with whom we're communicating via the arm-length test, and whom we're treating.

As therapists, it's spherical vision that saves us—this vision and the ability to recognize the soul of a human being offers us orientation in the energetic chaos.

This doesn't mean that we always have to clear up the energies and the identity as the first step, but by asking for the number of energies, we know what to expect. By trusting the *innerwise* test cards and letting ourselves be guided by them, we can clear up identity issues in the quickest possible way.

Frequently, clients approach us with crucial questions: whether or not to keep a child, or whether or not to separate or change jobs. Any such question can only be tested and clarified when there is just the client's own soul field left; prior to that, any response is mostly useless.

If the client has five energy fields, each of the five can answer when using the arm-length test; the therapist just doesn't know which one is responding. Therefore, re-establishing the identity of the client concerned takes absolute priority in the treatment.

Manipulation can occur from two sides:

1. People themselves manipulate others, steal parts of their energy, thereby acquiring fields, "hunting trophies" so to speak.

2. People are being manipulated—other parts are implanted as anchors, energy pipelines or dumpsters.

If the identity switch comes from energetic manipulation, this opens up the opportunity to therapeutically utilize this state of having a foreign identity, as there's free access to the manipulator. Those who impose their identity on others in order to steal energy, thereby automatically allow access to themselves. And this is precisely what we can utilize to end the manipulation. This can lead to situations where the client can sense who caused this based on the false identity; we can ask the client to sense the underlying motivation and take a closer look at the one who caused it so that this won't recur in the future.

In this state, we can also draw healing cards for the manipulator and give them directly to the foreign identity in order to end this manipulation.

Those who play also have to deal with the possibility of losing the game. That's life.

The Self

What is the Self, the "I"?

Paracelsus called the human ether *archaeus,* referring to the part of the world ether, or *spiritus mundi,* which flows through the human being.

This personal ether is bound to the soul of a human being, which gives this ether its particular characteristics.

Thus, the Self is an energy, but it is also what fills this soul's life with meaning and corresponds to the purpose of this soul.

The Self is not the character or personality of a human being, as it cannot be described by certain behaviors or by the masks that people put on in their lives.

"My car, my house, my wife" aren't terms that describe the Self either.

We can see it in people's face and eyes when they have their own identity; then their eyes are clear, and their soul is shining through them.

We can hear it in someone's voice, as then it's authentic, and we can hear the soul.

We can see it in people's bodies, in the way they walk, as their soul pervades their body, through and through.

When there's a problem with our identity, we can perceive disharmony.

Having our own identity is the prerequisite to inviting divine providence into our lives and preventing life from turning into a struggle.

The ego

For many years, I tried to eliminate my ego with yoga and emotional therapies, in line with esoteric fads, as I thought that my ego stood in the way of the path of realization and enlightenment. For instance, when practicing a particular yoga position referred to as "the ego eliminator," I held my arms up above my head until I could no longer feel the pain. Defeat the pain and thus the ego—that's what I believed, so I fought my Self with all available means … until I realized that I was on the wrong path and that my ego was the most sacred and beautiful thing I had.

Giving up the ego doesn't bring us closer to realization and enlightenment; rather, it makes us as fit as possible to become soldiers, to fight in armies as God's warriors, to join sects or to live in ashrams.

The SELF is the expression of the Divine within me; and only through that, creativity can unfold.

The ego is not the problem; rather, it's people who believe they don't have one.

In Latin, *ego* means nothing other than "I," which is the SELF.

Human beings without a SELF are beings without willpower, who are no longer able to live their SELF, their soul purpose here on Earth.

The word *personality* goes back to the old Latin meaning of "mask," and the designation of actors who talk via a mask in their roles.

Thus, developing the personality serves to create masks; basically, it means learning how to smile even when feeling miserable.

There are two major approaches people can take on the path to realization, insight and enlightenment:

1. the path of eliminating the ego,
2. the path of living out the ego.

People who give themselves up, do so to follow somebody who hasn't done that. For the most part, they don't have much energy.

Leaders of religious communities are charismatic people who love their ego and have found their path. Sometimes, even centuries later, these "gurus" still attract people who believe they can follow the path of these individuals by giving themselves up. Yet they will never find their own path in this way.

If we decide to walk our own path, to respect and love our own Self, and to be wary of betraying it, we'll have plenty of energy and feel well nourished. We can experience life as flow, and live out the potential of the five basic energies (soul, structurizing, life, creative and love).

However, this also means not following the beaten track when we're on the clearing of life, in the middle of the jungle, but instead, taking a machete and clearing the way for our own life path.

Identity of a foreign soul field

In rare cases, there is, ultimately, only one energy field, and the statement "I am I" gets a "yes" response. Yet a strange feeling remains.

Now you can repeat the test using the first name:

"I am (first name)."

And it can be the case that this statement yields a "no" response.

What's going on?

Then test the statement:

"The soul within me is the original soul that I incarnated with."

If this statement also yields a "no" response, from my experience there can be two reasons for this:

1. At some point in your life (often when you were already in your mother's womb), your soul no longer wanted to deal with everything going on down here on Earth; it returned to the Light, and another free soul acquired your body secondhand. This raises the question of whether it was a fresh soul or the soul of someone who died and was caught in the intermediary world (for example, the soul of a sibling who'd died). And which soul is better for you? Therapeutically, there's often the option to bring back the original soul. However, the person concerned has to be ready for that.

   It also means that people have to look at their own issues again and resolve them.

   If people experienced a severe trauma on the spiritual level, it may be the case that they voluntarily give up their soul's identity. Then they select a spiritual identity, for example.

2. The identity was switched through black magic or advanced brainwashing techniques. (Try testing the identity of prominent politicians after they took office.)

In my own case, I was given the opportunity to experience this state twice. Once I missed a connecting flight and was stuck in a foreign city overnight without knowing any longer where I felt at home. My life suddenly seemed completely meaningless. I knew that remaining in this state meant that I would no longer be able to fulfill my life purpose and would turn into a threat to *innerwise*. As a last resort, one possible way out was suicide, as I wouldn't have wanted to continue living in this way. In that situation, I was saved by a prayer, a conversation with Papa. I had just read *The Shack* by William Paul Young and had finally found a way to relate to God, the big African-American woman called "Papa" in the book. This also put an end to an almost unbearable inner trembling. Another time, I received help from two therapists who readjusted me remotely over the phone.

Especially if you're happy with your soul and have found your soul passion, a soul-swap experience feels like being skinned alive.

"I am I," I am myself—this is the gist of life.
If you then have only the field of your own soul, and it's your original soul, not much can go wrong in life anymore.

11. The Principle of Healing

Healing—but when, who and where?

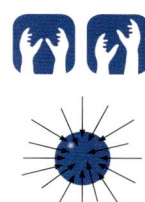

> ### Testing topics
>
> - By healing symptoms, I heal myself.
>
> - My symptoms are caused by issues and energetic charges from my life.
>
> - Energetic charges are my challenges and homework.
>
> - I imagine being a baby in my mother's womb.

"Thank you, illness, for coming to me.
You give me the strength to transform something
that I didn't have the courage to change before."

It would be so easy if we could just heal symptoms, but nature doesn't make it that simple for us.

True healing can only be achieved when we work on the issues and energetic charges that created the symptoms.

Symptoms don't come out of nowhere, just like we don't get a cold simply because we "caught" it.

Symptoms reflect the excess pressure valve when the pressure in the human system gets too high. From a logical point of view, merely closing the valve would be about the silliest thing imaginable, yet this is what modern Western medicine typically tries to do.

Energetic charges

Energetic charges are energies with a directionality, a focus, a purpose.

How are energetic charges created?

Energetic charges arise whenever events and energies haven't been resolved or cleared up, when they haven't been worked through and digested, and when they remain unforgiven—that is, we swallow our anger and tears and fail to achieve inner peace. In short, they're created when we aren't able to say "Thank you" for everything that we've experienced—the result being that these energetic charges lie dormant within us like time bombs.

There are also energetic charges of a different kind: those that our soul brings along when it incarnates. Some call it karma; for others it's the soul purpose and the tasks that the soul brings in.

Other types of energetic charges are those we take over from other people.

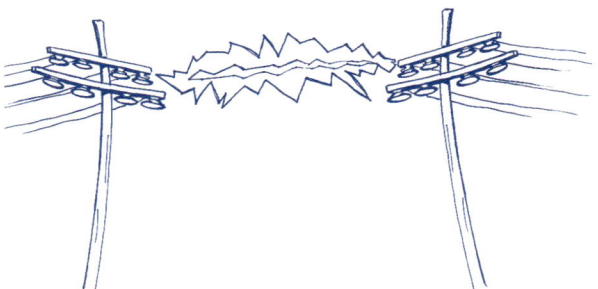

The principle of energetic charges

The purpose of energetic charges

Energetic charges aren't a form of punishment! They create experiences that are indispensable to us, because the meaning and purpose of our human existence is to experience life and thus expand our consciousness.

This growth requires challenges and tasks that we need to experience in order to overcome our inertia, to become active and change.

An illness isn't a punishment, but rather, an opportunity. We have both the responsibility and the choice to either surrender as a victim or seize the opportunity to clear up what lies unresolved—to let go of the old and allow for the new. By falling ill, the body says: "If you're not able to perceive the subtle signs, I'll give you more obvious ones." This is tantamount to "having to learn the hard way" if we fail to listen.

Basic energetic charges of the soul

We're not born perfect, as our separation from the Source is already an imperfection that creates a longing to be part of that Source again.

Personally, I don't believe in reincarnation; I don't believe that our soul has already had a previous life as another human being.

The way I see it is that we bring in energetic charges, a purpose and tasks into this life; that's why I've developed the model of the "divine stockpot."

At the end of one's life, what hasn't been resolved goes into a divine stockpot; then the individual soul dissolves into the One. Each newly created soul receives a scoop to put into its own grail and may make use of its life to "drink up its grail as it has brewed it," thereby doing something meaningful for the One.

It doesn't matter what someone believes in; the only thing that matters is recognizing that we have a soul, which doesn't reincarnate in a pure and innocent form, but already brings along its purpose and main tasks in life. The soul chooses its life, time and parents in order to be able to fulfill its tasks optimally.

Energetic charges from conception, pregnancy or birth

We experience the first severe traumas in our lives already before we're born. About 90 percent of all people weren't wanted unconditionally by both parents when they were conceived. And almost all people experienced some kind of trauma during pregnancy, such as relationship problems between the parents, fear of the unknown or medical interventions.

In addition, about 60 percent of all people have some sort of birth trauma. Working through these issues takes most people an entire lifetime; many never manage to clear the related energetic charges, which keep determining their life experiences.

The arm-length test reveals all these charges, making them identifiable and treatable.

The following statements can be used for testing:

- "Imagine your own conception."

- "Imagine being in your mother's womb."

If this causes stress, it's possible to determine the exact point in time when the stress occurred by testing the individual pregnancy months.

Energetic charges from life traumas

When we look back at our lives, there are always moments and events that still hurt even if they occurred a long time ago.

When we use the arm-length test to find out when an illness really began, we often find the cause months or even years earlier.

Cancer doesn't start on the day someone is diagnosed; usually, it's triggered by a severe emotional trauma 10 to 20 years before. And we don't get the sniffles or a cold just because somebody sneezed on us on the bus; rather, we've been in a state of rigidity for a few days already, which the body tries to break.

This also illustrates why we have to initiate the healing process where the original trauma lies.

When taking into account all levels of being—organic, biochemical, rhythmic, mental, emotional, energetic, spiritual—we see that the cause can be on all these levels, requiring tools that work on all of them to enable healing.

Charges that are taken over

My grandmother died from my grandfather's cancer.

Out of love, she took over the energetic charges of his cancer, thereby giving him the gift of a few additional years so that he could complete his life's work.

He followed her when he was almost 100 years old.

Apart from people, only some pets, such as cats and dogs, choose the option of taking over energetic charges out of love; and they also take over illnesses and energies from people.

In all other cases, people take over energetic charges for others in order to be loved. "If I do everything for you, then will you love me?"

Energetic charges can also be passed on to others through manipulation in order to control them or gain access to their energy; or when people themselves manipulate others, thereby taking over charges from them.

Healing

Healing doesn't mean applying cortisone cream to sore skin, thereby shifting the issue to the next deeper level, the lungs. For example, treating neurodermatitis in the wrong way can lead to asthma or chronic bronchitis.

Healing means resolving the causes of energetic charges on all levels.

The art of healing consists in directing the healing energies of our own consciousness to where they manifest their maximum effects.

Healing energies don't always manifest their effects in an equally strong fashion. It depends on how a question is phrased, as well as on the consciousness held as they're being selected.

An experienced healer can make all the difference.

12. The Principle of Illness

Illness as a sign of disharmony and rigidity

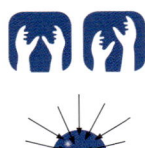

> ### Testing topics
>
> • Viruses and bacteria are mean and make us ill.
>
> • Why do the same 5 out of 100 people always get athlete's foot after going to a public pool?
>   a) Because they're dogged by bad luck.
>   b) Because they didn't disinfect their feet afterward.
>   c) Because they're too acidic, and their milieu attracts fungi.

Good health is harmony

How and when illnesses arise

Do we fall ill because of "mean" germs?
That's where our current Western conventional medicine comes from, fighting the germs with all available means.
Holistic medicine sees this a bit differently.
A healthy system is like a sine wave—harmonious and balanced.

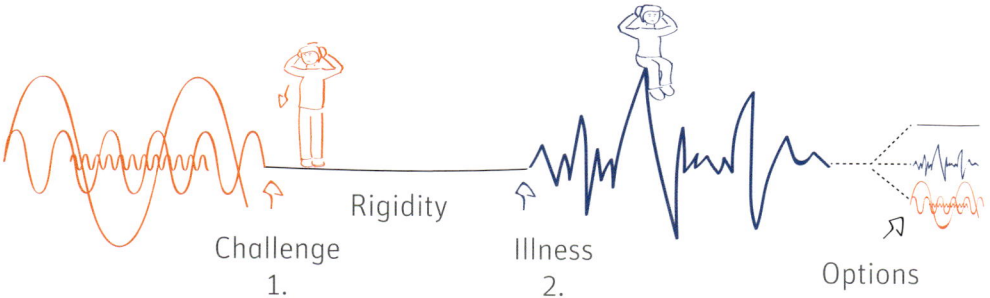

The path of illness

In the case of an irritating event or stress, this sine wave turns into what ranges from a clearly deformed or blocked curve all the way to a flatline—a partial or full rigor mortis.

This irritation often occurs on the energetic or emotional level.

It's not compatible with life and its basic principles.

Consequently, human beings try to free themselves and break up this state of rigidity.

Small children suddenly develop a fever in the evening, and in the morning they're fine again.

Adults are often blocked on multiple levels and thus no longer able to produce such a healing fever reaction.

The body then tries to unblock the system with diarrhea, the sniffles, a cough or another illness that manifests at the personal weak spots of that individual.

And those germs that are always present in the body help in the best way they can: streptococci cause a strep throat, for example; or *Candida* (otherwise producing vitamins for humans) cause a bowel irritation.

Should this seemingly turn good friends into adversaries?

Should deadly enemies suddenly emerge out of a peaceful symbiosis?

In our intestines, we have ten times more germs than cells in our entire body. From that perspective, this poses a permanent deadly threat inside of us—a constant terror alert.

Sterilizing measures don't help either, as killing all germs in our body would also kill *us;* all those helpers that take care of so many tasks for us would be gone.

But an accident or any other event that shakes us up is also an attempt to break this state of rigidity. The important thing is to create chaos; the rest can be straightened out later. This is the only way for our body to free itself from a blockage.

Prior to every accident or case of diarrhea or the sniffles, we find the body in a state of rigidity.

Often, the body manages to liberate itself and re-establish harmony through this measure of creating chaos at first.

Frequently, however, it doesn't; then an illness becomes chronic.

This shows how an illness does indeed start sooner than we may have thought so far.

In this way, first we're sick and tired of something, then we catch a cold. We're fed up, and what follows later is an ulcer; we swallow our tears and get a cough; we can't speak up and so we lose our voice; then we cast our vote, which is our voice, and end up with higher taxes.

The "mean" germs help us overcome blockages and states of rigidity.

This shows clearly that holistic medicine follows a different healing approach and uses other methods than Western conventional medicine does.

The goal is to remove the blockage and clear the subsequent damage that followed the rigidity in order to reach a state of harmony, and to empower the person so that the event that caused the issue doesn't have to recur.

This often requires changes in life, as the initial blockage was a sign, and was invited in because the earlier, "nicer" signs were ignored.

If we go against our intuition and continue in a job that we don't love, and which doesn't fulfill us; or if we eat or drink something that our body is allergic to or whose toxins it can't break down; or if we stay in a relationship because we don't have the courage to be honest with ourselves and our kids … then the signs will become more obvious.

Those who know the state of flow realize very quickly when it's no longer present. When people are used to earning a living in a creative way and cultivate life energy as a value, they will feel any irritation, and thus, any type of disharmony, very clearly.

With the help of the arm-length test, it's easy:

- "Yes" and "no" should produce a distinctly different response. If this isn't the case, the body is in a state of rigidity, and it's time to do something before it resorts to other means to help itself.

- The greater the difference between the "yes" and the "no" when using the arm-length test, the freer the self-regulatory capacity.

- But the breathing, our inner clarity, as well as how strong our energy field and voice are, also offer clues about our overall state.

13. Levels of Being and Stages of Illness

A broken heart also hurts

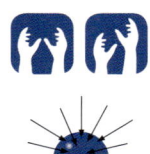

A broken heart also hurts

We're made up of eight major levels:
the physical, biochemical, rhythmic, mental, emotional, energetic, spiritual and unknown levels.

The physical level
This level comprises our structure—the organs, tissues and cells. Except for accidents, this level is the last one that's affected over the course of an illness. Often, it takes years for changes already apparent on the other levels to manifest on this one.

The biochemical level
The biochemical level encompasses all biochemical processes in the body. This includes organic functions, and hormonal and biochemical regulatory processes in the body.

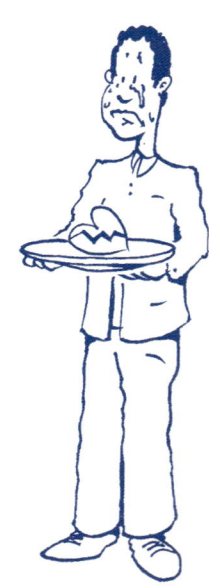

The rhythmic level

Our bodily rhythms include the heart, breathing, and cranial and craniosacral rhythms; as well as the sounds and vibrations of the regulatory plexuses and all organs and structures.
Each organ has a specific rhythm that determines its function.

The mental level

The mental level is the world of our thoughts, including the monkey mind.
It encompasses the inner voice that comments on everything, the loops that we get caught up in, as well as our acquired knowledge, which includes all limiting misinformation.

The emotional level

This concerns both the sum total and wealth of all our emotions, as well as the hurt that we've experienced on that level.

The energetic level

Our energy field that we perceive as the tingling, vibrating sensation; the flow in us. This level is both *the* war zone for energy vampirism and energetic manipulation and the level of the greatest ecstasy in life. Most problems and disorders take place primarily on this level (followed by the emotional level). From here, illnesses "eat" their way through the other levels.

The spiritual level

This is the level of our soul, our soul field, soul space and soul purpose or soul passion. It is the level of our fundamental tasks and programs.

The unknown level

This level offers access to everything we don't know yet or haven't realized yet, while serving as an invitation to discover it.

On what level is the problem, really?

When testing the body, we take all levels into account. Humans cannot be deconstructed into individual levels.

Problems or disorders often start on the energetic or emotional level, and with time, they also manifest on other levels.
For a therapist, the challenge is to look at all levels in their entirety; this is possible

using spherical vision. With the arm-length test, the levels concerned can be identified, as well as the point in time when the problem or disorder originated. Here, it's important to differentiate the original from the secondary levels.

If the heart shows stress in the comprehensive view where all levels are taken into account, the therapist then tests all individual layers to identify those that are currently affected. These are the levels of manifestation.
Now the therapist asks on which level (and when) the heart problem originated. In most cases, the heart is broken, the liver is full of swallowed anger, and the lungs are filled with unshed tears. These are the levels of origin where we find the cause.

When a patient has stomach problems, frequently the stomach itself doesn't reveal stress. It says: "It's not me. I myself don't have a problem, but the liver with all its anger is squishing my vessels. Have a look there!"
In Chinese medicine, we find the following diagnosis: The overpowering liver strangles the center. Precisely that would be the case here.

The Level Filter as a testing aid

I developed the following graphic representation to identify the level of origin, the cause, and the levels of manifestation—either by using intuition or the arm-length test.

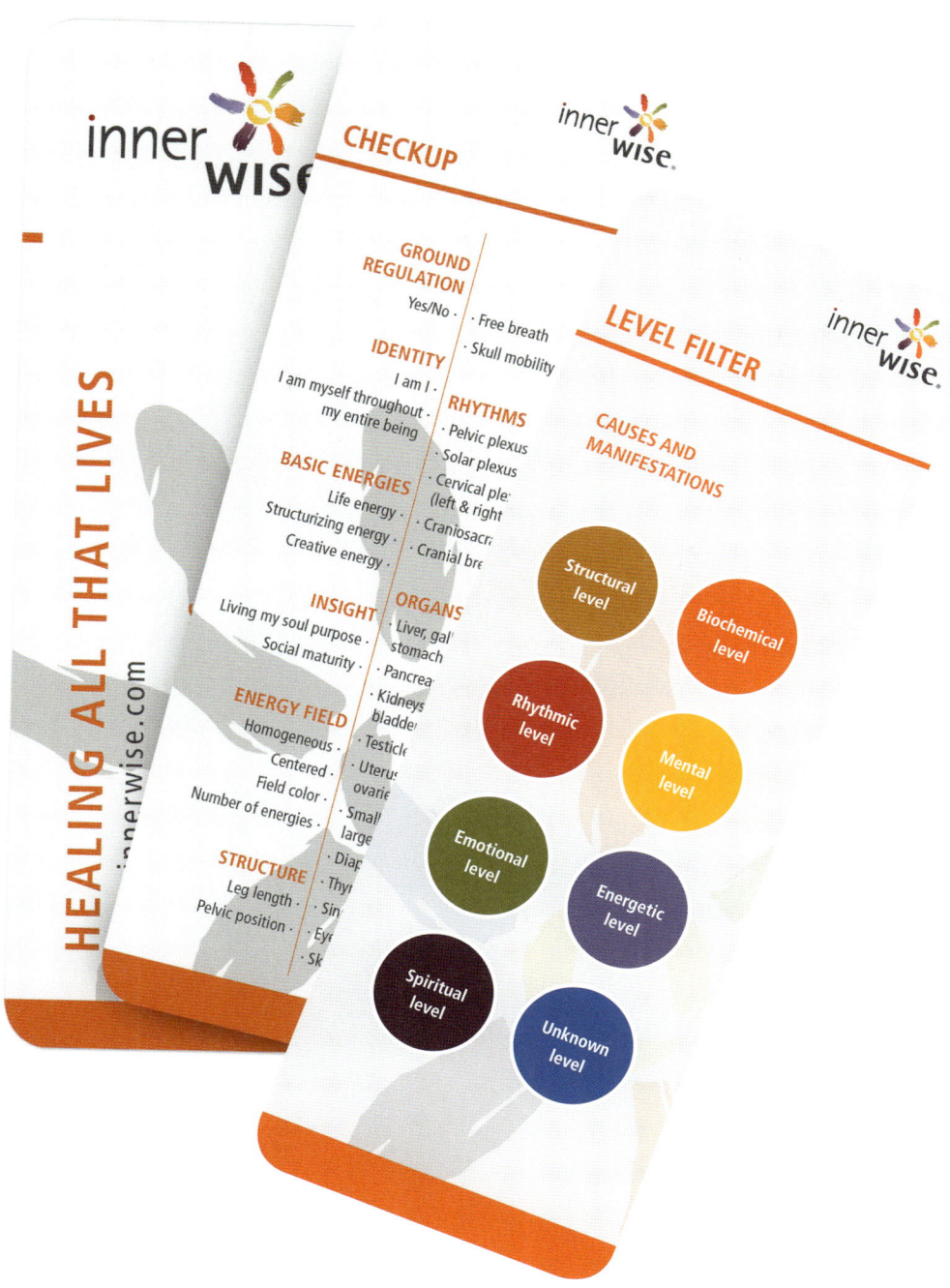

CHECKUP

inner wise

GROUND REGULATION
Yes/No ·
· Free breath
· Skull mobility

IDENTITY
I am I ·
I am myself throughout ·
my entire being

RHYTHMS
· Pelvic plexus
· Solar plexus
· Cervical ple
(left & right
· Craniosacr
· Cranial bre

BASIC ENERGIES
Life energy ·
Structurizing energy ·
Creative energy ·

INSIGHT
Living my soul purpose ·
Social maturity ·

ORGANS
· Liver, gal
stomach
· Pancrea
· Kidneys
bladder
· Testicle
· Uterus
ovari
· Smal
large
· Diap
· Thy
· Sin
· Ey
· Sk

ENERGY FIELD
Homogeneous ·
Centered ·
Field color ·
Number of energies ·

STRUCTURE
Leg length ·
Pelvic position ·

inner wise

LEVEL FILTER

CAUSES AND MANIFESTATIONS

- Structural level
- Biochemical level
- Rhythmic level
- Mental level
- Emotional level
- Energetic level
- Spiritual level
- Unknown level

HEALING ALL THAT LIVES

innerwise.com

14. The Principle of Vibration

Life is harmonious vibration and self-regulatory capacity

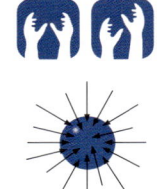

> ### Testing topics
>
> - During … percent of my life, my ground regulation was completely free, and I was in the flow.
>
> - During … percent of my life, I've been in a state of complete rigidity.
>
> - For … percent of my life, I've been in a state of partial rigidity, which has prevented me from living my full potential.

"Everything flows out and in; everything has its tides; all things rise and fall; the pendulum-swing manifests in everything; the measure of the swing to the right is the measure of the swing to the left; rhythm compensates."

The Kybalion

Ground regulation

The arm-length test is the best indicator for ground regulation and self-regulatory capacity.

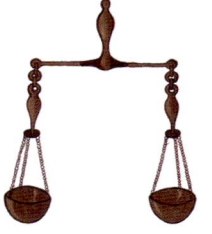
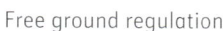

Free ground regulation

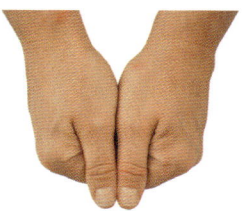

YES

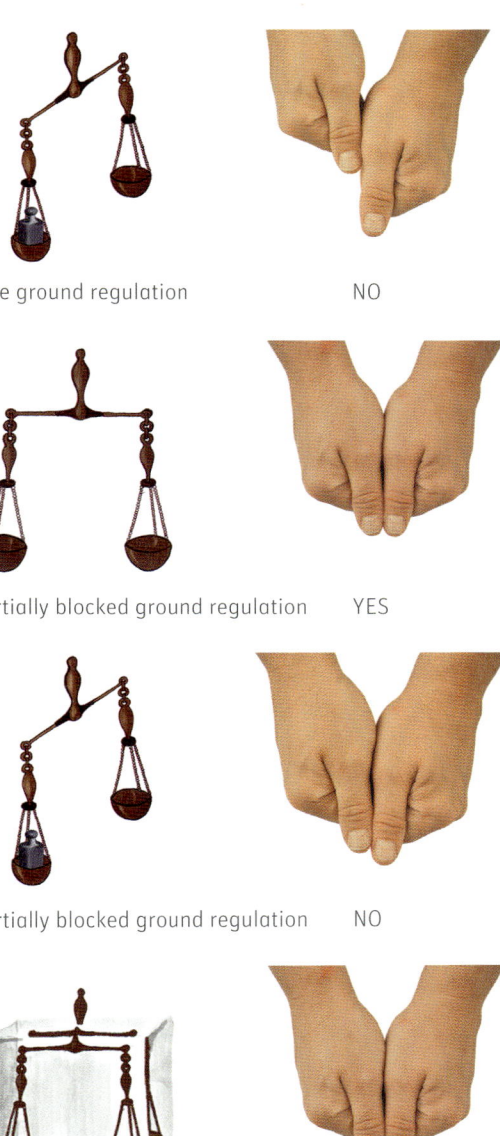

Free ground regulation   NO

Partially blocked ground regulation   YES

Partially blocked ground regulation   NO

State of rigidity   YES—NO

Everything flows—or not

Ideally, every system is in the flow.

However, many systems are partially or even fully blocked.

Blockage is a state similar to being frozen.

The body goes into a survival mode; the available life energy is reduced by half. People stay stuck in time in the very moment the rigidity set in. The perception of time has changed: "What?! Summer is already over? I didn't even notice …" Reaction time becomes three times as long, increasing the probability of an accident.

In the second half of the last century, the Viennese professors Alfred Pischinger and Felix Perger discovered the system of ground regulation. In this medical system, the openness of regulation, of our self-regulatory capacity, is the basic principle of health and healing. Holistic biological medicine is based on that. But this went against the interests of the pharmaceutical industry, which had just introduced the "magic bullets": antibiotics and cortisone. As a result, and also due to the level of comfort sought by many doctors who didn't want to try to understand the deep causes of medical problems or disorders, the system of ground regulation faded into oblivion.

Today, hardly anybody is still interested in the capacity of the connective tissue to transport information and substances and respond to stimuli, or in the impact of focal infections on the entire organism.

Consequently, this know-how was lost, and it wasn't the first time in history that this has occurred. The knowledge of Paracelsus, Aschner, Hufeland and many others is also almost forgotten. Yet these medical doctors and scientists had a more comprehensive understanding of healing than what's being taught today in our universities. They didn't know the genetic code, but they understood life.

Regulation refers to a system's capacity to respond to a stimulus in an appropriate way.

Ideally, it's totally free.

Imagine that you're driving a car and it starts raining:

Free ground regulation

If your windshield wipers clean the entire windshield, you can still drive in a relaxed manner at a high speed.

Partially blocked ground regulation

If, however, the windshield wipers are partially blocked and clean only a part of the windshield, your concerns or fears will increase, and you'll move closer to the windshield to be able to see more, and avoid running over someone's feet.

State of rigidity

If the windshield wipers stop working completely, you can once again relax and wait for your end to come, or you can stop and wait as well.

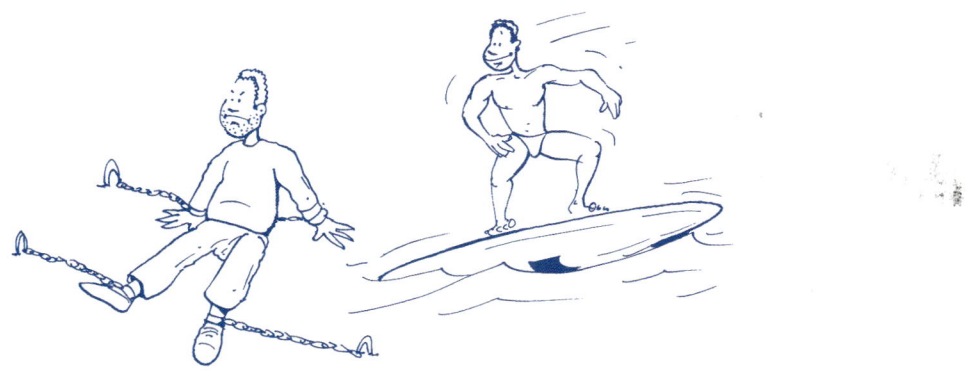

Imprisoned or free—you always have the choice.

The more open our ground regulation is, the more easily and quickly we can react, adjust and find solutions. The more blocked we are, the lower our self-regulatory capacity is.

We're like trees in the wind that can adapt to the environment, and which swing back and forth and aren't uprooted as a result of inner rigidity.

Our inner rhythms are also linked to open ground regulation. These rhythms include the heart, the cranial and craniosacral rhythms, the rhythms of our lungs, all our organs and our autonomic nervous system. And, in turn, the entire fine-tuning of our body is linked to our rhythms. If they become weaker or stop completely, we're no longer finely tuned organisms that function in a consistent manner, but instead, an accumulation of individual fighters for survival who can't communicate with one another.

Each organ does what it considers right, but no one coordinates with the other organs as part of the team. In time, all organs "derail," leading to functional irregularities and damage. Problems arise if this state of total blockage lasts for two to three weeks. Damage to organs can already be detected using the arm-length test.

However, the diagnostic tools of Western conventional medicine can't detect this, as they often only recognize long-term damage. Seeing something in an ultrasound requires a size of about 0.2 inches, which corresponds to approximately two to four million cells. Liver and kidney values only increase when half of the organ's functionality has stopped.

X-rays only show inflammations underneath the teeth once more than half the bone has been eaten away. Even with the best intentions, we can't call this early diagnostics.

In addition, Western conventional medicine merely examines the biochemical and structural levels. This type of diagnostic approach won't detect a broken heart or a liver full of accumulated anger.

When the body is able to react to stimuli, we can reveal any kind of stress by using the arm-length test, whether the issues are on the spiritual, energetic, emotional, mental, rhythmic, biochemical, structural or unknown levels.

The kinesiological procedure I studied is physioenergetics, according to Raphael van Assche.

Just as in any kinesiological procedure, diagnosis starts by carrying out some pre-tests in the client to determine his or her testability. The most important pretest is to check whether the client's arms differ in length during the arm-length test when saying "yes" or "no."

The bigger the difference in arm length between the two statements, the more open the self-regulatory capacity.

The more open a client's ground regulation is, the more—and also the more clearly—he or she can respond to questions using the arms.

It's like the random access memory (RAM) of a personal computer (PC). If it's small and many or large programs are running, the PC crashes. With infinitely large RAM, this won't happen. A completely open ground regulation is like an infinitely large RAM.

With the support of *innerwise*, we can fully reopen our self-regulatory capacity again, allowing for unlimited testability.

15. The Principle of Resonance

Teasing is a sign of affection

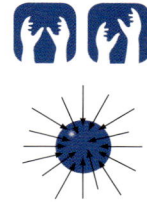

> ### Testing topics
>
> • Based on resonance, I've attracted all experiences in my life myself.
>
> • I am fully innocent and have nothing to do with my experiences.
>
> • Everything in my life has been a mere coincidence.
>
> • Everything in life serves as a mirror for myself.

Why is homeopathy good but not perfect?

When a woman describes her dream partner's age, size, weight, skin color, first name, profession or preferred type of music—why doesn't that tell us anything about their love for one another?

Why are most men unable to buy their beloved girlfriends or wives the clothes they like?

Because there is resonance.

Everything in life is based on resonance:

• the music we enjoy,
• the partners we love,
• the paintings we appreciate,
• the remedies that really help us,
• our favorite cafés,
• the issues we attract and allow to occur, and
• the ailments we take on.

If we take a D100 homeopathic remedy, but in fact, we needed a D153 because it's precisely this potency that's in resonance with the issue, the remedy cannot have an optimal effect.

Resonance means that by perfectly matching two pieces of information, the greatest possible effect can be achieved with the least possible effort.

And that's exactly what we want. The idea is to offer information that fits precisely what is needed regarding a certain issue or topic, thus changing something quickly and effectively.

But how can we identify the remedies that can offer this exact resonance?

This is only feasible with the help of our intuition.

And to do so, we need to learn to trust it again.

This is precisely what the arm-length test is for. It's a way to double-check to see if our feelings have made the right decision.

When we realize that we're touched and influenced by another person's issues, this happens based on our resonance with them, and is a good sign that we still need to look at these very issues in ourselves.

16. The Principle of Cause and Effect

Karma, or the divine stockpot; coincidence or fate; and self-fulfilling energetic charges

> ### Testing topics
>
> - I've never lived before.
>
> - My soul already existed as another human being in the past.
>
> - Within me, I hold memories and energetic charges of other people who lived before me, even if it's not clear how they got there.
>
> - Everything I experience has a meaning and is a gift.

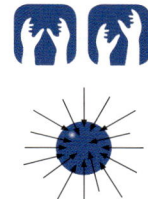

"Every cause has its effect; every effect has its cause; everything happens according to law; chance is but a name for law not recognized; there are many planes of causation, but nothing escapes the law."

The Kybalion

Are there past lives?

One of the most frequently applied esoteric principles is that of past lives and karma. I stopped believing in it, as I experienced and witnessed more and more abuse in this area. Almost always, karma is used as an excuse for irresponsibility and a lack of willingness to change.
"I cannot act differently now, because I experienced this or that in a past life."
"I was a princess in a past life and thus still want to be treated accordingly. I have the right to be huffy." "I can't change that; it's my karma."
In many people, the theory of past lives has created a feeling of guilt over what they believe they did in the past, and this guilt blocks them in their current lives.

I believe, and have also experienced, that we're born with charges. These charges contain experiences from past lives.

However, this doesn't automatically mean that these were lives my soul lived itself. It only means that we continue to work on what has been left unfinished from past lives to resolve these issues further.

Here you will find a text I wrote for *A Course in Healing* that describes it well:

The divine stockpot

What if there were no past lives, and if our souls didn't continue to exist after we die?

Some believe in hell, others in heaven, after we die; atheists only believe in dust, Hindus believe in karma, and modern esoteric people believe in reincarnation.

I have no clue which of these beliefs is really true, but one day we will all experience it.

My father was a philosopher and encouraged me to think about things. It's in this spirit that I would like to invite you to reflect on these concepts in terms of thesis and antithesis.

Karma, past lives and so on—are they really what we think they are? Through past-life regression, we can gain access to our past lives:

- when we used to live,
- who we used to be,
- where and how we incurred guilt,
- what we didn't do because we were too cowardly,
- and with whom we shared various experiences.

Then, we can attempt to clear some karmic charges; or at least, we'll have good excuses for bad behavior in *this* life.

As you continue reading, chances are you'll find that you can't use these excuses any longer. You may find that knowing how saintly or royal you were in a past life doesn't make your behavior in <u>this</u> life any more noble. Then even the statement: "I think we met in a past life" may actually be no more than an esoteric pickup line.

So … what if there was no individual karma?

Instead, what if we offered all individual experiences to the One after we died and let them go completely? The meaning of our human existence would then only consist of having experiences on all levels—physical, mental, energetic, rhythmic, emotional and spiritual.

These experiences and maturation make up our true fortune, not the wealth we accumulate while on Earth.

And who said that life on Earth was always going to be nice and easy? Pain, fear and loss are as much a part of life and learning as happiness and abundance are.

If you now think of all you've lost and experienced, all your feelings of guilt or negative experiences, you can leave your victim role behind and tell yourself: "I've become rich—rich in experiences."

And since we can't hold on to anything, it's likely that we also lose these riches when we die.

When we're back in the Light, we're free from all human burdens. And when we're back in the Light, we're an integral part of it, not an energy-saving lamp.

There, our human suffering doesn't exist; there's no pain. In the Light, we can recover and prepare for the next journey.

In this Light, everyone is equal: the prostitute, the pope, the atheist, the Satanist, the homeless person, the millionaire, the murderer—everyone, without exception.

Those who believe in hell will have to wait until their next incarnation on Earth in order to re-create it anew for themselves.

In the Light, we are perfect and complete, one with everything. We are free.

We are like a drop of water that after death returns to the great water and becomes part of it. This drop of water never existed in this exact consistency before, and will never exist in that form in the future.

We will again become one with ALL THAT IS, and all that is individual dissolves. This includes the past, the future and even the soul itself.

Of course, you can refer to ALL THAT IS by a different name, such as the great water, the Light, God or Allah. Everyone according to his or her own preference.

When another drop separates from the great water, this separation from ALL THAT IS again turns it into something individual, and a new soul is born.

It's as if ALL THAT IS took a break from itself and went on an adventure to once more go for the full experience.

As a newly created individual, still completely pure and innocent, we then proceed to the divine stockpot, which contains the experiences and lessons of all human beings who ever lived.

From there, we then take a big ladle for our personal bowl. Some people who are very hungry for life seem to take a particularly large scoop, or even two.

The stockpot is like a secondhand store where every soul has to find the right clothes.

Thus, the stock bowl contains the tasks and contracts for *this* life—that is, roughly the circumstances, a new name, a new face and a new past.

Sounds like a witness-protection program.

It thereby holds the basic energetic charges that we bring into this life.

Since it's composed of the experiences of numerous people, we're able to remember different aspects and times and carry the charges of many others within us.

This means that our soul doesn't drag around specific karma forever.

Our soul hasn't experienced the past belonging to the new identity, but we have absorbed it with the stock.

We're not a special soul, nor are we a particularly old, wise or even young and inexperienced one—there is no incarnation of a special person. Rather, we're just a part of the Light that has to eat the stock it has brewed—that is, face the music. Even though Cleopatra *did* once exist, you may confidently stop believing that you are her reincarnation, but of course, if you learned this during a past-life regression, your ego is probably getting a real kick out of it.

It won't make wrinkles and love handles look any sexier, though.

Thus, I say good-bye to any karmic excuses or pretexts, to spiritual vanity, to living in the past and to all forms of spiritual classification systems.

Welcome to a world where you're responsible for everything you experience here on Earth. You are the creator of your own reality.

Is it all a coincidence, or what?

At a friend's house, lightening struck a tree in front of their home. Two days before, my friend and his wife considered buying the house they were renting despite the fact that it was located in the flight path of a major airport under construction and that all local residents had been offered quintuple-glass windows for free. He'd planned to replace the IT equipment he needed as a graphic de-signer in six months, but now the insurance would cover it.

Is everything a coincidence?

When everything is in the flow and goes well in the *innerwise* system, includ-ing things related to the team of mentors and myself, the number of visitors to our website rises immediately. Also, the sales ranking of *innerwise* books on Amazon is directly linked to the energetic situation of the system. When it's optimal, resonance is high—that is, many people feel that it resonates with them.

Is everything a coincidence?

A 17-year-old woman experiences repeated inflammation and pain in her lower abdomen. Between the age of 5 and 12, she was raped on a regular basis. Her first boyfriend was violent and abused her physically. Her mother, aunt and grand-mother had been raped as well.

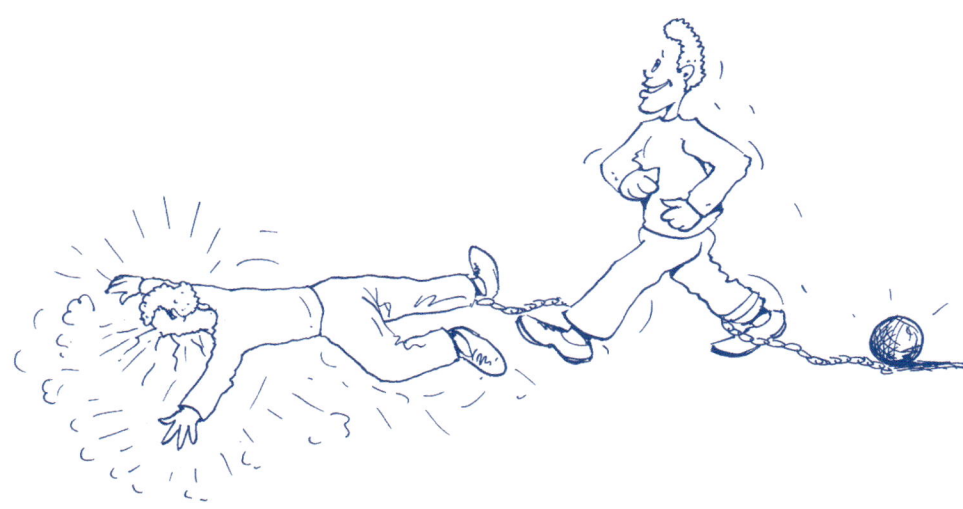

Is everything a coincidence, or what?

Ouch! This is going to hurt!

No, none of those situations are coincidences.

And one of the greatest gifts for therapists is to realize how everything in people's lives is connected so that they can intervene at the right juncture.

Issues can only be resolved where they originated.

If we want to resolve an issue, we first have to determine exactly where it came from—its source—and then resolve it right there, with the very person, and in the very time, concerned; we can't resolve it in the now.

17. The Principle of Polarity

It's all within us, and it's not just Light

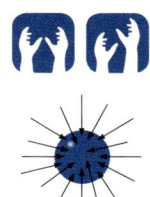

> **Testing topics**
>
> - I am authentic.
>
> - I smile although I feel like crying.
>
> - I let processes happen.
>
> - I'm grateful for all challenges.

"Everything is dual; everything has poles; everything has its pair of opposites; like and unlike are the same; opposites are identical in nature, but different in degree; extremes meet; all truths are but half-truths; all paradoxes may be reconciled."

The Kybalion

Nonduality and duality

Those who raise their heads above the gray masses to seek the light will also have to face the darkness—the darkness within themselves and without.

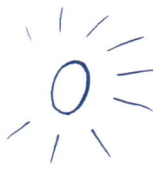

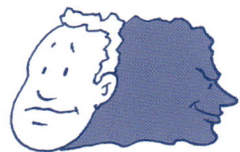

"I'm a pure channel of Light, but don't you ask me about my mom."

Thus, the polarity of light and darkness becomes the driving force of evolution. "I'm pure light"—an often-practiced form of self-sanctification, but only by those who don't want to face their own darkness. Neither wearing white clothes all the time, nor constantly babbling mantras, nor a sanctimonious channeling of angel messages shortens the way.

We walk the path to realization and enlightenment by living authentically, by letting processes happen and then resolving them.

People who've experienced bioenergetic work, according to Wilhelm Reich and Alexander Lowen, for example, and the potential of movement in combination with hyperventilation, know that under the surface, darkness lies dormant in every human being. Issues of the past also lie dormant in nice, modest people; and as they do bioenergetic work, these issues can be released with an amazing force by screaming or hitting something. With all this swallowed anger, they may then try to smash a wood block with their bare hands.

The energies that are released in such a process are nothing foreign—they're part of us. Once they've been released, we can experience the miracle of healing. In this way, I was able to correct 1.5 diopters of my defective vision in both eyes, a condition that had been caused by a birth trauma.

The second aspect of duality involves "learning aids" and support from outside. Testing the stability of your energy field requires being exposed to extreme energies. Naturally, you may also fall flat on your face at times and lose your flow in the process. However, it's precisely those situations that show you where you can keep searching and where the next potential for growth is.

When you're in the flow, these challenges will come to you by themselves. You only have to take them on with gratitude and grow with them.

The best and, to me, dearest therapists I know have all experienced the highs and lows of life, enabling them to understand and provide guidance to others.

"Where there is the greatest light, there is also the greatest darkness."
—Anonymous

Without duality, life would be boring, and we would no longer grow.

18. The Principle of Love and Partnership

About love and the desire to possess — games people play

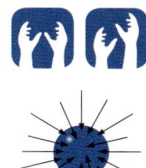

> ### Testing topics
>
> - I need my partner.
>
> - My partner needs me.
>
> - I get … percent of the energy I need from my partner.
>
> - I give my partner … percent of my energy.

What do we love about each other?

Love is only possible on a soul level. This means that we can only love one another when we can sense the other's soul. If there's a problem with someone's identity, let alone another soul has influenced or taken over that person, a treatment can lead to an interesting awakening. I've seen a number of couples where one of the partners didn't have his or her own identity, or where the soul hadn't been present during the entire relationship. Although the couple had been living together for many years, the two didn't really know each other yet.

Love for one another, and the resonance that goes along with it, can also suddenly vanish when one of the partners loses his or her identity.

I experienced this myself with a partner where my feelings for her disappeared from one day to the next. Deep inside, I knew all of a sudden that we were no longer a couple.

Using the arm-length test on this woman yielded the following responses:

- I am I. – No.
- Is your own soul present? – No.
- Since when has it been no longer present? – For four weeks.

- Did you give it away voluntarily? – Yes.
- Do you want it back? – No.
- Is living with another soul field easier for you? – Yes.
- Was your soul severely traumatized at some point? – Yes.
- Do you have the strength and willpower to want to heal this trauma? – No.

For many years, this woman carried a spiritual name, also living this identity, and now she'd returned to this pattern.

Consequently, I could no longer feel love for her, as I was in love with her soul that she had now rejected once again.

There was nothing more to say.

Every human being is responsible for him- or herself. I couldn't save her, nor did I have the right to do so. Only if she gains the necessary experiences and wants her own soul back, can I support her.

Love and relationships

When I met my first partner again after many years, she said to me, "I love you, but I don't want anything from you."

My first thought was that she didn't want me, that I wasn't good enough.

But then I was relieved, because she explained that she still loved me but didn't want to possess me or use me.

Most people want something; they want to possess or use others, or they want security. When people are newly in love, this may not be obvious yet. But as the initial ecstasy of feeling *one* vanishes, such motivations rise to the surface.

Love begins to die as dependencies arise, and as it turns into mutual dependencies and a relationship where each partner identifies with the other rather than with him- or herself.

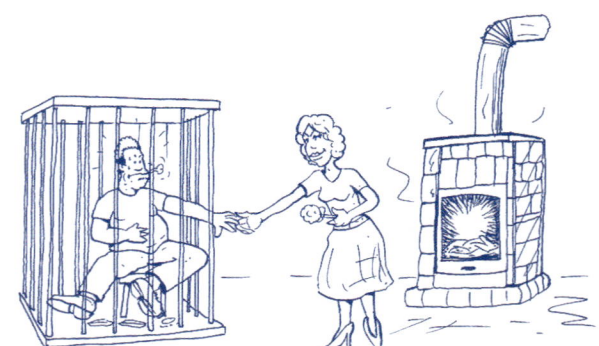

If Hansel doesn't watch out,
he'll land in the oven.

The soul pie

People often resemble pies that have been partially eaten; they hope they'll become whole and complete again by uniting with other incomplete pies.

Together we're ONE, says the rest of the apple pie to the remaining pumpkin pie. However, just like different pies that are lumped together won't make up one whole and complete pie, neither do couples. It's just an illusion as we fall in love with somebody.

Naturally, being ONE involves more than feeling like a whole and complete pie. The more whole and complete a pie is, the more connected it is with "the One," the divine source; and the more whole and complete the soul is.

And that oneness with the Source is what everybody is looking for—some also call it paradise.

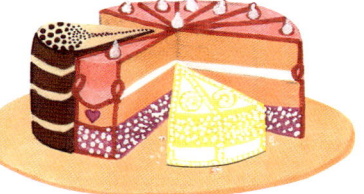

When people are asked to draw their soul pie intuitively, including the fragments of their own soul, the pictures can often look quite scary: the pie plate is largely empty; and often pieces of the pie are drawn in a different color or crosshatched differently. These are fragments of partners or ex-partners who are still being utilized.

Together we're one; together we're complete.

All shares of the pie that are no longer on the plate have transformed into the pain body.

And any part that isn't on the pie plate is no longer nourished on an energetic level. All pieces that have become part of the pain body are constantly hungry and suck energy wherever they can. We typically find this in "victims."

Two half spheres or two full spheres

Consequently, "together we're one" doesn't work, leaving as the only option to become whole and complete yourself so that you no longer have to "need" your partner.

And when you get to that point, it may happen that your partner says: "You no longer want anything from me—don't you love me anymore?"

Creating a hyperspace

Through their love, souls who are in love with one another create a love field that surrounds them. Love is like a hyperspace, created from a whole and complete soul that hasn't yet experienced duality. It is a grace of Creation—perhaps the solace for finiteness. As long as love is new and clear, it's all good and wonderful. When a couple separates, however, the traumatized and charged-up hyperspace remains. Energetically, the two people stay connected—even over decades—unless they dissolve this field, this space.

This can be easily done with the healing breath, for example, which I developed.

Imagine your ex-partner, and concentrate on the love field that still connects both of you.

First breath
Inhalation: Breathe in your old love field completely.
Exhalation: Breathe it out fully into the Source.

Second breath
Inhalation: From the Source, breathe in your energy only.
Exhalation: As you breathe out, fill up your soul space alone with your breath.

Apply the healing breath until you can no longer see your partner in front of you, and the field that formerly surrounded you has dissolved; do this until you're both free. In this way, love can also turn into friendship.

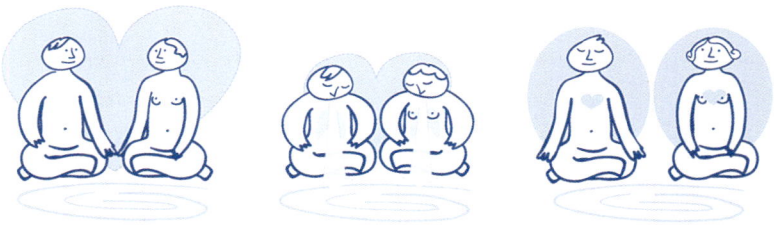

Releasing partners with the healing breath

Joint issues

With a couple's joint soul pie—the fields that connect both of them—some issues are almost always transferred to the other partner. The two partners start to feel responsible for one another and consciously or unconsciously begin to carry their partner's issues. In couples' treatments, I see time and again that one partner is carrying the other's issues. When an issue is solved in one, symptoms disappear in the other. That's why it's always necessary to test whose issue it really is.

Dependencies

Just as there is "Alcoholics Anonymous," there is also "Co-Dependents Anonymous." And most likely, the number of co-dependents exceeds that of alcoholics. Through mutual dependency patterns in relationships, partners attach the other to themselves, transfer their own competence over to the other and give up their autonomy. The following test questions will help you determine your degree of co-dependency:

You are my partner; you belong to me:
- A Fully applies.
- B Partially applies.
- C Doesn't apply.

It's me, always me, who takes responsibility for us:
- A Fully applies.
- B Partially applies.
- C Doesn't apply.

I prefer doing things with you rather than alone or with others:
- A Fully applies.
- B Partially applies.
- C Doesn't apply.

Since I've been with you, I've lost touch with more and more friends:
- A Fully applies.
- B Partially applies.
- C Doesn't apply.

I'm not always honest with you because I don't want to hurt you:
- A Fully applies.
- B Partially applies.
- C Doesn't apply.

I'm jealous:
- A Fully applies.
- B Partially applies.
- C Doesn't apply.

Your body and sexuality belong to me, and my body and sexuality belong to you:
- A Fully applies.
- B Partially applies.
- C Doesn't apply.

For your sake, I will gladly give up something that's important to me:
- A Fully applies.
- B Partially applies.
- C Doesn't apply.

19. The Caretaker's Principle

I would do ANYTHING so that you feel better

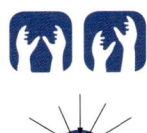

> ### Testing topics
>
> - I want somebody to take care of me.
>
> - I like taking care of others.
>
> - By taking care of others, I help them.
>
> - By taking care of others, I harm them, because I take over and thus shoulder a part of the responsibility for their lives.

"A problem shared is a problem halved."
The elevation of caretaking and turning it into a value is largely responsible for much unnecessary suffering.
For those who are taken care of, easing their burdens lessens their need for change, thus prolonging their suffering.
People taking care of others compound their pain, which is destructive for the caretakers and prevents them from dedicating themselves to their life purpose. Instead, these people declare caretaking as their life purpose, hoping that Heaven will reward them.

Mine, yours, ours

On average, 30 percent of all problems and disorders aren't our own; instead, we've taken them over from, and carry them for, other people.
"On average" means that there are also people where this percentage amounts to 95, and others where it only makes up 5 percent.
Therapists deal with the problem that issues can only be resolved where they originated—this means that they didn't start in the caretakers themselves, even if the issues they carry have already made them ill.

With caretakers, therapists can only work on encouraging them to stop taking care of others as a preventive measure. The issues and related energetic charges that they've already taken over and are carrying remain.

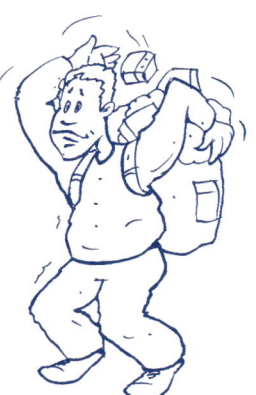

I like to bear the burden for others–I'm a caretaker.

Our own issues versus those carried for others

For a therapist, it's key to identify whose issue something really is.

If it's not our own issue, it can be that of our partner, a friend or a client. It can come from people way back in our lives, and even be passed on through the generations.

For example, an issue going back to someone's grandmother, which originated during World War II, can still cause problems in members of the family today.

With the help of the arm-length test, it's easy to determine whom an issue belongs to. Sometimes, however, a therapist may not think of testing for it.

Yet at the very latest when the treatment goes around in circles, and issues that were seemingly resolved come back into the loop, it's time to question whether the therapist is working on the right person.

Why do we carry issues for other people?

One reason could be that we may have never experienced unconditional love and hope to receive substitute love by taking care of others, or because certain issues are forced upon us from the outside through energetic manipulation. In addition, we often bear the imprint of society, in particular that of the corrupted Christian religions as a result of the Church's obsession with power.

"Who am I, and if so, how many?" This is the best way to describe this topic. With the help of the manipulation test card 8 (explained in more detail in the related chapter), it's possible to identify what kind of manipulation has been used, and treat it.

How do we resolve issues that have been taken over from, and are being carried for, others?

With *innerwise*, it's not a problem to work with people who are far away or who died a long time ago.

Energies can move and be placed, independently of time and space. This enables us to bring the energies (like target coordinates) to the time and place where they're meant to manifest their effects.

With our consciousness, we can determine when the remedy is supposed to act. Working with a 40-year-old man, for example, we can send the energies to the point in time when he was 5 years old and let them manifest their effects there.

In the same way, we can give them to the soul of another human being, whether he or she is still alive or not.

What matters is giving these energies as a gift from the heart and without intention.

If there's any form of intent, the energies won't be accepted by the souls.

Guided by the testing system, the therapist tests healing cards for this soul and hands them over to the client to pass them on from his/her heart.

All clients who do so can see with their inner eyes how the remedies are accepted, and how the souls react with a sense of liberation and relief. If these are souls of people who already passed away, this can sometimes enable them to finally leave the intermediary world and return to the Light.

20. The Principle of Victimhood

I love my drama; I need my drama

> ### Testing topics
>
> - I'm innocent; I'm a victim.
>
> - I'm the creator of my life.
>
> - I alone can change my life.
>
> - I'm grateful for all experiences.

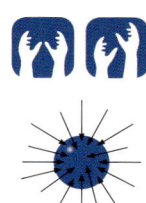

Many people are victims; at least, they feel as if they are.
A victim's purpose in life is to suffer and to make others responsible for his/her pain.

When I used to work at a pain-therapy clinic, one of the first questions I asked my patients was whether they'd applied for disability benefits, because if they'd filed a claim based on an illness, this desire for financial security would be endangered by any form of relief or healing. For this reason, the rule is: "Come back when your disability pension claim has been closed; prior to that, we can't help you." This would cause some frustration, as the patient didn't really want to be healed in pain therapy; rather, he was looking for another confirmation of his incurable pain for his disability pension claim.

Many people benefit from their illnesses: they get attention; they no longer have to work at jobs they despise; their migraine headaches, for example, may serve to help them avoid sex; or they've finally found their life purpose: the illness. Now, they always have something to talk about and can count on pity.

There appears to be some sort of a consensus in society that things are always the fault of others.

Over 90 percent of all people voluntarily behave like prisoners at least occasionally, or volunteer to be gagged.

It seems to make life so easy: "It's not my fault, so I don't need to change anything. If I don't need to change anything, I don't have to grow up."

From a therapeutic perspective, it's pointless to console victims and keep handing them tissues.

This won't resolve or change anything. Naturally, people feel better at first, when they've been able to cry on someone's shoulder and delegate the blame. "You're the only one who can still help me!"

At the same time, they drain the therapist's life force if he/she lets this happen. After the session, the therapist feels drained and may have even taken over part of the problem. And the client has recharged him- or herself like a vampire. Expert victims visit two to three therapists per week and nourish themselves quite well in this way.

And these therapists let it happen—so they can only blame themselves.

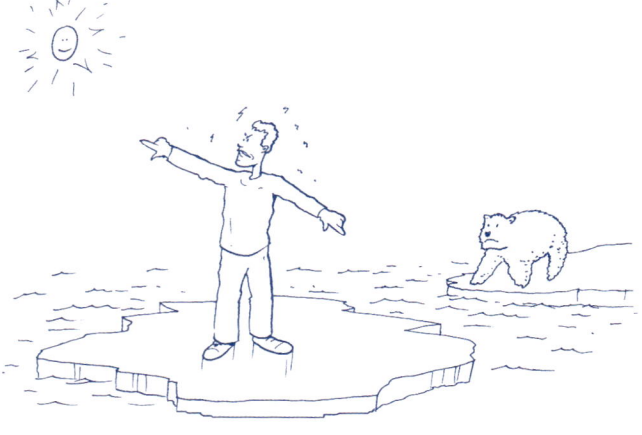

Sun, it's your fault!
When I get off of here, my lawyer will sue you!

In my own case, I've lost the motivation (as a medical doctor) to work with people who behave like victims, and have stopped listening to whose fault it all was a long time ago.

"Because my grandmother … ," "and my mother … ," "and especially my husband … ," or "But you can't do … !"

Or, "When I finally earn a lot of money … ," or "I've always had to take care of my children, and even now that they're grown up and have their own families, I still have to take care of everything and have no time at all to live my own life …"

People who want to take so little, or no, responsibility for their lives get one or perhaps two chances in treatment with me. I tell them openly what I see and hear, and also point out how their excuses for bad behavior and their clinging to continued suffering causes me a massive energy drain. If at that point, they still continue their games, I put an end to the treatment and ask them to go home.
Deep inside, people who see themselves as victims aren't willing to take responsibility for themselves and their own lives.
If they have that type of attitude, no therapist can help them.

The alternative to victims are doers—proactive people who recognize that they've created their lives themselves and are the only ones who can change them.

People don't have to run around with bitter expressions and drooping mouths—that's not part of the big plan.

21. The Principle of Self-Responsibility

Have I really created all of this myself?

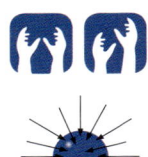

> ### Testing topics
>
> - I am responsible for everything happening in my life.
>
> - I suffer, but I can't change my life.
>
> - I've attracted all experiences myself in order to learn from them.
>
> - I am ready to change EVERYTHING in order to live a healthy and happy life again.

I've created my life myself.
Only I can change it.

I love to be a doer; almost all of my friends are, and also my kids have become doers.

I can't stand depriving people of their right to make their own decisions.
"You have to take better care of yourself. Don't work so much. Someone has to take care of you." After hearing these words, I broke off all contact with my partner's parents.

"Put on warm clothes, I'm cold!"
Who doesn't know this type of drivel?
Doers take responsibility for their lives and enjoy doing so.
They realize their compromises and put an end to them, even if others don't like it, but doers aren't responsible for other people.
Doers try to live as authentically as possible and to inspire their children through love and leading by example.

Doers create—however, not for the sake of others—but because they enjoy what they do. They feel a joy that victims can only come close to during orgasm: a joy that makes all cells dance; and which creates an energy field that unites with the infinite and is connected to a sense of freedom, such that even a single moment of this joy makes one's life worth living.

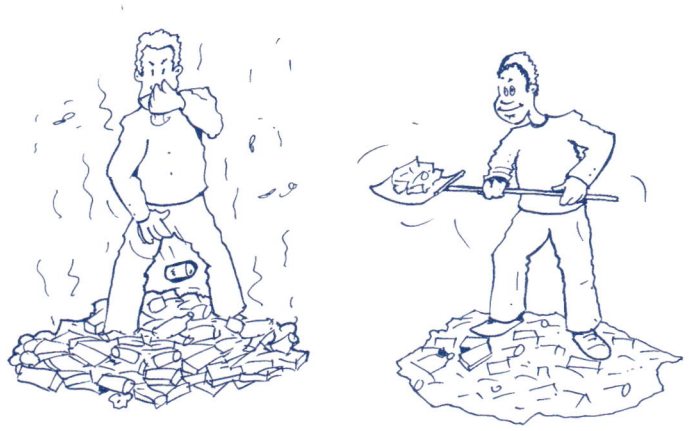

"Mom! I don't want to grow up."

22. The Principle of Life

A short guide to the game of life

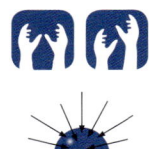

> ### Testing topics
>
> - I want to know beforehand what kind of presents are waiting for me.
>
> - I enjoy growth and let processes happen.
>
> - I love my drama; I need my drama.
>
> - Fragments of my soul have separated due to traumas.

Presents come to you after you let go

Many of us would prefer that things be different, but that's life.
When we clean up, resolve things, make decisions and put an end to compromise, we receive presents.
This requires courage that many people lack.
When we're struck by illness, it's high time to stop everything in life that no longer fits, independently from societal values, commitments or promises.

When you fall ill, put an end to any compromises and live your dreams before it's too late.

I live my dreams, even if this means disappointing others.

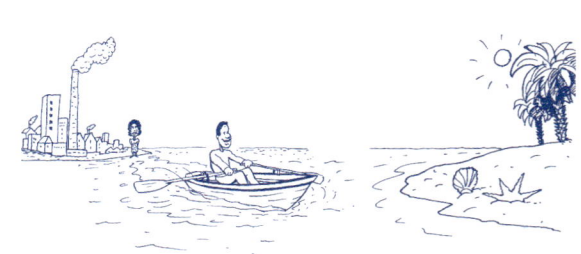

Flow is fun!

Ever since I started to follow the principle of flow and have made sure I'm in the flow myself—that is, I've kept my identity clear, my field stable and am living my soul passion—I've been experiencing so much joy and divine providence in my life. The struggle is over. All I need comes to me; it's offered to me and I only have to accept it.

Life really can be so beautiful!

Letting processes happen

Things might also hurt at times, and that's okay. Sometimes they may even hurt so bad that one questions life itself.

If I met someone who's about to jump off a building, I would tell him or her the following: "Well, then jump, I'm going to leave because I don't need to watch this. It was nice meeting you." In that very moment, those who want to commit suicide are being called upon to take full self-responsibility and can no longer use this threat to cry for help or blackmail others. This encourages these individuals to rethink their decision, and gives them a chance to change their minds and grow up.

We can't save our partners or friends from their processes either. We can only be honest with them and trust that they'll grow with the challenge.

Neither do I want anybody to save or adopt me, or deprive me of my right to make my own decisions.

I'm entitled to my own processes and growth.

There's plenty of energy, but not everyone has access to it

Just about everybody could enjoy plenty of energy; however, it requires finding and living your life purpose, your soul passion. In return, you have access to un-limited energy, and energy vampirism is no longer necessary.

How trauma affects the soul

Lighter trauma hurts the body, emotions and energy field. More severe trauma hurts the soul. It leads to the separation of soul fragments, which then disappear through "escape tunnels" into the dimensions of Being, into an n-dimensional space.

"I can't stand this any longer, I'm going to bail out."

But such wounds don't have to stay open or leave ugly scars forever. The art is to recognize that parts of the soul are affected and to retrieve these fragments. Since they can be anywhere in dimensional space, finding them would be like searching for a tennis ball in the cosmos.

The easiest way to find them is to follow them through the escape tunnels, as those lead to them directly.

As we breathe in pure energy from the Source during the healing breath to fill the escape tunnels, it touches these soul fragments, and we can retrieve them using the healing breath. They only need to briefly visit the spa at the Source before they can be reintegrated into our being.

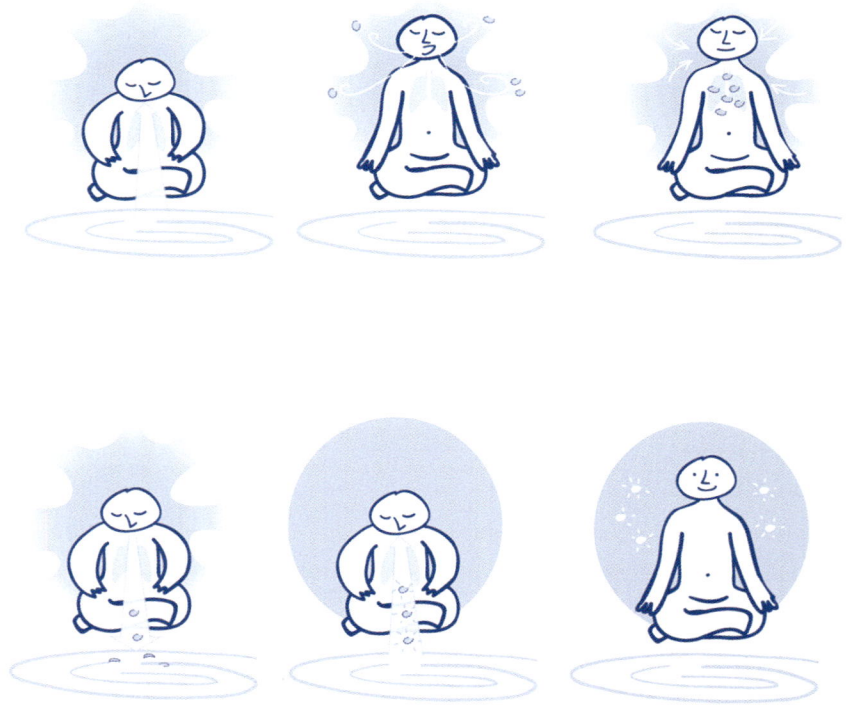

Healing the soul with the healing breath

THE HEALING BREATH: Healing the soul

Visualize all channels through which you've ever lost parts of your Self, your soul, in your life.

Immerse yourself in the energy of the Source of Light, the symbol on page 199. Imagine the infinite healing space, your soul space and the Source.

First breath
Inhalation: From the divine source, breathe in pure energy.
Exhalation: As you breathe out, fill up all escape tunnels of the soul fragments that separated, all the way to the end with this energy, this light.

Second breath
Inhalation: From the escape tunnels, breathe in the energy, and thus, all soul fragments.
Exhalation: Breathe out all retrieved soul fragments into the Source.

Third breath
Inhalation: From the Source, breathe in your healed soul fragments.
Exhalation: Re-integrate all soul fragments back into your life as you breathe out.

Repeat the healing breath until your soul is complete again and the escape tunnels are empty and have disappeared.

Healing the past through forgiveness, acceptance and through healing the soul

For a long time, I tried to resolve traumas through forgiveness and acceptance, yet the results were merely satisfactory. Only retrieving the parts of the soul that had been lost due to traumas brought about the successful outcome I was looking for. "Thank you for the experience" only accomplishes half the job.
The remaining half is accomplished by healing the soul.

The journey of the soul

Here, I'm describing the journey of the soul as it appears most congruous to me today:

Duality is created by the One, like a drop separating from a great water.

This corresponds to the expulsion from Paradise in the Bible.

For the first time, a soul has been created—something individual that was separated from the One. At this point, the soul still has maximum completion and perfection.

However, sin now comes into play (the story of Cain and Abel). Figuratively speaking, this corresponds to "loading up" with karmic charges.

I no longer believe in past lives; however, I can imagine the divine stockpot, with every soul taking a scoop of this stock into its own grail.

The stockpot includes all the unfinished business of those who died that was part of their life or soul purpose. Thus, the soul already holds specific charges, losing its perfection.

As the next step, the soul chooses the optimal situation and the right parents in order to be able to fulfill its tasks.

And so it is born.

At the end of its life, it returns to the Light, or dissolves again in the great water. All its unfinished business goes back into the big stockpot. There are also souls who remain stuck in the intermediary world and don't reach the Light.

In Spain, for instance, it's common practice to stay with someone who has passed away—that is, to hold a wake over the corpse until the soul has returned to the Light. The Spanish people still know that a lot can happen on the way to the Light. Souls who died suddenly or too early due to an accident or trauma often remain stuck in the intermediary world. There's also the possibility of light channel manipulation (explained in more detail in the chapter related to test card 8), which prevents the souls from returning home.

Thus, the soul comes from the Light, incarnates and usually returns to the Light at the end. It becomes one with the Light again, ceasing to exist.

23. The Principle of Enlightenment

Fear of death or fear of life?

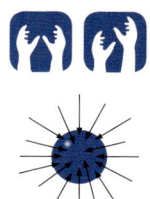

> ### Testing topics
>
> - I'm afraid of death.
>
> - I'm afraid of life.
>
> - I already died a long time ago.

Death is the fastest way to enlightenment. Life, however, can be the most wonderful way to enjoy it.

Why are people who are ill afraid of death?
Often, they've already been dying their entire lives.

When we die, we're like a drop of water that returns to the great lake and becomes one with the water. We turn into Light again, bask in infinite love and are released from duality. Why does that sound so terrible and make most people afraid of it? It's simply paradise …

True and ongoing dying is a life that isn't carried or fulfilled by one's soul passion. That's what people should be concerned about, and they should do whatever they can to find and live their soul passion.

Their true fear is passing on without ever having truly lived.

Those who live their soul purpose, can also leave the human body and duality in peace, because they've accomplished what they incarnated for.

This is not meant to encourage suicide, but to finally start living!

Remembering that I'll be dead soon is the most important tool I've ever encountered to help me make the big choices in life. Because almost everything—all external expectations, all pride, all fear of embarrassment or failure—these things just fall away in the face of death, leaving only what is truly important.

Remembering that you are going to die is the best way I know to avoid the trap of thinking you have something to lose. You are already naked. There is no reason not to follow your heart.

Commencement address delivered by Steve Jobs
at Stanford University in October 2005

24. The Principle of Manifestation

Creating your life yourself, for beginners and advanced practitioners

> **Testing topics**
>
> - Anything that I don't control goes wrong.
>
> - The glass is half full.
>
> - The glass is half empty.
>
> - My negative focus (negative basic attitude) is … percent.

The conscious mind and the unconscious

There are two major forces working within us: conscious and unconscious forces. Both create our reality. The key question is the share they each have in it.

Distribution of power

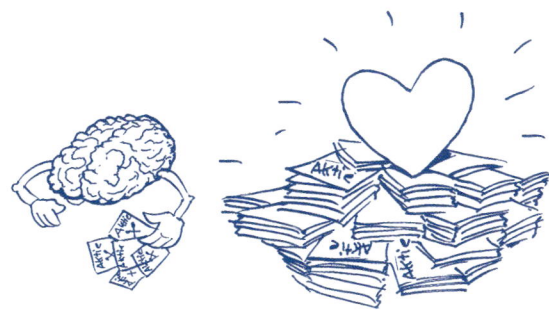

With one percent of the shares, the conscious mind doesn't have a say.

Most people believe that they can create reality with their conscious mind and willpower, and they fail miserably. We can write "I love you" 1,000 times on the mirror but we won't love ourselves an ounce more.

The greatest wish expressed by anyone who's ill is to be healthy. The arm-length test reveals, however, that it is precisely this idea that causes all people a great deal of stress.

Usually, the unconscious has a 95 to 99 percent share in the power of creating reality. This leaves only 1 to 5 percent for the conscious mind, one's willpower.

In a few very conscious people, the share of the conscious mind increases to more than 20 percent.

This distribution of power is a disaster, as all therapies and personality-development strategies that focus on the conscious mind are, thus, largely doomed to fail because they're directed at the wrong addressee.

The negative focus

The reason for this unequal distribution of power is to protect human beings from themselves.

If all negative thoughts had a strong manifestation potential, humanity would have already been wiped out. The negative focus—that is, the share of negative thoughts in *all* the thoughts we have—often exceeds 80 percent.

It's only when the negative focus is reduced substantially that it becomes safe for the conscious mind to attain a larger share in creating reality without endangering the human.

Chronically ill people have a negative focus of nearly 100 percent—what good can come of that?

The positive focus

A positive focus stems from radical liberation and forgiveness. It doesn't have to be this way, since the positive focus of children is often still high when they're born. Most of the time, however, adults aren't able to sustain this gift in their children.

As a result, we need to heal our traumas as we grow up in order to regain the lightness of Being.

Be unrelentingly honest!

Forms of manifestation

There are three ways to manifest something in life:

Flow and divine providence

We can simply let things happen and let divine providence unfold. This requires, however, being in the flow, living our own identity and embracing our soul purpose, our soul passion. It's the easiest and most wonderful way to live our lives, but it requires a great deal of work in advance.

Manipulation

We'd prefer not leaving anything up to chance; instead, we'd rather remain in control of what's happening. Those who can't trust themselves don't trust others either, and resort to all sorts of manipulation—including pressure, blackmail, fear, bribery, aggression, control and the withdrawal of love and affection—to ensure that what happens is what we *think* should happen, whether it currently fits into the bigger picture or not. Nothing is worse than relying on chance, as it could lead us to somehow fall short.

"Trust is good, control is better." Stalin said that—and sent millions of people to concentration camps.

The most common form of manipulation, however, is *self*-manipulation.

By expressing fear, we attract the events we're most afraid of.

Fate

Whatever happens—whether good or bad—is viewed as fate.

"I broke my leg—that was fate." By thinking like this, we give away self-responsibility. Our energy field is chaotic, and so is the course of our lives. The human being as a typical "victim" is the result.

It's still a long way to divine providence, requiring a radical shift in growing up.

25. The Principle of Manipulation

Energy vampires are everywhere

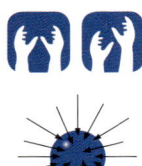

> ### Testing topics
>
> - I manipulate through,
>
> - or have experienced manipulation through:
>
>   – blackmail
>   – jealousy
>   – drama
>   – victimhood
>   – the withdrawal of love and affection.
>
> - … percent of all my contacts with other people
>   are totally free of manipulation.

During all my years of energy work, I was given the opportunity to learn about many different forms of manipulation between people, and I would have rather done without that knowledge. No matter which method was used, two key questions always remained in the end: *What is the goal of the manipulation?* and *Which role does the manipulator play, and what is his/her responsibility?*

In my view, manipulators are always responsible for what's happening. However, in many cases they're puppets of other forces that work through them.
At any rate, manipulators benefit from the manipulation and must resonate with the energy they're allowing to unfold through them.
The goal of any manipulation is always the most precious thing that human beings have to offer: the light of their soul, heart energy, love, life energy. This is the ultimate goal of any energetic manipulation.

Manipulations can occur on any level:

- On the physical level, through all forms of physical violence or all sorts of drugs or toxins.

- On the unconscious level, through frequencies, dreamtime manipulations, drive and sexual codings, dependencies or addictions.

- On the mental level, through brainwashing, propaganda, thought content, thought fields or drugs.

- On the rhythmic level, through foreign rhythms or the modulation of people's own rhythms.

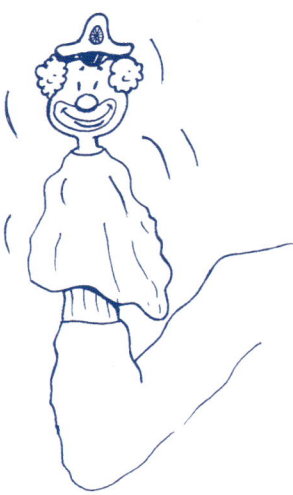

You do what I want!

- On the emotional level, through anger, rage, aggression, greed, envy, stinginess, lies, ruses or fears.

- On the energetic level, through oaths, pacts, initiations or maledictions.

- On the spiritual level, through soul fragmentation and separation, ruptures of the soul field, soul-field duplicates, energetic corrosion, techniques involving a hydra or nebula around the soul field, or light channel manipulation.

The application field for manipulation is immense.
And manipulation is always based on an inner lack of some sort that's compensated at the expense of others.
It's the eternal battle of darkness versus light.
5 percent of all people are dark inside, 5 percent are white, and 90 percent are gray.
The problem is that gray is a lighter form of dark. This means that only 5 percent enjoy true clarity, while 95 percent of all people use manipulation.
This is frustrating, and largely limits one's choice of friends.
It's always a pleasure to meet people who don't manipulate or play games, who communicate in a pure way and who are honest and authentic.
As I said before, it's time that we evolve from the *Homo sapiens* to the *Homo integer*.

The following is a list of different forms of manipulation compiled by workshop participants. They were asked to complete the following sentence: "I manipulate by or through …"

- forcing my help onto others
- pity
- expectations
- arrogance
- judgment
- complaining
- influencing others in subtle ways
- being offended
- suffering
- a "Take care of me" approach
- a "You don't love me anymore, do you …" approach
- aggression
- creating dependencies
- wanting to be the center of attention
- blackmail
- playing the protector
- being hard of hearing (my grandpa understood every dirty joke; otherwise, he acted as if he was hard of hearing)
- black magic
- secrets
- provocations
- the withdrawal of love and affection
- denying sex
- constantly talking ("verbal diarrhea")
- illness
- lies
- dishonesty
- avoiding confrontation
- the compulsion to help
- gossip
- temptation, seduction
- gifts that have an intention
- being hurt
- sex
- sarcasm

- deception
- remaining silent
- bribery

So we can see that almost anything that happens between people can also be used to manipulate others.

As long as people are filled with so much fear, we'll have to deal with the topic of manipulation.
Manipulation needs fear: we manipulate *out* of fear and can be manipulated *because* of fear.

How can we create a world free of manipulation when the average human fear factor is between 60 to 80 percent?

We can keep cleansing ourselves from manipulations, or recognize the ways that we manipulate others and stop doing those things. But as long as fear has such power, these behaviors will return.
This only leaves one way out: reducing our inner fear.

26. The Principle of Honesty

Perhaps I'll be brave enough tomorrow

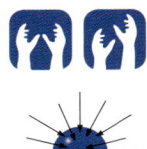

> ### Testing topics
>
> • I am unrelentingly honest.
>
> • I always say what I think.
>
> • I don't do anything to harm myself.
>
> • I always express my honest opinion,
>   no matter how the people around me react.
>
> • I don't compromise myself in any way.
>
> • I don't lie to myself or others.

If you can respond to all these statements with a clear "yes," I bow to you.

As for myself, I do my best to be honest in all situations, but I don't manage to do so 100 percent of the time—yet.

Sometimes I simply feel that there might be a better moment to say certain things, or I still want to let my thoughts mature a bit and get a bit clearer before I express them.

When I say something, however, I'm only responsible for myself, and not for other people's reactions.

I have to trust that they are adult, self-responsible and able to deal with unembellished realities. Nobody needs to be protected.

Honesty doesn't start with expecting honesty from others, but with living honestly yourself.

This may inspire some to do the same and make others shy away, but it's no loss if they do so.

Any form of dishonesty in life has an immediate effect on our life energy—it drops.

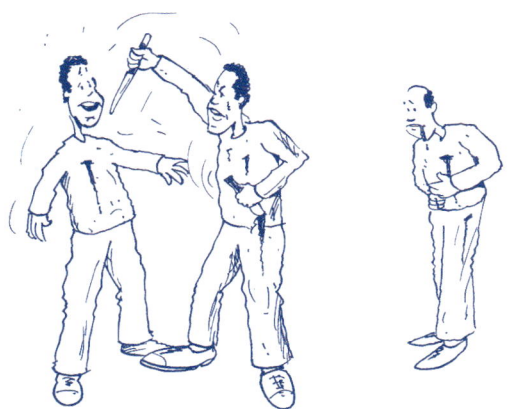

With lies, we hurt ourselves and others.

For therapists, it's important that they're able to tell their clients everything they sense in them. Therapists don't need to protect their clients—no matter whether they perceive sadness, a state of rigidity, a feeling that someone's feet are stuck solid in cement, a missing identity, or even when pointing out certain areas in the client's body that don't feel good.

The core of living life with integrity is honesty and authenticity.

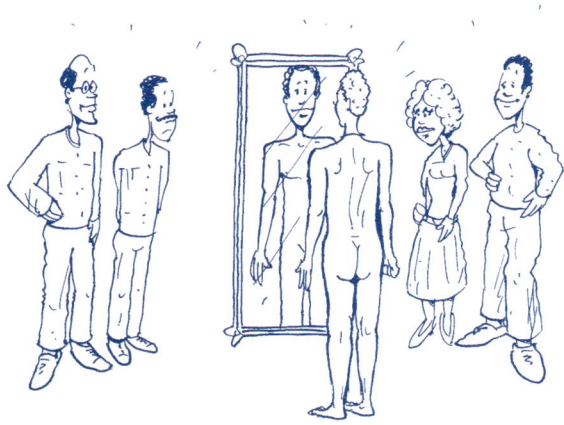

Feel free to look at me if you want; I have nothing to hide.

27. The Principle of Correspondence and Analogies

Easy learning for lazy people: once you understand one, you understand them all

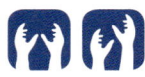
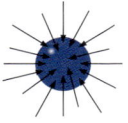

> ### Testing topics
>
> - Whatever I've understood on the small scale, I find again on a large scale.
>
> - Once I've understood my own life, I can also understand any other life.
>
> - I can work with buildings.
>
> - I can work with organizations.

"As above, so below; as below, so above."

The Kybalion

Everything we can observe in people, we can also find again in any other living system, whether it's animals, buildings, teams, systems, organizations or states.

This makes life quite easy: once we've gained a profound insight on one level, we can also apply it to any other level. This is also the criterion for the truth of any insight—it has to be applicable to everything else in order to be true.

For this reason, it's possible that
- designers who use *innerwise* to develop logos and products first work with their clients so that they are clear on what the final design should look like;
- a physician coaches companies without fully mastering business lingo;
- veterinarians treating animals also work on the people and buildings that are part of the animals' environment.

Thus, it just takes a short time to analyze an organization, and no longer several months. "I'll take an inner look at the organization." That is, you look at the fields and resulting images and already have an overview. *innerwise* practitioners have practiced identifying with other people and systems. They feel them inside themselves and as images on the outside. This enables them to analyze objects independently of space and time and grasp the big picture and how it's all connected, without having to work through or lose themselves in the details.
The fields always give us the big picture.

Manipulations are another example.
We can find the same basic forms of manipulation in people, systems and even states and religions. Once we've understood and recognized them in people, we can identify them everywhere.

Flow is the optimal state for human beings, as it is for landscapes and organizations.
Everything can be translated from the small to the large, and vice versa.
Thus, working with *innerwise* is always a journey of discovery.
Everything is alive!

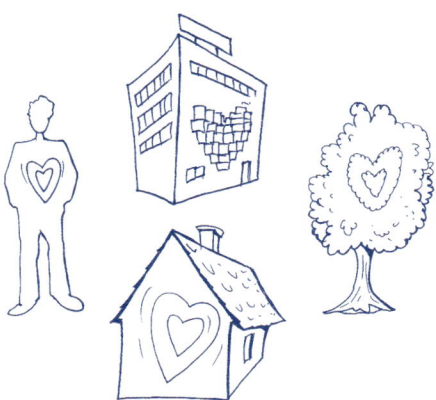

What we see on the small scale, we also find on the large scale.

28. The Principle of Sensitivity

I can see something that you can't see

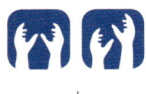
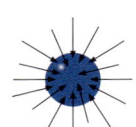

> Testing topics
>
> • I was hiding behind an armor.
>
> • Everyone can tune in and feel someone or something.
>
> • Everyone can see.
>
> • I am willing to be vulnerable again, and in return, will be able to use my senses again in the way they're meant to be used.

"Everyone who keeps his voice pure … will see things that are invisible to others, and hear things that are inaudible to others."

Pythagoras (edited translation)

While classical medicine ponders whether hypersensitivity is a treatable illness or not, this ability to use our senses in the way they were meant to be used constitutes the prerequisite for energy medicine.

As therapists, we're delighted once we've managed to fine-tune our perception again with a lot of work so that we're able to feel and also see emotions, thoughts and energy fields.

Then, however, the world is no longer what it used to be. You lose your innocence and naïveté, as you can now see connections that cannot be perceived by the average person, or rather, those who tend to be blocked and are therefore inclined to explain the world to themselves differently.

Children are usually born as highly sensitive beings but lose these abilities during the first years of their lives, as there aren't adults around them to confirm their perceptions of reality.

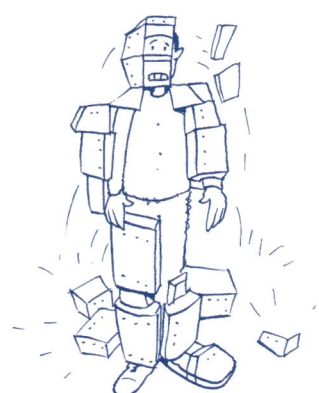

"I don't need this armor anymore."

In my workshops, I've seen time and again that everyone can still feel and sense things, yet most people don't trust their perception. In our workshops, we often start out by forming a circle and perceiving and sensing one of the participants, who's standing in the middle. The participant's stance, posture, emotional state, blockages, pains, energy field, reactions to certain situations—is all actively sensed by the rest of the group. But they also tune in to how that person felt five or ten years ago, how he/she feels at work or when being with his/her partner.

Then all of the participants share their perceptions, and it's amazing how precise they are and how much they match.

You can't hide much from highly sensitive people. They see you.

They can also see the fields and energies of buildings and systems, and sense people remotely. For example, you're thinking about a friend and you know how he/she is doing. The same thing then happens almost all the time with all the people you love. And yet you can't, and may not, prevent them from living out their own experiences. You will still have to learn to stand by and watch—to know yet say nothing. Anything else would deprive these people of their right to make their own decisions. You can only help them recognize issues and see how certain things are connected by asking targeted questions, such as: "Who are you right now?

Are you yourself?" "What's sitting in your heart?"

In treatments, this is a blessing,

But in your daily life, this can almost turn into a curse. With your seemingly "de-ranged" perception, you face plenty of perceptions as a therapist. You've successfully removed the filters that used to protect you. Now, however, you have to learn to also process all your sensations. This requires your nervous system to perform well. Then again, you'll create a different environment for yourself; you will no longer subject yourself to certain influences that aren't good for you. You recognize the intentions and games going on between people. However, in our usually dishonest world, this doesn't really make life any easier.

There's that saying: "Fortune favors fools."

Those who don't realize anything won't be touched by anything either. And we can still resort to Alzheimer's as the ultimate form of oblivion. Then, we can once again walk around with permanently happy smiles on our faces.

29. The Principle of Process Work

Life—I want it all!

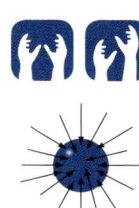

> ### Testing topics
>
> - I'm afraid of processes and try to avoid them.
>
> - I try to protect my fellow human beings from process work. For this reason, I don't always say what I think, or do what I'd really like to do.
>
> - I'm considerate of other people, thus failing to consider myself.

Who actually said that life has to be beautiful all the time?
Very often, life means just letting things happen, and allowing whatever is coming to just come.
Life is an unfolding process.

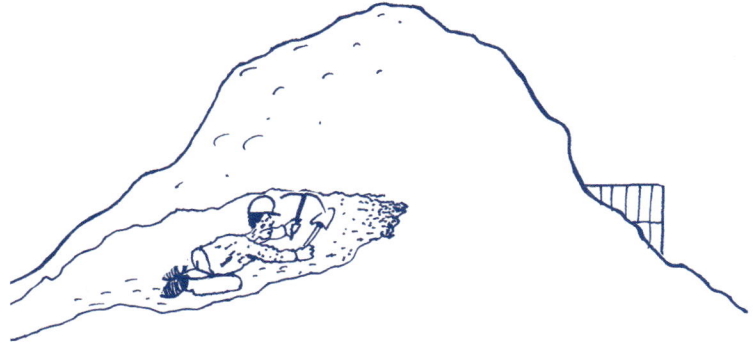

I love my process work.

I was able to gain the greatest insights and take the biggest steps once I'd looked at my own issues in depth, and once my greatest challenges had pushed me to the limits of what I thought I was able to bear.

It's not a terrible thing if we're hurting some times—if we cry, or even if we reflect on the right to commit suicide.

The only thing that matters in process work is that the processes can take place and evolve, and that people don't get stuck in them—that is, that a process doesn't turn into a drama in which the victim part of a person comes out stronger than before.

Let processes happen, allow the pain to surface, discover how things are connected on a deep level in your life, but don't drown in the process.

And grant this right to everybody else, too.

People are sanctified after they died, if they are sanctified at all.

White clothes worn during one's lifetime as a substitute for sanctification often hide something. And after being sanctified, people actually don't need them; then, they don't need any clothes anymore.

Learn to see what's inside people; look at their eyes and see if they shine. Find the soul of a person and see its perfection and completeness.

Process work in treatments

When working with *innerwise*, many well-hidden issues can be touched. The healing cards and the energies coming through them enable us to go directly into the resolution of issues. The energies take over the hard work, and a process is no longer a struggle.

Process work after treatments

In the days following a treatment, cleansing processes can take place; it's possible that other issues can come up once more, and we may be able to see things more clearly, dropping our blinders. The healing symphonies that are "composed" during a treatment help people go through process work without getting stuck.

Not everyone experiences a cleansing of some sort (such as thoughts, emotions, dreams, images or secretions) after a treatment; only about 20 percent of people do. If the garbage piles up high, clean-ups are necessary. We have to do them at some point if life is supposed to be fun and joyful—particularly if a state of rigidity has lasted for weeks or months and the body has suddenly woken up from a deep sleep. And after a hundred-year sleep, our mouth won't smell like roses— rather, it'll be time to brush our teeth!

"Oh God, what a mess!," says the body in dismay as it awakens from its paralyzed state. Then the big cleaning begins.

With the arm-length test, we can determine whether cleansing reactions are to be expected and how long they'll last.

When patients call me after a treatment to tell me that they've started to have reactions, I test how long these reactions will last and tell them, for example, that they'll be over in two days. That way, they know what to expect and can deal with it in a positive way.

And if something additional is needed, the arm-length test can reveal that remotely.

30. The Principle of Forgiveness

Others maybe, but not myself!

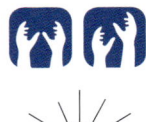

> ### Testing topics
>
> • Thank you for ALL of my experiences.
>
> • Thank you, … , for helping me grow.
>
> • By forgiving other people, I don't assume responsibility for them.

There's a little story about two angels who meet in Heaven and tell each other what they've learned during their lives as humans.

One of them says, "I experienced everything. There's just one thing I didn't do—I didn't learn to forgive." The other angel replies, "If you like, I can help you experience this next time around."

"You would do that for me? You're a true friend, and I love you," the first angel responds.

Then the other angel looks deep into his friend's eyes and says, "Please don't forget that you asked me to do so."

Attempted murder

The woman is still shivering. Eight days ago, her ex-partner tried to kill her. During the night, he entered the house they'd both lived in until eight weeks ago, using a copy of the key, and tried to strangle her with a rope.

He moved out after they ended the relationship due to his problems with alcohol and his violent outbursts.

Ever since the attempted murder, the woman can no longer be by herself; she's filled with fear and panic and sleeps at a friend's home.

When I asked her what she used to love about her ex and why she continued to stay with him for the last two years despite the already difficult and partly violent situation, she replied, "Because of his dick!"

This response even shocked me.

During the testing, it turned out that she was frozen in a state of rigidity—that is, in a state of shock, with her arms differing in length.

After this was cleared up with the help of the *innerwise* cards, the layer underneath became apparent: the difference in her arm length kept increasing, revealing an emotional panic reaction.

Then I tested her identity.

To the statement "I am I," she responded with a "no."

To the statement "I am my ex-partner," she responded with a "yes."

I tested where in her he was energetically present. The testing revealed that it was in her midsection, referring to the space where they would meet, the space of their sexual intercourse.

So I drew *innerwise* healing cards for her until she was completely rebalanced.

Then I picked cards for her ex-partner, which she gave him energetically like a gift, without any intention.

Then I prepared an energy disk for her environment, as the attempted murder was still present as a trauma, keeping her stuck in her victim role in this field.

The one-hour treatment yielded the following results:

The woman could imagine facing her ex without fear; standing in front of him, looking him in the eyes and thanking him for all the experiences they'd had together, whether those were positive or negative.

She could even imagine being by herself again and leaving the window open at night while she slept.

She could imagine accepting her house and garden again as her home, and as a place where she could feel safe and good.

She could imagine giving her ex-partner a present: a job ad that she'd cut out of the newspaper. This was the greatest present she could offer him, so that he could stand on his own feet again and be happy.

She could also imagine opening up to an intelligent and strong partner with clarity. She left it open whether this would be a man or a woman.

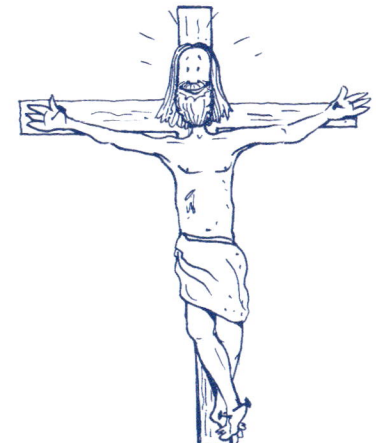

Thank you, God!

31. The Principle of Taking the Stage

Everyone according to their own beliefs

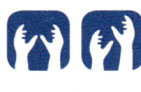
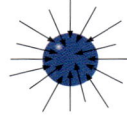

> ### Testing topics
>
> - I only pass on my own insights.
>
> - I pass on the insights of other people.
>
> - Other people know and can do it better than I can.
>
> - I'm willing to stand onstage, assuming 100 percent of my responsibility for myself and my life.

Everyone according to their own beliefs
It has been said that this is what Jesus said. He hardly meant the later interpretation of these words by the Church as an institution of power that used him by proclaiming to believe in him, Jesus.

But it's always the same problem with people in the second row—those who don't live their own lives but who instead latch themselves onto other people. These are individuals who don't live with their own connection to the Source.
Therefore, beware of taking advice from people who haven't found their life purpose yet. Beware of spiritual teachers who recite the words and chants of their masters and demand that you also learn them by heart.
Common to all of them is a claim to power that serves to compensate for the lack of meaning in their own existence, which is being maintained through all forms of manipulation.
Human existence only becomes meaningful once you live up to your soul's potential.

Belief corresponds to what the heart says, to the unconscious. Belief doesn't come from the mind.

All people who are ill want to be healthy in their minds, using their willpower. However, the unconscious, doesn't want to. With its power of manifestation, it has called in the illness as a learning opportunity, and to push people to change something unhealthy in their lives. Illness as an opportunity for transformation for all those who need strong and clear signs—for all those who don't trust their intuition enough or are no longer able to hear its voice.

Find yourself, trust your feelings and perception, and live your life. However, this requires that you have your own identity, that you can respond to the statement "I am I" with a "yes." Otherwise, you're once again living the life of somebody else.

Thus, "everyone according to their own beliefs" means everyone according to their own hearts, everyone according to their unconscious programs.

Be on your life's stage.
Even in the first row, you're only a spectator.

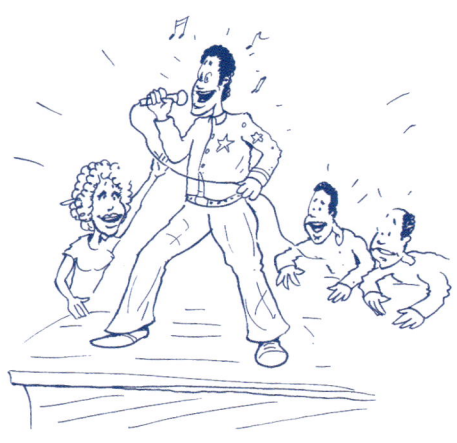

Not the second row!
Not the first row! The stage!

32. The Role of the Therapist

From being a know-it-all to being a student

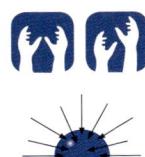

> **Testing topics**
>
> • I heal.
>
> • Healing occurs, and I am allowed
>   to be present.
>
> • The healing doesn't matter to me;
>   I only help other people heal themselves.
>
> • As the therapist, I know it better.

It's no longer the healer who heals other people.
Therapists no longer have "helper syndrome," try to save others or even shoulder their burdens.
Neither are they channels for healing energies.
They don't sacrifice themselves for other people.
They aren't the all-knowing doctor.
In short, they're neither saviors, nor healers nor sages.

Yet what remains?

Therapists are empathetic, loving people who keep learning, discovering and being amazed.
Therapists—or let's call them coaches or simply practitioners (basically everybody who uses *innerwise*)—have a wonderful opportunity to learn a bit more about life and to experience the beauty of life again while offering that opportunity to others.

The tasks of therapists include:

- humbly practicing a neutral view—spherical vision;
- allowing themselves to sense something unknown on a very deep level;
- embarking on journeys of discovery and understanding how cause and effect are connected in life;
- experiencing the magic of how old charges and issues clear up with the support of energies and sounds, and how this serves to transform reality instantly.

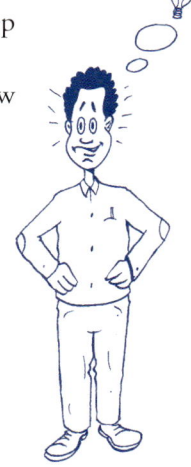

I'm given the opportunity to learn and even get paid for it—that's great!

Using *innerwise* is like a deep meditation that connects us with the beauty of Creation.

When therapists have less energy after an *innerwise* treatment than before, they've done something wrong.

They've let their clients play victim games, have tried to shoulder their clients' burdens and haven't allowed them to take responsibility for their own lives.

The purpose of *innerwise* is not to confirm the knowledge people have acquired through books or have learned by heart, but to learn how to read the only book really worth being read—people themselves.

Every *innerwise* treatment reveals new information on how things are connected. I will stop doing treatments when I realize that I'm no longer discovering anything new. Then it will be time for a new calling. But I haven't reached that point yet.

The therapist composes a healing symphony

The *innerwise* testing system, which guides the user intuitively through the treatment, takes the therapist from one core issue to the next in the most efficient way. Through the *innerwise* cards, the healing frequencies are made available, and their sounds are maintained during the session.

The *innerwise* system takes over all the hard work.
And therapists don't need to channel the energies themselves.

In many cases, it's much better this way, as energies can often be mixed with a therapist's projections; or the sources that are used aren't pure and clear. Unfortunately, this often leads to manipulative trespassing by therapists who work energetically.

The *innerwise* system was created, and has grown, over a period of 20 years with the support of people from 20 different countries.
It's under constant observation by a team of therapists, and when there's the slightest sign that something needs to be changed, we analyze it and make the necessary modifications, if need be.
Over all these years, I've taken very seriously any and all feedback from practitioners that has indicated disharmony.
innerwise is a dynamic system that evolves constantly. I don't know if it will ever be completely "finished."
The quality of time undergoes permanent change, and staying present in the time window requires continuous evolution.

For this reason, in the spring of 2011, I completely reworked the 4,200 remedies that had been created over the past 15 years, and also exchanged 1,000 of them. This was possible by inserting a disc into every large *innerwise* Cardsystem, which updated it.
This works almost automatically, similarly to what Mac users are used to with their computers—easily and smoothly.

innerwise **is a living, wise being that offers therapists the opportunity to grow.**

33. The Principle of Energy Density

Some stars shine brighter than others

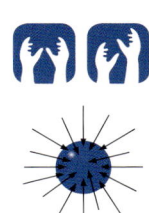

> ### Testing topics
>
> - I get … percent of his/her energy from the following person.
>
> - This energy makes up … percent of the amount of energy I need.
>
> - I lose … percent of my energy to the following person.
>
> - The … percent of energy I give away corresponds to … percent of energy to the other person.

1. **Why is the energy of some people high and concentrated, and weak and thin in others?**

If all energy were the same, 5 percent of one person's energy would match 5 percent of another's.
But it's not at all like that; also, if that were the case, energy vampirism would no longer make any sense.
Then, the "empty" grandparents would have no interest in recharging themselves from the newly born grandchild (of course, unconsciously in most cases).
Five percent of one person can mean 80 percent for another.
It's possible to test this when you feel you've lost energy to somebody else, whether voluntarily or not. You can test what percent of your own energy you've lost (for example, 7 percent) and how this corresponds to another (for example, 27 percent).

How does this difference in energy density come about?

2. **If the smaller share of the human's conscious mind in manifesting life serves to protect him from self-destruction through negative thoughts, and if there are also people in whom the conscious mind and the unconscious participate equally in creating life, then what is the difference between these people on higher energetic levels?**

3. **Why is the soul presence and glow of some people stronger than that of others ... as if the Divine has expressed itself through some people in a stronger and more direct way than in others?**

4. **If we were all little princes, would our home planets always be the same size?**

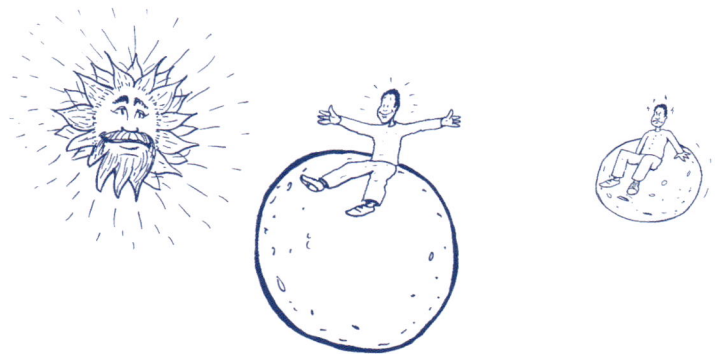

By living my soul purpose, I get closer to
the Source and have more energy.

I've established a simple theory to find conclusive answers to all these questions. The more we keep a positive focus and have positive thoughts, the larger the share the conscious mind can have in creating reality, and the closer we are to the Source, the Divine.

And the closer we are to the Divine, the larger our soul space, our home planet, becomes.

And the closer we are to the Divine, the more concentrated, dense and clear our energy is.

Thus, it's all up to us and in our hands how much divinity we want to sense in ourselves, and how separate or how connected we want to feel.

At this point, here's a hint as far as choosing your partner:

Always look for a partner where one percent of your energy corresponds approximately to one percent of his or her energy.

With a greater gradient, there will always be energy-draining and inferiority issues in the relationship, even with the best of intentions.

34. The Principle of All and Nothing

How the Dual is born out of the One

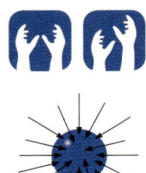

> **Testing topics**
>
> • I like to follow others.
>
> • Gurus are great, and know the way to the Light better than I do.
>
> • I only follow my own path.
>
> • I have the courage to live my truth.

Here we are, back to the big questions, just like we were at the beginning of the first part.

How is the Dual created? Where is the Dual in the One? Why do many people become energetically darker? Which role does living your soul purpose play?

What is the quintessence? Is enlightenment attainable? Where is the One? Where is God?

The long quest has been successful and has led to a simple graphic that explains the All and the Nothing, or all and nothing (see next page).

The Dual is an infolding within the One. The One fills up the infinite space; and in this One, there are countless blisters, infoldings or spaces of duality. They all look like apples.

The world ether, the *spiritus mundi,* flows into them and becomes individual soul energy. This individual soul energy flows into the apple through the life channel and creates the island of life in the center, life's stage.

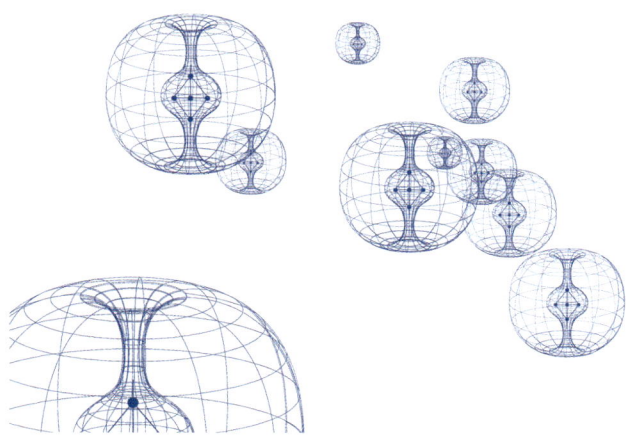

The ONE folds inwards, creating the DUAL.

In people who find and embrace their own soul purpose and connect to their soul energy, this channel of the island of life opens to the bottom, and the transformed soul energy flows as love energy out of the apple and back into the world ether. For those who try to follow another person's life or purpose, the channel turns into a dead end.

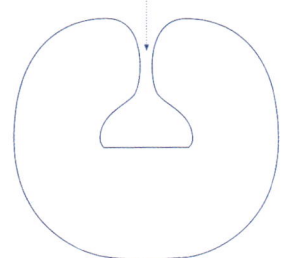

A dead-end street—
this path leads to continuous dying.

But let's take a more detailed look at the clearing of life.

It's the original playing field for the big game, the grand scheme of life. That's where all people start their search for their soul purpose.

There are paths leading away from that clearing where other people have already walked successfully; there are swords lying on the ground to clear a new path in the jungle surrounding the clearing.

Shall I take the beaten track, or clear my own path through the jungle?
But which path is the right one? Which one will lead me to the Light, to enlightenment?

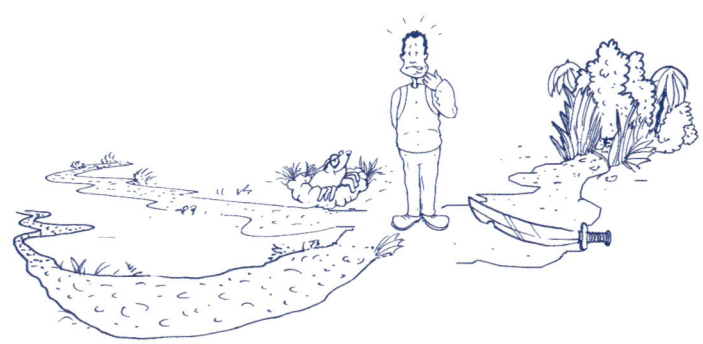

Shall I take the beaten track,
or clear my own path through the jungle?

It's only those people who are looking for and finding their individual soul purpose who are even approaching the Light. This is the quintessence.
Those who try to cop out and follow the purpose of others are running after a mirage and automatically go into the darkness.
We all have our own soul purpose, and only living that passion will bring us closer to enlightenment. Living our own soul passion nourishes us, and connects us with an infinite source of energy.

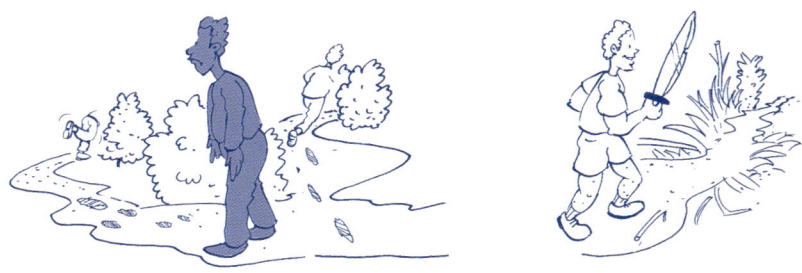

We all have a choice: walking our own path and staying fresh,
or following others and looking old.

If we follow someone else's path—be it a master, guru, partner or whomever—we cut off our connection to our own source of energy. What remains is only asceticism, and restricting ourselves so that we consume as little energy as possible, and/or energy vampirism.

These people acquire a dark aura and learn all forms of manipulations in order to be able to survive—from playing the victim, the need to control others or aggressiveness—to manipulation on the soul level.

Once we've taken the beaten track, it's difficult to turn around, as the hope to finally find our soul passion lurks behind every turn.

However, we can never find it there. This means that we have to turn around, return to the island of life, and look for our own path and dare to take off into the unknown and trust only ourselves.

Most people only manage to do this after they've experienced a great loss, or when their own life is at stake—in short, when they have nothing to lose anymore.

But even then, 95 percent don't understand the signs and let this opportunity go by.

Besides the abundance of life force, the surest sign of walking our own path is that what we do, we do for ourselves.

For example, I didn't write this book to please readers; I did so because I enjoyed writing it. Doing this work is part of my life passion.

And if it inspires others along the way, that's wonderful.

Another sign that we're on the right path is when we experience divine providence in our lives … when life is no longer full of effort and struggle.

35. The Creation and Sources of *innerwise*

Larger than life

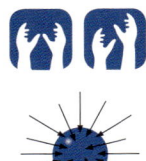

> ### Testing topics
>
> - *innerwise* is authentic.
>
> - The integrity of *innerwise* is
>   … percent.
>
> - *innerwise* benefits … percent of
>   all users.
>
> - *innerwise* harms … percent of
>   all users.

Simplicity

"It can't be that simple." Yes, it can. Simplicity is a sign of quality.
It took 20 years of development work to find this simplicity and clarity.
All aspects of the *innerwise* system and all processes need to be experienced. This is the only way to regain authenticity and simplicity.
A new idea was followed by intense analysis, and then trying it out and delving deeper into the topic and examining it from all perspectives. That's creative chaos! For some developments, this took years; for others, it was just a matter of days. At the end, however, when I had the feeling that I'd understood the topic and was able to integrate it into the grand scheme of life, it was suddenly really easy again.

For me, the parameter for the degree of maturation of something is its applicability to all situations. If it applies to people, it also has to be applicable without restrictions to everything else that is alive.
This is the criterion for truth. Animals, plants, trees, systems, organizations, ideas, projects, and so on, are also alive.

This has been the true "endurance test" for *innerwise* over the last years. People in more than 20 countries coached and worked with everything possible—whether illnesses, states, situations or projects. They probed the realm of possibility and limits that pushed us to keep searching.

I refrained from seeking any recognition from official science, the approving nods of eminent personalities, studies or titles (my doctoral dissertation landed in the trash after I'd completed it successfully) or publications in renowned magazines. The only thing that matters to me is how effective something is in practice.

The basics

• My grandmother loved me unconditionally.

• My grandfather served as a living example of decision-making ability and inspiration.

• My mother showed me perseverance and the love of work.

• My father was a philosopher who set an example of free thinking and expressing ideas outloud.

• Complications when I was born (birth palsy) gave me the strength to walk my own path, even alone if need be.

• My position as the middle child gave me the gift of continually looking for my position.

• My work as a nurse offered me the gift of empathy.

• My medical studies provided me with background knowledge.

• Growing up in eastern Germany showed me the beauty of human depth and simplicity.

• The fall of the Berlin Wall brought me the gift of freedom.

• My work as a physician at different medical clinics offered me the opportunity to recognize limits.

- Thanks to Traditional Chinese Medicine, I learned to look at everyone and everything individually.

- Neural therapy, focal infection research, and professors Pischinger and Perger gave me the gift of understanding ground regulation.

- Physioenergetics showed me the possibility of testing and energy treatments.

- Homeopathy showed me the effectiveness and difference in the quality of energetic information.

- Craniosacral therapy helped me understand the body's rhythms.

- And the many other healing methods offered endless inspiration.

- The crop circles have a special place on this list as a type of earth energy acupuncture and a geometric library of wisdom. If the questions were clear, I always found the answers there. Their perfect geometry holds everything in encoded form; we just have to read it.

- And last but not least, the energy sources that I can simply call divine.

The only true source of *innerwise* is experiencing life, and life itself. I referred to information in other books only after I'd recognized something myself, in order to compare it to the insights of others and be inspired.
The only true sources have been, and still are, the treatments and people I'm asked to work with, who challenge me and offer me further insights.

PART II

Internal and External Tools

Overview

I believe that healing through spiritual methods, in a non-material way, has a future of undreamed-of possibilities. And I believe that their range will gradually grow above and beyond what we—rightfully or not—call "functional" today, and also encompass everything organic.

I see the dawn of a new age shining forth before me when certain surgical interventions, such as those on internal growths or tumors, will be considered mere patchwork. We will feel absolutely horrified that our knowledge of healing methods was once so limited. Then there will hardly be any room for conventional remedies. Far be it from me to demean modern medicine and surgery in any way; on the contrary, I greatly admire both. But I've been allowed to glance at the enormous energies inherent in people, and at those of external sources, which, under certain circumstances, flow through them, and which I can only describe as divine—powers that can not only heal functional, but also organic disorders, which turn out to be symptoms merely accompanying emotional, mental or spiritual troubles.

Prof. Dr. med. Carl Gustav Jung, 1875–1961 (edited translation)

Internal Tools

Practicing *intuitive healing* requires learning the necessary tools. It's like learning how to juggle: At the beginning, you'll drop the ball here and there, especially if your mind doesn't calm down. But at some point, it will become second nature to you, and you'll be able to juggle many balls with ease.

All human beings have these abilities and skills within them, yet they're often buried under mountains of traumas and inner protective mechanisms.

None of us is perfect. I've also been walking my own path step by step, and still do—following the principle "learning by doing."

In this way, *intuitive healing* is open to everybody who wants to use it. One doesn't have to be enlightened first to be allowed to experience it; rather, it supports us on the path of love and insight.

There's always the space to let the necessary inner processes occur, even if they're very painful and our environment has a problem with them. One of the highest values is to be honest with, and take responsibility for, oneself, as well as for one's own path.

In addition to the internal tools that exist within every one of us, only waiting to be awakened and discovered, I've created many external tools that make intuitive yet precise work possible, and which make using *innerwise* really easy. These include therapeutic systems with healing cards and test cards, geometric structures, and amulets and discs as memory media for the healing symphonies that are composed during this work.

Being Able to Love

Being able to see the completeness and perfection of the soul in each and every human being is the first prerequisite for working therapeutically with people. To see this completeness and perfection—even if it's not immediately obvious—means to be able to love that person. People can't develop what we don't trust they can.

Whomever we're facing—whether they have stinky feet, weigh 400 pounds or are murderers—it's our task to see and recognize the beauty and potential of their souls and not block the treatment because of our own inner judgment.

Here, spherical vision is the most essential tool in attaining a state of neutrality.

Spherical Vision

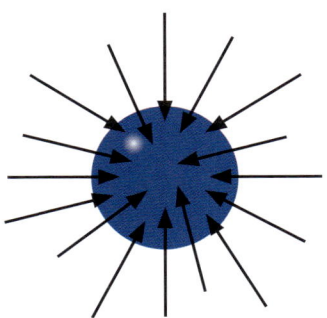

Spherical vision is the biggest challenge for all users.

Our range of vision is the biggest challenge, and it's also a pre-condition for energy work.

We usually look at something from our own perspective. This also means that we compare what we see with what we've experienced so far, evaluating and judging it internally.

Better, worse, the same; oh yeah, I'm already familiar with that; oh well, nothing new; not again. … This prevents us from having a neutral and independent perspective, from recognizing the full beauty of something and opening up to something new without bias.

We can also compare this to looking at a bouquet of flowers. We actually look at only one part of a flower, yet we think we're looking at the entire bouquet.

Consequently, everyone looking at this bouquet will describe it differently. Also, the bouquet will look different depending on the angle from which it is viewed. This may be okay for an interior designer who will arrange the bouquet in such a way to make it look its best. For a therapist or coach, this view is the final blow.

Many years ago when working with a patient, I noticed a weakness in the technique. Using the arm-length test, I asked myself whether I was done with the treatment. The answer was "yes." Yet I had the feeling that something was still missing in the treatment. Then I imagined being a woman and asked myself again. This time, the arm-length test showed that the treatment wasn't finished yet. This was a sign to me that I had to leave my individual perspective to obtain reliable results.

I've developed a type of vision where it doesn't matter whether I'm a man, woman or a child; whether I'm European, African, Asian or from the Moon—the test results are always the same.

I look at somebody from above, below, right and left—from all directions at the same time.

Thus, I don't miss any problem that still requires work at this point in time. Not all issues reveal themselves in all directions. It's possible that a heart problem can only be tested from the left side, or that some other issue is only visible and testable in certain sectors. When using the arm-length test while moving around a person who's lying down, we will find these sectors.

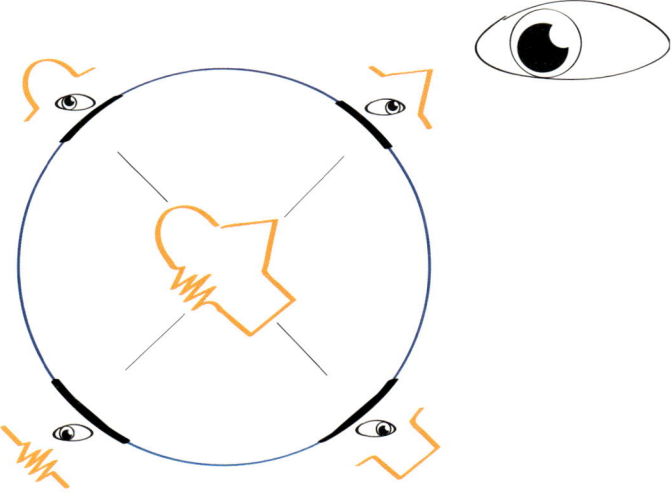

For some issues, we need a certain perspective in order to see them.

In the same way, it can happen that we can't hear particular words coming from certain directions. We can test this with one person standing in the middle, and another going around this person in a circle, while whispering something at the same volume. Such a blind spot or area results from a situation where, at some point in our lives, we were addressed from this direction, and this situation was coupled with a very negative experience. Consequently, this spot or area is blocked out. "Nobody will ever hurt me there again." And we put on protective armor.

When applying spherical vision, we're able to see everything, no matter where we stand, or who and what we are. We can even analyze and then work on situations remotely.

The easiest way to learn spherical vision is to imagine being in the middle of a large group of people who are standing around you in a circle, and being able to see yourself through the eyes of all of them simultaneously.

You can also imagine being the Earth, all stars are eyes, and you're able to see yourself with all these eyes at the same time.

Then everything becomes visible, and it's no longer possible to hide.

With our normal view of something, the arm-length test can only be about 80 percent reliable.

For diagnostic vision, this is unacceptable, even if it's still better than any lab or imaging diagnostics that often reveal health problems only when half of an organ's functionality has stopped.

With spherical vision, we can achieve 100 percent reliable testing or close to it, depending on our individual testing quality.

Spherical vision also helps prevent projections, which are quite common for therapists: therapists see their own issues in patients, thereby manipulating them.

Spherical vision also prevents the phenomenon whereby patients and therapists switch roles during treatment. Unfortunately, this is not that rare and leads to the patient manipulating the therapist.

No matter which therapeutic system we use, spherical vision always determines the quality of our work.

Those who coach companies or projects, for example, drown in their tasks and make the worst mistakes if they don't master this type of vision.

You will find the spherical-vision symbol before each exercise in this book as a reminder to apply it.

The Arm-Length Test

This is not some esoteric fad, but rather, a neurological reflex, with the muscles relaxing on one side of the body while contracting on the other. This is why the arms differ in length.

It's a response by our muscular system to stress. Here, the brain controls our muscles via a neuropeptide, the substance P, at the speed of 1,500 meters (about a mile) per second, in ways that make strong muscles, like those in our arms, suddenly become weak.

Let's get started.

☀ Stand up and let your arms hang loosely at your sides. Relax your shoulders and arms.

☀ Now bring your hands together in a relaxed manner in front of your body, right at its center.

☀ Turn the backs of your hands outward so you can use your thumbnails as a measuring tool. When you're in balance, your thumbs are at the same height.

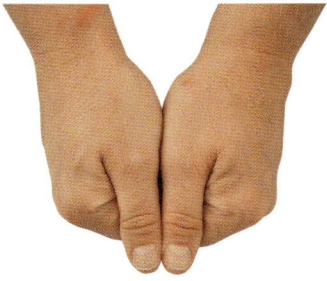

Arm-length test: "yes" or balance

☀ Bring your arms back to the sides of your body and remember to apply spherical vision.

☀ Say "yes" and once more bring your arms together in front of your body. Again, they will be equally long.

* Relax your arms again and let them hang loosely at your sides.

* Now say "no" and bring your arms together in front of your body.

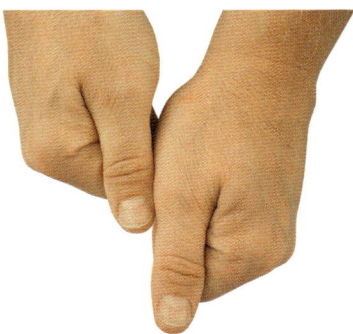

Arm-length test: "no" or stress

This time, your thumbs will not be at the same height. There will be a difference in length, except if you're caught in a state of rigidity.
This will be explained in more detail in the next chapter.

* Your body says "no." It's stressed when it says something negative. Now practice this once more with your eyes closed.

I often close my eyes when I want to sense something, as one can often see better this way.

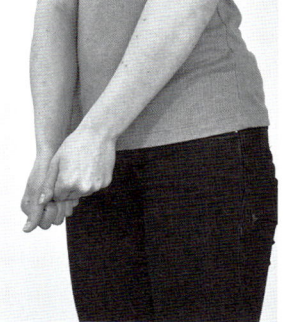

Arm-length test: position of both arms

At the beginning, the difference in the length of your arms during testing can often still be fairly small: 0.5–1.5 inches. The more relaxed you become and the more you practice, the greater it will be. Even differences of about four inches aren't uncommon. Just relax, and your answers will be totally clear.

With time, it will no longer matter to you how your thumbs respond because you will trust your body. You will have become a perfect tester.
In this way, you can talk to your unconscious through your body:

- Think of something positive and your arms will be of equal length.

- Think of something negative and the length of your arms will differ.

Your stress and lie detector is always with you.

Testing: Real Situations

Regular Test

☀ When you say "yes" and test, your arms are equally long.

☀ When you say "no" and test, the length of your arms differs.

You're able to test!

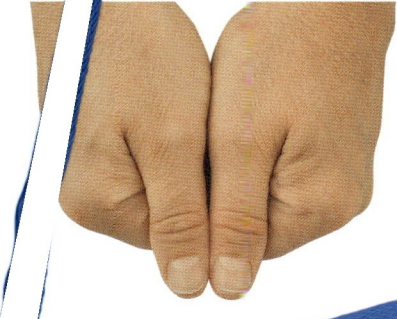

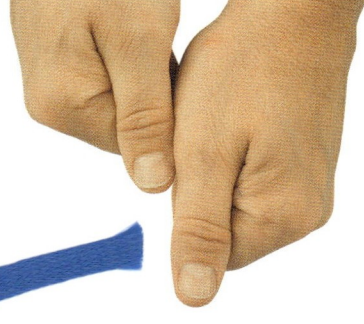

Arm-length test:
"no" or stress

Initial stress

✺ When you say "yes," your arms differ in length. You're out of balance. One side of your scale already has a weight on it.

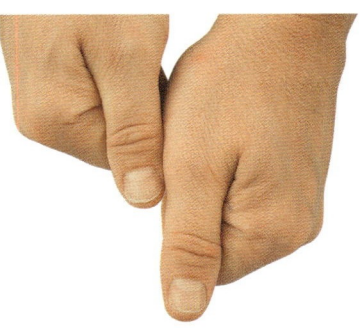
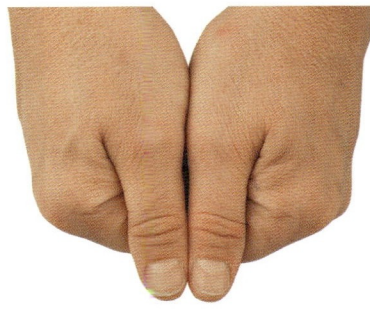

Arm-length test shows "no" or stress response with "yes" statement

Arm-length test shows what seems to be a "yes" or balance with "no" statement

✺ With "no," you're now adding a weight on the other side. The scale looks like it's balanced, although there are weights on both sides. For those of you who are more mathematically inclined: two "no's" equal one "yes."

The first thing to do is treat yourself!

✺ Use colors, essential oils or herbal teas. In the next chapter, I will show you even more options.

Blockade or rigidity

☀ You're frozen! Either in balance or in stress.

☀ Your arms no longer respond when you say "yes" or "no." They remain the same—either equally long, or their length differs.

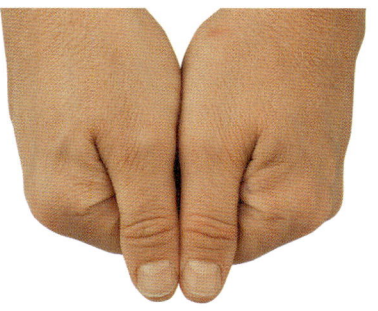

Arm-length test shows "yes"
or balance with "yes" statement

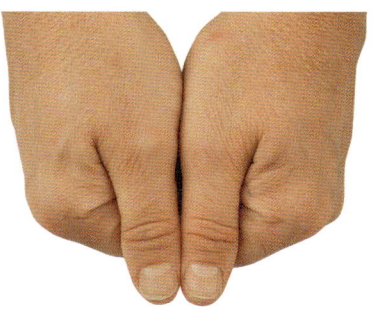

Arm-length test shows "yes" or
balance with "no" statement

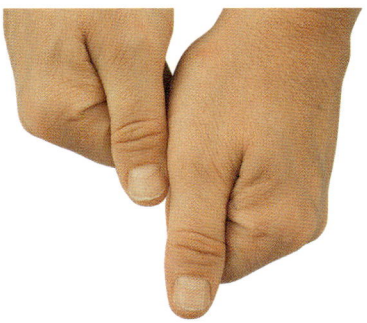

Arm-length test shows "no" or
stress response with "yes" statement

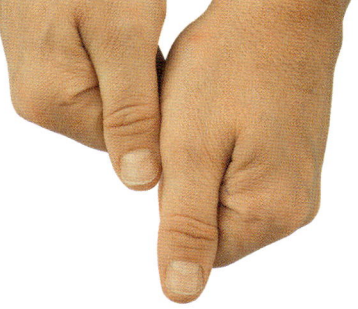

Arm-length test shows "no" or
stress response with "no" statement

The first thing to do is treat yourself!

Response options when using the arm-length test

The arm-length test can do more than just show a "yes" or "no." It can also express a small "no" or low stress, or a big "no" or high stress. And it can reveal allergies and panic.

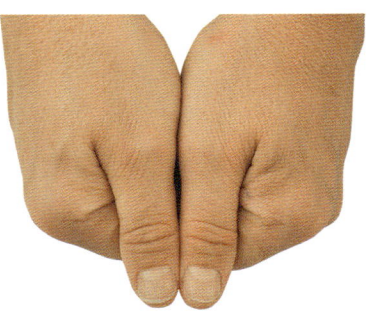

Arm-length test: "yes" or balance

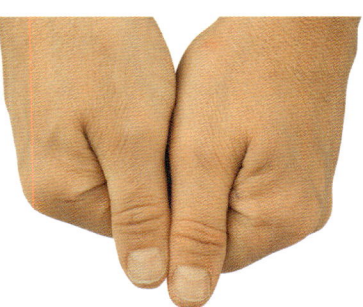

Arm-length test: small "no"
or low stress

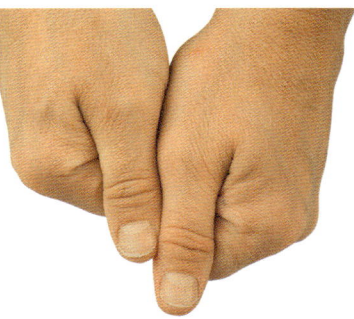

Arm-length test: medium "no"
or stress

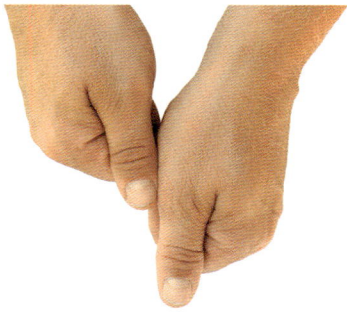

Arm-length test: big "no"
or high stress

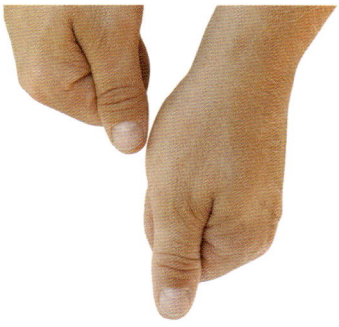

Arm-length test: huge "no"
or very high stress

Allergy or panic

The difference in arm length will keep increasing as you repeat the testing several times in a row. The cause can be an allergy or an emotional panic.

- It's an allergy if you're testing food, shampoo, a dental filling or any other material or substance to which you might have an allergic reaction.

- It's panic if you're thinking of a situation that causes a panic reaction in you.

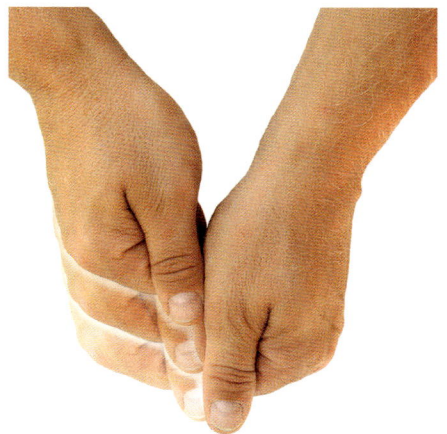

Arm-length test: allergy or panic response

Yes/no or balance/stress

How do I assess the response of my arms? This depends on what you're testing:

- **If you test statements** such as "I do … ," then equally long arms indicate **"Balance. This is good for me."**
  Arms differing in length, however, mean **"Stress. This is not good for me."**
  With such statements, you can already test reliably as a beginner.

- **If you test questions** such as "Should I do … ?" or "Does … harm me?", assessing the response of your arms depends entirely on how the question is phrased. The test can only reveal a **"yes" or "no."**
  If it really harms you, your arms are equally long. Your body says "yes."

Testing questions is an option that I recommend to those who are already confident in using the test, and who consider in advance what a "yes" or "no" response to that question means to them.

Assessing the test response

When testing statements:

- Equally long arms: **Balance. This is good for me.**
- – Arms differing in length: **Stress. This is not good for me.**

When testing questions:

- Equally long arms: **Yes, this is correct.**
- Arms differing in length: **No, this is false.**

Intuition

"I began to realize that an intuitive understanding and consciousness was more significant than abstract thinking and intellectual logical analysis."

Steve Jobs

We can only see the true nature of people or things with our heart. Our mind analyzes immediately; it judges and compares.
If we understand ourselves to be instruments recognizing a higher force, and wish to let its intelligence unfold through us, our intuition is our divine autopilot.

Feeling and inner sensing are broader and can move more freely in more dimensions than our mind.
A flying eagle sees more and grasps a bigger picture than a hunter even with the best possible binoculars.

The *innerwise* system is used purely intuitively. That's why children can use it successfully even when they're only three years old. Kids are still free to discover *innerwise* with their senses. Adults often have to let go of their conditioning, value concepts, protective armor and the monkey mind telling them how things should be, before they can open up to the full potential of *innerwise*.

This is my tip:
Forget the head and trust your heart. Trust your first feeling and the words and images that arise within you.
The second feeling, word or image that is checked by the mind, trimmed to fit and then released, is worthless.
When working with other people, always say whatever comes up in you, what comes through you. Have the courage to do so. The patient can always do something with it and feels that the therapist sees and understands him or her deep inside.

Imago—Images—Imagination

"The spirit is the master, imagination the tool, and the body the plastic material."

Paracelsus: De morbis invisibilis

Analytical psychology refers to *Imago* (Latin plural: *Imagines*) as unconscious visual memories that were formed in early childhood and that influence a person later in life. These images primarily relate to people.

Over the last 20 years, we have developed a kind of virtual systemic constellation work that is referred to as *innerwise* Imago, recognizing and expanding this concept as created by its founding father, C.G. Jung.

While conducting virtual systemic constellation work, we move freely in time and space. We see rooms or spaces, energies, people and systems as constellations and images. Using the healing energies, we can easily transform and clear up these images.

Whenever I'm in a confusing situation, I look at the related images inside myself or actually sit down and draw the situation on a piece of paper. This makes all forces at work visible, as well as the position of all people involved and other invisible influences. These drawings can be easily combined with the arm-length test:

Is the person here in the picture? Is anyone missing? How tall is the person? Is there something on this drawing that doesn't belong there? …

innerwise Imago is highly effective process work that patients often perform themselves. With the support of *innerwise*, the therapist provides guidance to ensure that it goes smoothly and that the charges clear up in the end, thus transforming the field and making real changes possible in the lives of all involved.

The time it takes varies. Anything is possible—from one or two minutes up to a half-hour. You never know where these journeys in pictures will lead you. But throughout all these years, we've always found that the issues *can* be resolved.

The fundamental principles

I've never met anybody who wasn't able to apply this technique or couldn't see any images.
Many people don't trust their images; therefore, it's the task of the therapist or coach to encourage and support the client. This requires a quiet, relaxed atmosphere; you need a healing space.
The setup or design of the room is less important; what counts much more is the therapist's ability to create a supportive field so that therapist and client are surrounded by a bubble of time- and spacelessness.

No representatives
As opposed to family constellations, there are no representatives assuming roles in the Imago work with clients; instead, the clients see all the images themselves. This precludes the common problem of representatives remaining attached to their roles, because they take on an external field, often a soul, when assuming that role, and they allow those souls to show themselves through their bodies, their emotions and their voices.
For projects and situations, the client draws the Imago, so there are no human representatives either.

Patient and therapist go into the image that arises and often see the same images.

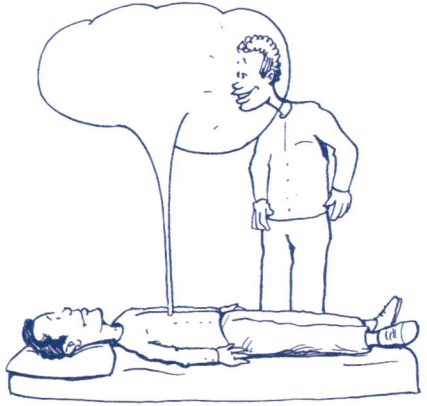

A good movie can hardly offer more suspense!

That way, the therapist/coach is best able to guide the patient or client and see more, as he or she maintains the overview.

The virtual size of the people involved indicates their level of responsibility.
If a child is the tallest person in the virtual image, he/she bears the main responsibility because his/her parents aren't, although it's their job.

Parents/couples should be equally tall (virtual height).
Only then can they be on the same level.

*Parents should be in the middle and face one another, looking in each other's
eyes and hearts.*
Couples standing next to each other are like brother and sister. It's not possible to
look into each other's eyes or hearts, or to kiss each other or make love. That's why
they should face one another and be able to open up to each other and engage.
Even if they're separated, they're both responsible for their children as parents, and
this is only possible when they communicate on the same level.

*Children should always be smaller than their parents and be able to move
around freely.*
They're free from responsibility. For this reason, they don't need to stand in the
middle or in a set place.

Grandparents don't belong in the same room as the core family.
They're still in that room if they don't trust their children to be parents themselves.
In such a case, accompanying the grandparents lovingly back to their own room
is the right way.

Fixed positions in the room
At the beginning, people are often sitting at a table. This symbolizes fixed roles,
rules and a lack of flexibility. It's important that people can move around, so letting them get up allows change to happen.

Any furniture, carpets or objects have to be removed from the room.
First, one should always have a look underneath and into everything; this may
reveal the lover in the armoire, the family secret under the carpet or a message
under the chair. After that, it's best to throw each piece out of the virtual window
into a big fire and burn it. But don't force anything. If a girl is hiding underneath
the red couch because her grandfather is standing in front of her with an erection,
one can't just remove the couch; first, the grandfather has to be accompanied
home where he can take care of himself.

First, try to encourage change verbally; if this doesn't suffice, use healing cards.
During Imago work, I always try to guide the patient verbally:
"Can you ask your mom to come closer? Could you both remove the armoire from the room? …" If this can't be done with ease, I use healing cards.
Never work *against* any resistance. First, clear the resistance using healing cards; then continue working.

Never give children responsibility for others in your Imago work.
Here's an example of serious abuse during family constellation work, as it should never ever happen:
In a family constellation according to Hellinger, a woman wasn't able to resolve her situation. Consequently, the facilitator asked the person then representing her 12-year-old daughter to stand behind the mother and support her.
In real life, the daughter built up a great deal of anger against her mother over the years to come; she took drugs and moved out at the age of 16. When the daughter was 21, I cleared up this spiritual abuse with the help of *innerwise* and released the daughter from the responsibility that she needed to support her mother. On the same day, the daughter contacted her mother. The daughter still showed cleansing reactions for two subsequent days, and then the relationship between the two was clarified and they could open up to one another again.

The laws of time and space no longer apply.
It's not that important when and where the Imago work takes place. People who have passed away are as much a part of the work as those still alive. A trauma that was experienced 50 years ago can still be resolved in that past moment, radically transforming the now, as well as the way these past 50 years are felt and experienced in hindsight. On a soul level, those who passed away in the meantime still receive the healing energies, and it often helps them to finally leave the intermediary world and find peace.

Determining the kind of Imago work by identifying the patient's age during the process
The easiest way to determine the kind of Imago work that should be carried out is to test the patient's age during the Imago. This reveals whether the Imago work should be done in the core family where the patient is still a child, or whether the patient is already an adult regarding this issue or whether other specific Imago work should be performed.

What is allowed, and what isn't?

It's not permissible to force something where there's resistance. The images have to transform with ease, which is possible thanks to the healing cards.

Sometimes patients don't want to look at a certain issue. If, however, the testing system and arm-length test confirm that this issue should be worked on, it's up to the therapist to convey this to the patient. Actually, it's only about convincing the client's mind, as the unconscious has already said "yes" through the arms.

It's part of therapists' jobs, and it's also their responsibility, to work out of spherical vision, free from any personal interests or perspectives, and to only do what feels "right"—in tune with the bigger plan and with clients living their soul purpose.

Additional inspirations

1. Who stands where? Who is not in the room? Describe the room. How is the light and the air? Which pieces of furniture are in the room?

2. What is under the carpet? Open the floor flap and look inside? *My father is sitting there holding a piece of paper in his hand.* Let him read out loud what it says on this paper.

3. Imagine a room with the women of the last seven generations.

4. Draw your project.

5. Draw your company on this piece of paper—just intuitively, the way you feel it.

6. Where are you? Where are the products and the staff? Where is the name? Include everything in your drawing.

innerwise Imago techniques

Visualization

Usually we use visualization in our work.

Here, the clients see images, and therapists immerse themselves in the clients' images.

The hand theater

Sometimes it's important to quickly get an overview of a situation. For this purpose, you can virtually put the situation in one hand, and look at it from all sides with your eyes closed. In the second hand, you can put the situation in a different timeframe for comparison, or another person, which will reveal relevant interactions. Often, it's also important to add the parents on the second hand and identify the energetic links.

Drawings

For system Imagos, it's highly recommended to always work with drawings to be able to grasp the complexity. After the first balancing work with healing cards is done, the image is drawn anew; the new drawing often looks very different. This process is repeated a couple of times until all are satisfied with the outcome. Here, the system is treated via the image, and the healing cards are placed on the image itself. At the end, the result of all the healing frequencies is copied to an *innerwise* disc and given to the system in order to function as a sound system.

Different kinds of *innerwise* Imago

The now

This is the current state, a situation or a project.

A specific age

With the arm-length test, we can identify the optimal age to resolve and heal an issue. This also determines whether the client will be in the child or adult role during the Imago work.

A situation

Situations can be grasped best by drawing them.
All you need is a sheet of paper, a pen and a frame that stands for the system or the situation. Then, all elements are drawn intuitively in the frame and the arm-length test provides all necessary details as you go along.

An organ

The uterus and the heart are the favorite organs, but naturally, organ Imago work can be done with *any* organ.
"Imagine your uterus is a room and describe it. What color is it?"
"The room is black and heavy; it's filled with something sticky."
"Could these be the energies of former lovers?"
"Yes, that's what this is; but only of two of them."
"Give them these healing cards and thank them for the experience."
"Now, the room is getting brighter and lighter."
"What are the walls like? What is over there on the left wall?"
"There's a hole."

"And when you look into that hole, what's hiding in there?"
"At the end of the corridor is the child I aborted 17 years ago."
The Imago work continues until the room is bright, beautiful and feels light.

Systems, projects and organizations

Systems are the ideal objects for drawings. In light of their complexity, they're quite special and challenging. Therapists or coaches who know how to work well with people using the Imago approach, who've gained plenty of experience and who particularly like multitasking, will enjoy the opportunity to be really creative. They'll have to think of everything—from the boss to the products, buildings, sellers, investors and clients—all the way to the cleaning staff. Changes in energetic situations and relations have an effect on everybody, so the coach has to be able to maintain the overview and know and feel what is happening at point Z when changing something at point A. It's best when those ordering or contracting a particular job—who always have to be the ones bearing the responsibility for the system—make the drawings themselves. For this kind of Imago, I recommend specific training offered by the *innerwise* Institute, where you learn to live up to the high level of responsibility required in this work.

Examples of *innerwise* Imago work

Draw your family

A therapist had problems with her 14-year-old daughter, as well as with her relationship with her partner.
I asked her to draw her family. The image clarified the situation: the partner was no longer next to her in the middle, but appeared in the top left part of the image. The 14-year-old daughter had taken his place and was disproportionally large. The younger brother hadn't just withdrawn in life, but also in the drawing.
The cause of all this was a third child who had died early and who still blocked the entire family constellation.

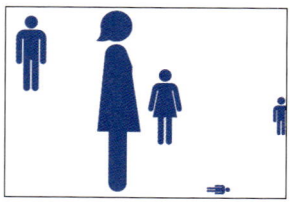

Initial situation

After healing cards were given to this third child, the 14-year-old daughter could take *her* place, the partner could take *his* place in the middle next to his wife, and the boy could come closer.

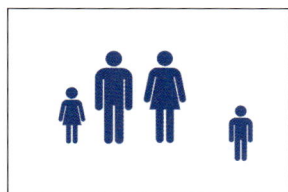

Intermediary step

But the image still didn't feel good; something was missing, which we balanced using healing cards. Consequently, the woman and her partner changed places, and there was stable harmony among all.

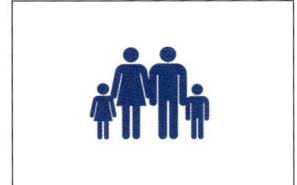

Final situation

The children sensed our energy work immediately from afar—a distance of over 1,600 miles by air—and the family dynamic changed as of that day.

The 14-year-old had been so rebellious because she had taken over her father's responsibility and thus, his role, who hadn't been able to overcome the death of the third child. This adult position of responsibility had completely overwhelmed the girl.

"Close your eyes and describe what you see."

A mother comes in with her six-year-old daughter who's suffering from severe renal insufficiency and is supposed to start dialysis soon.

Working with the mother, I ask her to close her eyes and describe the family room.

"I am standing in the middle. With the right hand, I'm holding on to my first husband (the father of the six-year old daughter), and with the left hand, I'm holding on to my current partner. If I wasn't holding on to these men, I would fall over.

"I'm facing the partner I was with between these two men. My daughter is lying underneath him; he had raped her."

(In real life, the man she is facing in this image still lurks behind street corners.) With the first *innerwise* healing cards, the image changes. The daughter can get away from this man and seek shelter behind her mother.

With the next healing cards, we try to get this man out of the room but can't manage to do so. It's only when I ask the patient to invite the mother of this man into the room as well that it's possible to bring mother and son out of the room with the help of the healing cards.

In this very moment, the woman can let go of both men she was holding on to. With the support of a few additional healing cards, she can turn to her current partner, take her daughter into her arms and carry the newborn baby together with her partner.

After that, the kidneys of the six-year old daughter are healed, and today, she is in perfect health.

"Imagine that you're five years old. Now describe the room of your family."
"I'm standing in a corner; my grandmother is in the middle of the room, and my mother is sitting on a chair next to her mother-in-law."
"Where are your father and your brother?"
"I can't see my father, and my brother is hiding in another corner."
"What is the room like? What kind of furniture is in the room?"
"The room is dark, and there's an old stove attached to the wall."
"Look what's inside the stove."
"There's nothing in that stove."
"Then take the stove out of the room."
"As I'm pulling the stovepipe off the wall, a photo appears that was hiding there."
"What do you see on this photo?"
"My grandmother's family at a grave."
"Ask your grandmother who is buried there."
"She says it's her brother who was murdered."
"Give these healing cards to your grandmother so that she can give them to her brother's soul."
"She is doing it, and he's taking them. Now, the entire room is turning very bright, and my father is standing in the doorway."
"These healing cards are for your grandmother so that she can finally trust that her son is able to take care of a family."
"Now my grandmother is leaving the room and going back to her own room.

And my father is coming into the middle of the room. My mother is getting up, and my brother is coming over to me."

"Are your parents now equally tall?"

"My father is still taller."

"These cards are for your mother."

"Now they're equally tall and are looking at each other."

"How are you children doing?"

"We're playing and are happy."

Imago from a client's perspective

Preface by the therapist

A mother came to see me (see description of session) after I had worked with her daughter. The daughter was 21 years old and had been in a psychologist's care since the age of 14. *Background:* Her mother's ex-partner had physically abused her over a long period of time, which led to the mother's separation from the man. Since she was nine years old, the daughter had been sexually abused by her uncle (her mother's brother). Since then, there hadn't been any contact with either uncle or grandmother, as both had accused the child of lying. Currently, the daughter has a boyfriend who hits her, but she says she can't leave him as she's not able to be by herself.

So far, the psychologist has only worked with the daughter. I recommended that she also work with the mother, even if the daughter is already grown up.

Since both sessions, one with the mother and one with her daughter, the daughter has been able to stay by herself in her apartment and doesn't call her mother for every little thing. She has largely reduced her contact with the abusive boyfriend. The mother is no longer so heavily concerned about her child and can let her grow up.

Since the mother had such beautiful images during the session, I asked her if she could write down her session for this book.

The client's Imago experience: my safe haven

I was walking along a long, narrow corridor, but I had no idea how I'd gotten here. A few seconds ago, I'd still been deeply engaged in conversation with a woman who had asked me to lie down and close my eyes. I was putting one foot in front of the other with keen anticipation of what would happen next. Gray-green tiles covered the walls of the corridor, which had smooth and robust flooring. Above the tiles, the wall was whitewashed, turning into a vaulted ceiling with bright neon tubes lighting the hallway. It seemed like a very long corridor of a hospital, but I wasn't completely sure, as a heavy, old wooden door appeared at the end of this hallway that didn't fit at all into the picture of a hospital.

I was prompted to open the door and look at what was hiding behind it. The door should have made a creaking sound as I opened it, yet I didn't hear anything. It was very quiet all around me. It wasn't an unpleasant, heavy silence; rather, it was almost sacred. As I reached out to turn the doorknob, I already found myself in a grotto. Directly in front of me, a single bright light at the end of the grotto made it possible for me to see something within this space. In the back, a wooden, antique-looking coffin stood on top of what looked like an altar made of polished stone. The setting reminded me of a closed shrine that only I had access to. As I was looking around, I noticed the walls made of gray stone; in the presence of this lit altar, they faded into the background. Somehow, I didn't manage to walk farther into this sacred space.

Silently, the door closed behind me, and now I was all alone in the grotto. I heard a voice say, "Who is lying in this coffin?" My mother, is what came to my mind. But only when the voice prompted me to take a look into the coffin did my legs start to move again. Slowly, a feeling of trepidation arose in me; I was afraid to see who was really lying in the coffin. But I felt that there was no turning back; the only thing I could do was go forward and see what I needed to see. Somehow, my curiosity also made this an exciting adventure. Where was it going to lead me?

When I arrived at the coffin, I could see that the lid wasn't closed. Carefully, I peeked inside, feeling some anxiety again.

I closed one of my eyes, pretending to myself that by doing so I might not have to see everything that was hiding inside, but it didn't help. Even closing one eye enabled me to see what I needed to see. As I saw the face of the deceased person, I felt relief on the one hand and total surprise on the other—I hadn't expected that. It wasn't my mother in the coffin, but my son's father, whom I hadn't been in touch with since my son was born. During the three years of our relationship, which had occurred an eternity ago—over 17 years before—this man's behavior toward my daughter and me had been marked by violent outbursts and physical abuse.

He was lying there the way I had known him years ago: with his smooth and flawless face and tall, strong body. And he was wearing a dark suit.

At first, it seemed that he was only asleep, but then I realized that he was indeed dead. His skin appeared waxen, his eyes were closed, and the corners of his mouth seemed to be drooping slightly. There was something peaceful about this image, and for the first time in many years, I felt liberated from the pressure that the mere mention of his name had often caused in me. He had no power over me anymore because he was dead. I felt neither sad nor euphoric, nor did any of the bitter feelings arise that had been connected with him. It was good as it was. I turned around to leave this space, which appeared to be a viewing area for his coffin in a funeral home. But the voice said to me: "No, you aren't the one who has to leave this room—_he_ has to. It's _your_ safe haven."

I was perplexed. How was this supposed to work? I wasn't going to be able to carry the coffin out of this grotto by myself. Before I could think further and come up with a strategy, the heavy wooden door opened, and a few men in livery uniforms entered. Without looking at me—in fact, it seemed that they hadn't even seen me—they took the coffin, closed it with the lid that was lying beside it and silently carried it outside. The massive wooden door closed without a sound, and now I was really alone in this room. I turned again toward the stone altar and the flickering light behind it. The source of light was a torch stuck in a support attached to a wooden wall. "Did something change in this space?" I heard the voice asking me. Slowly, I started to glance around the grotto. The walls and ceiling were no longer solely made of gray stone. In between, they glittered and sparkled like a thousand gems, diffusing the grotto's darkness.

I almost felt as if I were part of a story by [Austrian writer] Adalbert Stifter, visiting dwarves inside a mountain. Yet something about how I felt about my safe haven disturbed me. Although it was beautiful, I felt that this was not really my place. Despite the breathtaking view of the sparkling gems, I felt depressed. This room had no windows to look outside, and no door except for the one through which I'd entered; but for some reason this door no longer seemed to offer a way out.

The voice prompted me to take another careful look around the grotto. "Are there still any dark corners anywhere?" Instinctively, I walked over to the wooden wall with the torch. As I was approaching it, I realized that it was only a narrow wall made of boards; on its backside, the almost round space of the grotto continued. As a matter of fact, it was dark behind this wall, and an earthy smell reached my nostrils.

Suddenly, I noticed a small, simple wooden door with dark iron fittings, which was set in the stone wall behind. Without much thinking I knew that through this door I would be able to get out of this room into the open. I pushed the handle and here it was: my domain.

I was standing on a little hill, looking out into a small green valley. The path in front of the door I had just stepped through meandered down a rolling hill. The grass was high, and it smelled like a colorful, flowery meadow. I briskly walked toward my real destination: a quiet pond. On the right side of the pond, there was a huge tree with spreading branches, both flexible and sturdy. At the foot of the tree, I sat down in the soft, fluffy grass. It felt like a bunch of little green pillows snuggling against my skin and offering a cozy cushion for my behind. My back was leaning against the rough trunk without finding it hard, feeling the tree's support. I had all the time in the world.

I soaked up this environment, which never ceased to delight me. The pond was surrounded by gentle green hills with countless paths meandering through them, all leading out of this lovely little spot. The most beautiful thing, however, was the blue sky above me *that was reflected in the pond's water. The sun was shining, radiating a gentle warmth from the sky, and at times, a light breeze wafted over my arms. I was almost completely engrossed in this pleasant feeling when the voice jolted me out of my reverie. I still had a mission to complete here.*

The voice said, "Can you see somebody in this landscape? Are there any other people here?" I got up and walked to the bank of the pond. Yes, there was someone there: my brother—in the past he had abused my trust, and my daughter. He was an intruder in my domain, and I didn't feel good at all when I realized this. Helplessly, I was facing this fact, as well as my brother, when the voice asked me: "How was your relationship with your brother in earlier times?"

Tears started to flow out of my eyes and onto my cheeks. "It was very good; we stuck together," I replied. The voice said, "Look your brother in the eyes and forgive him for what he did. To forgive doesn't mean to approve, but to give him back the responsibility for what happened. Then cut the connection to your brother and let him go." Suddenly, I realized that he was standing right in front of me; thin white strings were connecting his body to mine, with little hooks attached to my body. I unhooked one string after the other, but my brother didn't move. He let it happen. He didn't say or do anything. It was as if he was paralyzed. His eyes were dead, and his face was totally rigid. After I'd released the last tie, he fell backward into the water like a wooden log. He didn't try to swim or reach the safety of the bank—nothing. He had turned into a lifeless piece of wood that was drifting on the water.

But how was I supposed to get him out of here? I didn't want him to be here, not even drifting on my pond as a dead piece of wood. The pond didn't have a drain that could take him away. Once again, the voice came to help me: "Is there perhaps somebody else? Someone who could help you with that?"

As the piece of wood drifted to the right, I turned my head in that direction and noticed my mother. She looked at me angrily from a distance as she was approaching me. I felt threatened by her, recalling her accusations that my daughter and I were lying and that we'd destroyed the family by accusing my brother. And again, the voice asked me to also look her into the eyes and thank her for being my mother. Just like she had acted as a mother by trying to protect her son, I also acted like a mother, trying to protect my own children. Once again, tears flowed from my eyes. The voice said, "Your mother has no power over you anymore. You can free yourself of her and let her go in love. She is assuming the responsibility for her actions."

It felt good and it felt right. I was grateful to my mother for being my mom, even if I had missed a lot as a child. I realized that she hadn't been able to act differently. In a split second, I understood that the way it had been was important and right for my particular evolution.

My mother turned around and walked along the bank of the pond. Over and over again, she tried to pull the driftwood out of the water until she finally managed to do so. She stuck it under her left arm and with a bowed head, she slowly walked off toward the range of hills on the right. I gazed after her until she vanished between the green hills with her "prey" under her arms.

Now there was nothing left to disturb me in my beloved spot; I was able to discover things I hadn't perceived before. On the left side of the pond, a bit away from the large tree, there was a small wooden shack with my husband standing in front of it. He looked over at me, and I had the feeling that he wanted me to finally be with him.

But I wasn't ready to go home yet. It even bothered me that he was pressuring me in his overly caring way. I loved him, but I preferred that he take care of himself and simply let me have a bit more time under my tree.

I looked at him, and the voice said: "You're not responsible for me and don't have to worry about me. I can now walk my path alone. We're connected through our love, but without dependencies. We enjoy one another and our time together with mutual trust."

My husband waved to me and disappeared inside the wooden shack, which had grown into a cozy wooden house in the meantime without my noticing it.

A moment later, I heard him hammering away, singing a little song. I knew he was busy fixing his bike behind the house and was already looking forward to a nice ride.

I sat down on the bench that was now under the tree. From here, I contemplated my safe haven, feeling satisfied. "Have a look into the tree," the voice whispered. As I raised my eyes, I saw my children, first Jasmin then Flo, perched on the thick branches of the tree. They didn't resemble birds on branches, but rather two squirrels, looking down.

I hadn't sent them up there. They had sought shelter amidst the tree's branches, observing from above what was happening down here. I smiled at them with encouragement. This was the sign for them to get down off the tree, as they no longer had to be afraid of anything. Without my help, they skillfully climbed down, took each other by the hand and walked off intrepidly. Past our house, they chose the path through the hills toward their new home. I knew they would keep visiting us from time to time, or we would visit them. My safe haven was open to them, and now, since there was nothing to fear anymore, I also knew that they would enjoy coming back. I stayed under my tree for a little while, but then I knew it was time for me to go home. I knew that I could always come back here if I felt like it. As I was only a few steps away from our home, my husband walked out from behind the house and looked at me in joyful anticipation. He smiled at me, and our eyes met. A warm and incredibly calm and satisfied feeling filled my body. He put his arm around my shoulder, and we took off to visit our children.

Lisa

"To forgive doesn't mean to approve, but to give back the responsibility for what has happened."

Perceiving, Feeling, Sensing

Everybody has the ability to feel and sense! It's just that most people have to regain trust in the accuracy of their perception.
The easiest way to achieve this is to observe oneself and to feel and sense situations and other beings.
I practice this every day myself, just like a pianist who practices to maintain and improve his skills.

Put this to practice for the best results. The following exercises can also be found in my book *A Course in Healing*. They came out of many years of experience giving workshops, and I also invite those readers who already know them to read them again and feel and sense themselves.

Journey into your body

Welcome to the world of your body!
Stand up with bare feet. Relax your feet, your legs, your pelvis, your abdomen, your chest, your neck and your head, and imagine your favorite tree.
Feel its trunk, its branches, twigs, leaves and roots.
Feel the sap as it's rising in the tree, and imagine you're this tree and the sun is shining. You see the clouds coming, the rain is providing humidity, and the wind is moving you. Take your attention back to your body.

Feel your legs as they're standing on the ground. Sense if the load is on the front of your foot, on the heel or in the center. Sway a bit to the front and to the back and perceive what's changing. Compare both feet: Do both carry the same load? Is the pressure the same on both?

Now sense your shoulders. Take a deep breath and only pay attention to how your shoulders are moving, the up and down. Is it the same on both sides? Keep breathing, and compare the movements of both shoulders as you're taking a couple of deep breaths.

Feel your eyes. Imagine the little muscles surrounding your eyes from the back. Now move your eyes a bit and sense what these muscles connect to in your body.
How can you feel your eyes' movements everywhere in your body?

Feel the hair on your head and sense how the different hairs lie and stand with regard to one another.

Imagine a downy feather. With this feather, you're gently touching your body's middle line, starting with the highest point on your skull along the forehead, nose, chin, larynx, breastbone, navel, genitals, anus, sacrum, up the spine, neck and back to the highest point on your skull.

Let the energy circulate along this middle line of your body a few times without using a feather.

Become aware of your stance, feeling your thighs and their strength and muscle tension. Feel your knees, calves and feet. Sense the pressure in both feet.

Is it the same? Do both feet carry the same load?

Sway again a bit from your heels to the front of your feet and back, sensing any changes in your entire body.

Breathe in deeply through your nose. Did the inhalation feel the same through both nostrils? Breathe calmly and deeply, and sense how the air is expanding in your lungs. Does it fill both sides equally?

Take a really deep breath. As you breathe in and out, pay particular attention to the left and right sides of your chest—are both sides rising and falling equally?

Keep breathing calmly, sensing whether both shoulders are rising and falling equally as you breathe.

Breathe into your abdomen and pelvis. Feel how your breath is spreading out and filling up this area.

Breathe into your legs, all the way down to the soles of your feet.

Breathe into your head, eyes and ears.

Breathe into your arms and hands.

Inhale through your nose and exhale through your genitals (vagina or penis).

Inhale through your genitals and exhale through your nose.

As you continue breathing in and out calmly, pay particular attention to the right and left sides of your body. Do they feel the same?

Sense them on a deep level.

Hold your breath and stay focused on the left and right sides of your body.

Return to breathing in and out calmly through the nose, and now focus your attention on the front and back of your body.

Focus all your attention on your head.

All your cranial bones can move a bit; they dance with one another. You can feel the dance of each individual bone.

The energy glides down both sides of your head, and you now feel your jaw joints. You can feel the tension in these joints. See if the tension in your jaw joints feels the same on both sides; slowly open your mouth wide and then close it again. Pay attention to the movement—does it go down straight or veer to one side?

Feel all your teeth. Sense what each tooth is connected to in your body. Start with the upper jaws and feel each tooth individually. Take your time so that you can sense the energetic connections.

Feel the uppermost bone of your spine and sense how your skull is resting on it. Slide down with your perception, vertebra by vertebra, and sense the mobility of each individual one. Once you arrive at the tailbone, let it dance very gently. Does it want to dance in all directions?

Slide your pelvis a bit to the front and then to the back. Sense what's changing in your body as a whole.

Now you can sway again from your heels to the tip of your toes and sense what's changing in your body.

Sway to the right and to the left with your entire body and perceive how you're feeling.

Can you hear your heart? Feel it; feel its rhythm.

Feel the rhythm of your lungs, your breath.

Feel the rhythm of your skull.

Feel the rhythm of your liver; sense how it breathes.

Feel the rhythm of your kidneys, their breath.

Now you're ready to feel yourself anew and fully.

Sense the symphony of the different rhythms of all your organs, your entire body.

Breathe in and out of every part of your body, from the ends of your hair to the soles of your feet.

Take the time to give every part of yourself the most loving breath it has ever received from you.

Sensing emotions

Stand up and close your eyes. You're a drop of water falling into a lake. It's a very calm lake, and you can see the ripples you caused. They're spreading out across the entire body of water, which knows now that you're here; it takes you in and offers you an infinite space to experience—a space that feels safe, secure and familiar. You're home.

You can feel yourself, your breath, your stance, your entire body, your energy field and your aura. You will now embark on a journey through your emotions, and experience yourself as you go. On this journey, you will learn how every emotion affects your body and energy field. You will then be able to sense what someone feels simply by looking at this person's body.

✸ Take a look within and allow yourself to be filled with these different emotions:

You're loved.
You're feeling deep doubts within you.
Nobody loves you; you're alone.
You're filled with longing.
You're feeling happiness.
Envy
Anger
Disappointment
You're feeling your loneliness.
Your cowardices
Your fear
You're feeling guilt.
Desperation
Jealousy
Hatred
Self-doubt
You're deeply sad.
You're feeling love.
Desire
Passion
You're feeling afraid.

Scared
Lovesick
You're feeling vexed.
Gratification
Suffering
Fear of death
Feel a lie.
Disgust
Hatred
Arrogance
Gratitude
You're filled with empathy.
Joy is spreading to every cell of your body.
Bask in love.
Now you're ready to feel yourself anew and fully.
Take a deep breath and give every part of yourself the most loving breath it has ever received.
You're wonderful the way you are, and you're loved.

Fields of perception

We can perceive and sense things:

- in another human being or in a system
- in ourselves—as if we were that other person or system.
- on real or virtual stages: in the palm or freely in space.

In another human being or in a system

We stay fully centered in us while immersing ourselves in another human being or system. This allows us to keep our distance. This technique is applied by people who start to practice their sensing skills yet are still careful.

In ourselves

We may also call this empathy—the ability to feel someone or something.

We fully identify with another human being or system, feeling in ourselves how someone or something feels. It's a kind of merging. I always ask patients in advance whether I may tune in to them, as this involves contact on a deep level.

And it's as if we're allowed to learn sensing and reading life itself. It's the greatest possible adventure on Earth!

I manage to open up and engage on such a deep level in treatments about ten to fifteen times a day; it requires high concentration, since with identification comes analysis.

Stance, posture, emotions, breath, energy flows, blockages, fragmentation and separation, energetic links … it's a gigantic flood of impressions.

As you start using this intense technique, I recommend limiting it to three to five times a day in order to avoid being overloaded with impressions. Our nervous system has to practice handling so much information.

Then you can say: "Now I know how you're doing and how you feel."

This also creates the connection that guides us through the treatment and that is completely released at the end by copying the healing symphony that was composed.

In this way, we as therapists are also touched deeply and can discover and learn.

At the same time, it's evident that the therapist has to be clear and centered and in his or her own identity to be able to carry out such work. For this reason, the rule is: balance yourself before you work with others.

Otherwise, therapists run the risk of projecting their issues onto their patients, thereby abusing them, as many psychotherapists do.

It's possible that a treatment can also reveal a therapist's issues.

In that case, therapists have to briefly interrupt the treatment and balance themselves with the *innerwise* system—that is, draw healing cards, put them in their pockets and have a careful look at this very issue after the treatment.

A few times in my own case, I wasn't able to balance myself immediately when one of my issues came up. So I interrupted the treatment, went to the bathroom or had a glass of water or called other therapists for support. In such a case, I always communicated my feelings openly to the patient, saying: "This issue resonates with me, and I need a moment before I can continue working with you."

People were always grateful that I opened up to them so they could understand where I was coming from.

They'd sensed it anyway, and were then able to deal with my honesty. They were grateful for the trust I put in them and knew that the work I did would be of the utmost quality.

On real or virtual stages

There are people or situations one doesn't want to feel inside oneself, even when one has the best of intentions.

If this is the case, you can put your hand in front of your body with the palm facing upward and place that person or situation in your palm.

If necessary, you can also visualize wearing a glove to avoid touching those persons or situations if they're very unpleasant or dark on an energetic level.

Now you can look at the person or situation from all directions; in your other hand, you can put the same person or situation five years ago, for example, and then compare both. Or, you can place your partner, ex-partner, parents or children in the second hand and then observe the interactions.

This is also possible without the hands acting as stages, that is, just doing this exercise freely in space.

In this way, you can observe entire ancestral lines and related interactions.

The hand theater is a wonderful way to gain a quick overview of a situation. "I'll have a look …"

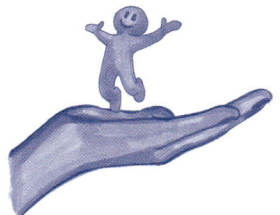

The hand theater

Core values in working with *innerwise*

Being one with the Divine and feeling the support

Those who work with *innerwise* become part of a large family. None of us is a lone fighter—that's not even possible in energy work. It's about discovering and growing together. The next steps in our evolution always occur in synchronicity for many people at the same time. It's like a collective journey of discovery. We're all connected to the time quality and through the global fields; and all those who use and love *innerwise* enjoy a special connection through its field. Thousands of new users have joined us since we went public after 15 years of development work and maturation, and since the German version of *innerwise*: *The Complete Healing System* was published by Allegria Verlag.

The family has grown, and the gratitude and love of all these people can be felt in the quality and field of *innerwise* and are thus available again to all of them.

Trust

Not fighting life but learning to trust that all is right as it is—these are simply necessary learning steps. There are no mistakes in life. We're just missing the big picture.
I can't climb a ladder step by step and then destroy each step I climbed and scream at it: "You were a mistake; I wish I'd never climbed you!"

Honesty

Toward myself, you and us.

You were a mista

Authenticity

Living honesty, being something instead of fabricating things.

"And the only way to do great work is to love what you do. If you haven't found it yet, keep looking. Don't settle. As with all matters of the heart, you'll know when you find it."

Commencement address delivered by Steve Jobs
at Stanford University in October 2005

The level of symptoms vs. the level of origin

Don't try to resolve issues on the level of symptoms—it's useless.
When your house is burning, you shouldn't turn off the fire alarm.
Symptoms are nothing but an alarm signal.
Find the cause; that's where you need to resolve it. Then, healing can occur.
If you only fix things at the level of symptoms, you create dependent people who come back every week and need "fresh makeup." This turns a therapist into a prostitute for victims.

Don't reactivate old dramas

It's a classic therapeutic path to reactivate life's dramas once more, hoping to be able to release them in this way. "What did your grandmother say at the time?" or "What did your uncle do to you?" During my first years of developing *innerwise*, I also did that. Tears were rolling out of my patients' eyes, and I hoped I had resolved their issue.

But soon I realized that reactivating old traumas doesn't heal anything. Often, this even reinforces the trauma. The solution is to merely touch on the issue gently without reactivating it.

I changed my approach, and now I just mention the corresponding age very carefully, for example, and only work on a solution-oriented basis.

For example, I might say, "Imagine that you're standing in front of your ex-partner and are able to look into his eyes and heart." And I always go a step further: "Imagine thanking him for all the experiences that you had together."

In the end, it's necessary to be able to accept all experiences in gratitude, and to also thank all those involved for making the experience possible.

It's not about saying "Thank you for the pain," but "Thank you for the experience even if the path to that experience was painful."

Good-bye, drama kings and drama queens

And there are many of them. They get attention and energy from the drama and from the suffering. They are little vampires who are intent on sucking the therapist's energy with their whining.

Therapists who let this happen, for instance, by listening to who or what is to blame for ten minutes, will be energetically drained afterward.

Honesty is the only way to handle this situation. Therapists should point out to these patients that such conversations are draining their energy, and then strongly encourage the patients to take responsibility for their own lives.

The therapist might say, "I don't want to hear all that. What was the gift that this situation had in store for you?" or "What did you need this experience for?"

I recommend that all therapists immediately interrupt any whining by patients, because it simply doesn't help. Some people have mastered the art of this approach, visiting one therapist after the other and feeding on the energy of each of them.

In such cases, it's easy to respond to the statement: "Yes, but I can't change anything about that" with "Well, then I can't do anything for you either. You'll have to live with that, not me. Good-bye!"

Usually, patients then stop their victim games, and you can start working with them. If not, I recommend stopping the treatment.

Over the past 20 years, I've sent fewer than ten clients back home without having achieved anything, and I only did so when I had the feeling they wanted to abuse me in order to validate their pattern of suffering. If you agree to a treatment under such conditions, patients are likely to call during the following two days, reporting on everything that had already improved. Two days later, however, you'll get a call saying that ever since the treatment occurred, everything got worse. It's the old game of the carrot and the stick.

The only way therapy can be successful is if people are willing and ready to behave like adults and assume responsibility for their own lives.

Preserving individuality

The right to an individual treatment

In addition to my medical studies at the university, I studied Traditional Chinese Medicine (TCM) for several years. This was a great gift, because in TCM, people aren't pigeonholed based on an illness, as is the case in Western medicine. Our medical system even establishes standards on how certain symptoms need to be treated. What medical nonsense, because we can't achieve healing on the symptom level. If that were the case, computer systems could just as well take over the treatment.

Symptoms are always an expression of personal unresolved issues. In Chinese medicine, we look for an individual's basic patterns; these are treated via a personalized prescription of decoctions of remedies, acupuncture and kinesitherapy. Consequently, TCM has proven its efficacy and has survived already for over 3,000 years.

If I want to go deeper as a therapist, rather than smoothing the surface, I have to fully open up to the person and engage, and uncover the real causes of current irritations or disorders through a kind of detective work. Causes can be current stresses or situations, or they may go back many years—even back to the mother's womb. Perhaps they're not even this person's issues, but those that he or she took over and is carrying for others. The causes can be manifold.

Along the same lines, we don't get infected by a trivial cold, with some virus or unclean hands to blame. People can be sick and tired of a situation; they can be caught in a state of rigidity, and then, the body tries to free itself from that. It could be that an intoxication is involved, and much more.

Opening up on a deep level and engaging in this journey of discovery is also why being a therapist is such a joy. Prior to each treatment, I can feel a bit nervous and excited, because I never know what will come up, and what challenges I will face.

It's all totally open. A treatment also reveals the gift that each individual has to offer whom a therapist has the privilege to work with: we're given the opportunity to learn and understand something new, gaining more insight and getting again a bit closer to enlightenment.

I've always sworn that I would give up my work as a therapist the day I stopped learning something new during a treatment.

So far I haven't reached that point yet.

Our individual life purpose

It's not our job to judge an illness. Everything has a meaning and a purpose. What *is* our job is to help people recognize this meaning and purpose and support them in changing their lives. A broken leg can carry the message to not continue on one's chosen path. A gastric ulcer can point to a lot of swallowed anger.

I once met a 24-year old man who was grateful for the cancer he had developed. He said: "This allowed me to experience and be forced to look at things I would have missed out on otherwise."

It's not our job to make it all smooth and nice for that person, to magically heal their symptoms; rather, it's about reestablishing flow and helping them find their way out of the multiple dead-end systems they got themselves stuck in.

Everybody can only heal him- or herself, and this often requires changing one's life. The illness or the symptom shows people the need for change and gives them the strength to go through with it.

Illness only means: "You can't go on like this," and since our experiences are our true fortune, we could also choose to be grateful for having gained another experience.

We all are free to suffer as much as we want or need to. As therapists, it's not our job to save anybody.

In my own case, I've already died many "deaths" in this life. As a child, I had to stay for weeks in a cast in the quarantine ward of a hospital, since they had no other free bed. I was only allowed to talk to my parents over the phone during this time. This experience also had its meaning and purpose—it gave me the strength to walk my path as a "lone fighter."

Your own energy supply

Always be sure that you have access to plenty of energy by enjoying your own clarity and finding and living your life purpose, your soul passion. Never use other people's energy—you're not a vampire, after all!

No spiritual racism

There are many spiritual hierarchies. "I'm an old soul, and you're only a young one; that's why I know everything better than you." "Your God is a woman? Mine is a man, and this is how it should be."

Pseudospiritual systems close to racism come right after fanatical religious and fascist systems.

"I am more enlightened than you!"

"Then keep masturbating" would be my response.

No classification systems

There are many classification systems that cause more damage than good—whether it's soul classifications, the different types of Ayurveda, signs of the zodiac or others. In the end, they're used more as an excuse for all that isn't possible than for what *is* possible.

"I'm a Taurus; I can't do this or that."

"Based on my soul's matrix, I'm allowed to be arrogant."

"I'm blond."

"This is my karma."

It would be more honest to say, "I don't want to do this" than hiding behind some kind of classification.

I believe and have experienced that all human beings have the full potential of their development within them. It's merely our cowardice and comfort that prevent us from living it out!

External Tools

They take over the "hard work" of energy healing. And that's a good thing.

Chronology of creative madness

1997	Creation of the first *innerwise* remedies
1997–2006	System of pellets, including 1,000 remedies
1998–2006	Test tubes comprising 21 topics
2003–2008	Crystals
2006–2011	Test discs
2006	*Cardsystem (healing cards pro)*
2006	*Medicine Wheel*
2008	Amulets, *Space* disc
2010	*Homo Integer*
2011	*Flowmaker*
2011	*Unconscious Mind Coach*
2011	*Heilapotheke* (in German; 2012 in English: *The Complete Healing System,* and Hungarian; 2016 in Spanish, Portuguese, French and Dutch)
2011	*Source of Light*
2011	The book *Der Heilatem* (in German) (The Healing Breath)
2011	The book *Ja/Nein – Der Armlängentest* (in German; 2012 in English: *Yes/No: Using the Arm-Length Test for Instant Answers and Wellbeing;* 2014 in Slovakian; 2016 in Spanish and Portuguese)
2011	*Quintessence*
2011	New testing system
2011	Multimedia e-book: *Ein Kurs im Heilen* (in German; 2014 in English: *A Course in Healing;* 2016 in Spanish and Portuguese)
2012	*Make Me An Instrument*
2012	The book *innerwise: Heilung für alles Lebendige* (new edition in 2016: *Intuitive Heilung/Intuitive Healing*) (in German, English, Spanish and Portuguese)
2013	System Test Cards
2013	The audio book *innerwise Meditationen: Der Heilatem* (*innerwise* Meditations: The Healing Breath) (in German)
2013	The audio book *innerwise Meditationen: Mutter Erde* (*innerwise* Meditations: Mother Earth) (in German)

2013	*IMAGO Game* (in German, 2014 in English; 2015 in Portuguese; 2016 in Spanish)
2013	*New Dimension* and *Integrity* test cards
2013	CD *Healing Sounds 1: Make Me An Instrument*
2014	The book *Besser schlafen, besser leben* (Sleep Better, Live Better) (in German)
2014	Hologram Amulet
2014	*Smile it away* stickers
2014	*Sleep well my love* stickers
2014	The book *Integrity is my way* (in German)
2014	The audio book *innerwise Meditationen: Der Fluss des Lebens* (*innerwise* Meditations: The River of Life) (in German)
2014	*Lebe: Das Heilspiel des Lebens/Live! The Healing Game of Life* (in German and English; 2016 in Spanish and Portuguese)
2014	10 Healers
2015	The audio book *innerwise Meditationen: innerYoga* (*innerwise* Meditations: *innerYoga*) (in German)
2015	The book *Heilmeditationen* (in German; 2016 in English: *Healing Meditations)*
2015	The book *Intuitive Diagnostik* (Intuitive Diagnostics) (in German)

The Higher Order

innerwise is not an individual system, but rather, it comprises different systems based on a higher order.

The *innerwise* rose

The first symbol was the *innerwise* rose that I drew in 2001. It represents the basic structure of the whole. It was created based on the flower of life; it's part of all the tools and also constitutes the metastructure.

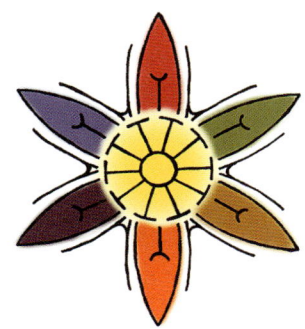

The *innerwise* basic geometric structure

The first system is the Healing Cards.
These are specific frequency patterns. They can be explained and you can look up their meanings and select them using a testing system.
They include *The Complete Healing System* with its test cards; the large card system, *healing cards pro,* with the large testing system; and the memory media—that is, crystals, amulets and the Space disc.

The second system is the Medicine Wheel.
A poster describing the paths to realization, insight and enlightenment, and the meditation of the three related paths: the energetic path, the physical path and the path of wisdom.

The third system is the Homo Integer.
Based on the Homo Integer symbol, this healing system works almost automatically. The healing energies are available as a field. They can no longer be put into words and instead of the testing system there is an intelligent structure. In addition to the Homo Integer, there is also the Unconscious Mind Coach as a card set; and the Flowmaker disc, the Gold and Silver Amulet and the Balance Card as memory media.

The fourth system are the healing meditations of the Healing Breath, Mother Earth, The River of Life, innerYoga and dance-fingers-dance.
A healing synthesis of meditation, focusing and breathing.

The fifth system is the Quintessence.
A card system based on number codes and geometric structures that can easily handle even major challenges related to manipulation.
This is an open system. Besides the 45 cards, the user can virtually create additional cards, if needed. Drawing the Quintessence test card indicates to do so.
For that purpose, test the amount of numbers that should be in the outer ring, followed by the actual numbers that should be part of it. The system takes care of properly arranging the numbers.

The sixth system is the symbol Make Me An Instrument.
Based on a 12-layer flower of life in three dimensions, this symbol represents the world's 12 dimensions. The 3-dimensional flower of life turns into a cube that we can enter virtually—a realm of harmony.
Number codes activate special functions within this holographic space.
The sixth system is particularly suitable for complex philosophical issues, such as time, the soul, sources, etc.

The seventh system is the Sounds of the Worlds.
The Sounds of the Worlds system offers an unlimited number of remedies based on music whose essence was liberated through frequency modulation and octaving.

The eighth system is Unison.
The only field representing the original idea of Creation of anything individual.
Unison can only be generated virtually through the hands of the user.

The ninth system is Live!
Live! represents an understanding of the architecture of Being and the forces at work, and allows for targeted effects.

The First System: The Healing Cards

Frequencies

The *innerwise* healing frequencies are at the heart of *innerwise*.

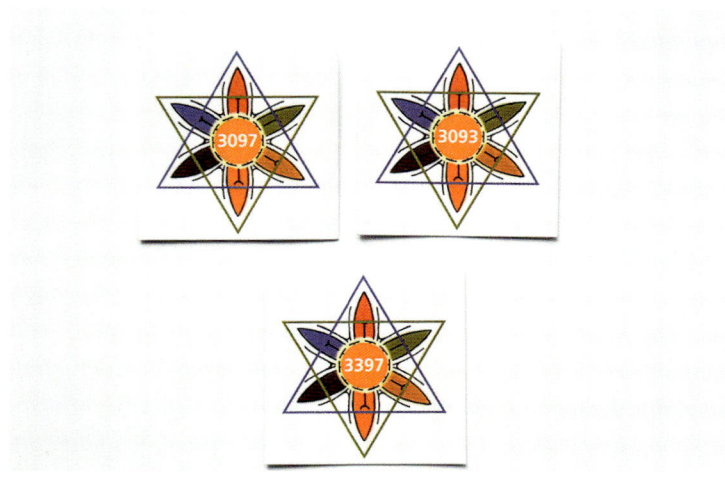

The healing cards—energy gateways

As a medical doctor, I learned, of course, and also believed, that it's the chemical substances that make remedies effective.

But over the last few years, I've been given ample opportunity to learn that this isn't true.

I produced blood pressure remedies energetically, and several doctors I befriended tried them out. The results were surprising: they were as effective as the large colorful pills.

Subsequently, I analyzed the energetic level and layer of the aura where Bach flower remedies, antibiotics, vitamins, painkillers, homeopathic remedies, and so on, were effective.

It was astonishing to find that often conventional medicine didn't affect the physical level either, but that it was effective in the energy bodies.

Another finding was rather frustrating: even the "esoteric" remedies manifested their effects only on certain layers. I couldn't find any remedy that was effective on all layers. However, since irritations and disorders can occur on all levels or layers—that is, in all bodies, we also need remedies that work on all of them.

These were the minimum requirements for the *innerwise* healing frequencies, together with the fact that every human being needs a different strength.

And as we've learned through homeopathy, the energetic quality—that is, the potentization, also plays a role. Yet homeopathy only offers a few potencies: D10, D30, D100, D200, D1000 …

What was I supposed to do if the patient needed the exact potency of D157 or D798, as those would be the resonance potencies?

All these factors called for new solutions:

Remedies that are effective on all levels and that have their own intelligence based on the essence of the particular remedy, adjusting their energetic power and quality to the user.

Remedies whose energetic and informational patterns can be combined and copied freely.

The first *innerwise* healing frequencies were created in my practice in 1997. The classical Bach flower essences proved to be weaker than other flower essences, so I potentized them anew. Using the arm-length test, I found the potency accord—that is, the series of dilutions—which was needed to lend them new strength.

I reformulated the series of Bach flower essences and found them to have a strength and clarity that had been unknown to me thus far.

Next, I worked on the crystal frequencies. At the time they were copied from selected crystals using Mr. Jahoda's "biocorrelator" device and then potentized in potency accords.

Over the next ten years, 4,000 additional healing frequencies were created. They became increasingly complex, and by linking them to the essence of the remedy, potentization was no longer necessary. Once the number exceeded 1,000, the treatment kit weighed over 40 pounds (which caused considerable problems when flying to give courses in Canada); and I decided to stop producing the frequencies in the form of pellets and chose instead to produce small paper cards. This has made it possible to fit the 4,200 remedies into a small laptop case.

Today, the following frequency groups are available:

Overview of *innerwise* frequencies

	From number:	to number:
Grimm's Fairy Tales	1	73
Orchid Flower Essences	74	93
Bach Flower Remedies	94	132
Australian Bush Flowers	133	201
Californian Flower Essences	202	304
Crystals	305	481
Elements	482	489
Colors	490	501
Organs	502	584
Vegetables	585	628
Taste	629	633
Spices	634	693
Plants	694	804
Trees	805	822
Sacred Geometry	823	830
Runes	831	854
Journey Home	855	862
Life Energy	863	864
Detoxication	865	894
Waters of Light	895	901
Chinese Medicinal Herbs	902	1311
Schuessler Tissue Salts	1312	1359
Nutrition	1360	1366
Vitamins	1367	1391
Amino Acids	1392	1412
Glyconutrients	1413	1420
Fatty Acids	1421	1455
Enzymes	1456	1461
Hahnemannian Homeopathy	1462	2514
Immunostimulants	2515	2523
Nosodes	2524	2623
Chakras	2624	2652
I Ching	2653	2716
Numbers	2717	2744
Spagyrics	2745	2828

	From number:	to number:
Chart Rulers	2829	2835
Paracelsus Remedies	2836	2919
Paracelsus Amulets	2920	2926
Alchemy	2927	2928
Osho Zen Tarot	2929	3007
Mayan Calendar	3008	3050
Astrology	3051	3068
Chinese Astrology	3069	3087
Fixed Stars	3088	3110
The Signs of the Zodiac	3111	3123
Sounds of Celestial Bodies	3224	3149
Nada Brahma	3150	3161
Thinkers	3162	3230
Tabula Smaragdina	3231	3243
Initiation Path of Thoth	3244	3265
Taken from Life	3266	3324
Systemic Therapy	3325	3360
Totem Animals	3361	3474
Holopathic Remedies—Remedies from Conventional Medicine	3475	3556
Snake-Venom Enzymes	3557	3567
Vaccine Nosodes	3568	3589
Essential Oils	3590	3749
Soul Remedies	3750	3759
Archangels	3760	3773
Sounds	3774	3801
Meridians	3802	3821
Elements of the Periodic Table	3822	3938
Colloidal Minerals	3939	3953
Emotions	3954	4004
Dance Rhythms (G. Roth)	4005	4009
Mary Magdalene Soul Symbols	4010	4039
Leela – Game of Life	4040	4111
Mother Earth	4112	4169
Places of Power	4170	4184

The big question is always whether remedies are even necessary. An energetic wave, energy passed on with Reiki or a prayer are also effective and no longer imply a dependency on any system.

This can be true, but when you take a closer look, people are connecting to a source of energy either directly or via a therapist.

And the question is, who is that source? How clean is it, and how free of any intentions?

I wanted to create a system that makes all energies available for everybody and in consistent quality, a system that enables the intelligence of the remedies' essence to unfold freely and makes them really easy to use.

innerwise symbols

From the start, *innerwise* was connected with symbols.

The main sources were the flower of life, crop circles and the golden ratio.

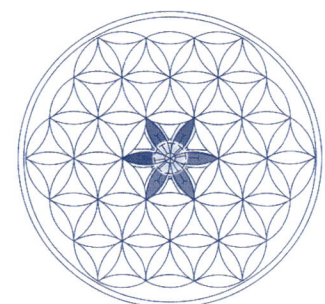

The flower of life—the geometry of Creation

The *innerwise* rose

I drew the *innerwise* rose during a workshop in 2001.

It's based on the flower of life, with the circle in the center symbolizing the source of energy of *innerwise*. The rays connecting it to the elements of the interrupted circle represent the connection of the individual users with the source. Individual users are autonomous and independent, as reflected through the interrupted circle.

The flower petals symbolize modesty in outward representation.

Being visible without going beyond the limits of the *innerwise* system. If our concept of flow is right, all comes to us at the right time.

The funnel between the flower petals stands for openness and for the new; however, there's a filter at the bottom of each funnel: it means that new ideas are never simply absorbed without being verified and tested.

The rose is the programmable structure. This implies that it's both visibly and invisibly part of all *innerwise* tools, and also makes it possible to copy energies to the amulet, for example.

The *innerwise* roses in all tools recognize one another, also preventing foreign energies from being introduced into the system.

The *innerwise* ONE symbol

It was inspired by the pineal gland, our third eye. This organ contains light-sensitive cells and today merely exists in rudimentary form, similar to a Greek temple. Thus, came the idea that it once provided access to the divine source.

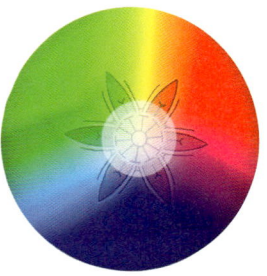

The *innerwise* ONE symbol

I put together two color-scale hemispheres, which create a white sphere in the center representing the divine source. On the outside, all colors are present twice, corresponding to the levels of duality of our existence.

All colors of life are in the outer part, while the white center represents the higher order.

This white part was graphically composed of 12 layers that correspond to a testing system, a structurizing system and a system of consciousness. And the *innerwise* rose in the sphere serves to connect it all.

This symbol was created in 2008 and is still the basis of the amulets and Space disc.

Source of Light

In spring 2011, an additional source of energy became accessible. We were on a seminar trip in Namibia, and I knew that it wasn't going to be possible to represent the next source through geometric structures, but instead, through living beings.

In a crystal museum in Swakopmund, clear/optical calcites were for sale. They were lying in front of me, and I knew that they were these beings.

I arranged the 21 crystals geometrically and lit each of them individually with a laser beam. This arrangement was photographed, and only the rim was adjusted graphically, changing it from gray to blue. The light field arose as the laser light was broken within the crystals.

Powerful support for challenging therapy situations.

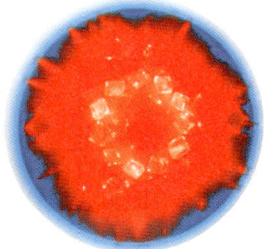

The *innerwise* Source of Light

Memory media

From pellets to amulets

In the early days of developing *innerwise*, I dissolved pellets and drops in alcoholic solutions that my patients could take at home for some time following the treatment. As a physician, I stretched the rules a bit, which *just* passed scrutiny from a legal point of view.

More and more people became interested in *innerwise* and wanted to work with it. Since even alternative health practitioners aren't allowed to give their clients energized pellets to take at home, what would designers, business consultants, energy practitioners or teachers do who wanted to work with *innerwise* in Austria?

We needed another solution, and this is how the idea of using amulets was born. Based on their geometric structures and symbols, the amulets were able to take in the energies of the *innerwise* remedies and broadcast them like a sound system.

At first, we used glass amulets. Geometric structures were shot into the glass using a laser beam. The glass amulets worked, yet they broke easily and were expensive to produce.

So we tried plastic amulets; unfortunately, they didn't resist aggressive sweat. In 2008, we found a usable and robust solution with brass amulets, on which we printed the symbols. For those who felt that amulets didn't go with their outfits, we created the Balance Card.

And for buildings, living and work spaces, as well as systems, we developed discs that serve as memory media for the energies and act like a sound system.

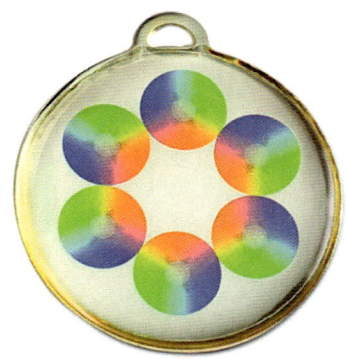

The *innerwise* amulet

It's become common use for anybody to insert a plastic disc into a device, press three buttons and then the disc contains music.

This is precisely how the amulets work, except that there is no blinking device—only the tangible energies of our hands for copying the music to the amulets.

Copying the healing symphony frequencies to the amulet

Place the amulet in one palm, lay the copy card on top of it and place the pile of selected healing cards on top of the copy card. Now hold your other hand an inch or two over the top. Close your eyes (doing so will allow you to see much better) and concentrate on your hands. Within a few seconds, an energy field will be created below your upper hand. It is the energy field that expands through *innerwise*. You only need to observe how it flows through the healing cards and the copy card into the amulet. You can feel it create a kind of energetic wave that expands from the amulet into the space around you. As an additional check, and to build confidence, you can place the amulet on your body and once again think about some topics or issues that have caused you stress. With the healing sounds in the amulet, those topics will no longer create stress.

Wear the amulet on a necklace or cord over your heart. If you feel that the energy is too strong during the night, sleep with it under your pillow.

To strengthen the effect, hold the amulet in your hand for a couple of minutes a few times a day, and meditate with it. Imagine your body, your life and your environment in their optimal state as you do so.

You can keep adding new healing symphony frequencies to the amulet without ever having to cleanse it. When issues no longer resonate with us, we won't perceive them as issues anymore.

Why do we store the energies after all?
Of course, we could also simply bring the healing frequencies into the person's energy field, but this won't have a lasting effect. After a treatment, people return to their old lives, where they'll have to make the necessary changes in order to feel better on a continual basis. Life will question them to see if they're really serious. Here, it helps to be able to keep hearing and listening to the individually composed healing symphony as support.

Storage or gateways
At the end of the treatment when the healing symphony is complete, it is transferred into a "storage" medium, such as an amulet, Balance Card or disc.
At least, that's what it looks like from the outside. In reality, these media act more like a memory, because neither the healing cards nor the amulets nor any other products contain any energy themselves. Rather, they are gateways through which we can receive the energy.
Therefore, only our individual connection to energy patterns in the field is transferred.

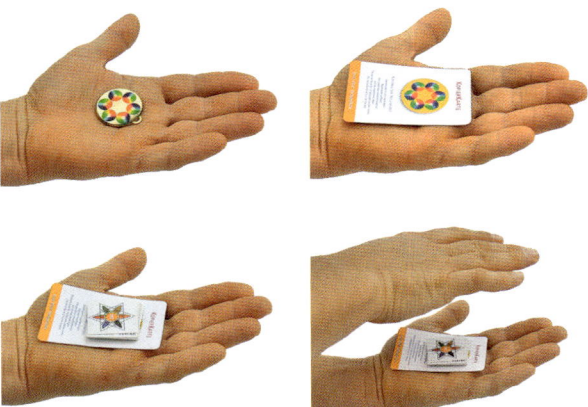

Copying *innerwise* frequencies

Do the memory media need to be cleaned up?
Since they're merely gateways that are based on the principle of resonance, and no energies are being stored, it is also not necessary to delete anything and cleanse the memory media after a certain amount of time.

Circles of *innerwise*
They were made of crystal glass and produced from 2003 to 2008. These highly effective products were created based on the flower of life. I had drawn the flower

of life in huge dimensions and elaborated on inner structures, activating structures within the flower-of-life structure as information and energy carriers.

Using a high-performance laser, we shot up to 300,000 single dots into small glass structures, creating 3D energy structures.

Due to the high internal tension, however, they could break easily, and it wasn't possible to include colors. Situations within the company that blocked its development arose especially for that purpose, and all of this led to the decision to stop production in 2008. Many people who loved these products are still sad about that.

In my own case, I threw out my stock of more than 30 development samples in 2010, staying true to my motto to live in the now and not keep anything from the past. When something is over, one should be able to let go of it no matter how valuable it is.

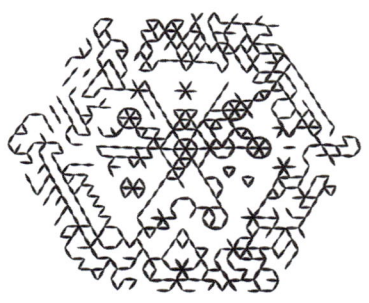

One of the geometric "Circle" structures

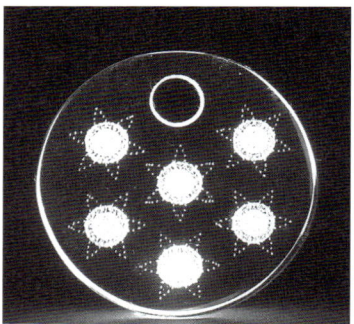

An *innerwise* Circle

The testing systems

The large testing system (see description starting on page 220) encompasses over 300 thematic complexes uniting the knowledge of various different cultures and times; as well as many years of experience, observation and research.

The intuitive use of the testing system makes it possible to immediately address the key points and work on them.

Thanks to the intelligence inherent in the testing system, it always shows just the topic or issue that needs to be addressed and resolved at that very moment in order to take the most effective path of healing.

Testing for all issues concerned at the beginning of the treatment would result in a long list. By letting the test cards guide us through the treatment, only a few topics will need to be worked on; the others are resolved by themselves thanks to the highly effective testing order.

Time and again, I experience a certain moment in a treatment where I feel deeply humble in light of the *innerwise* intelligence.

The Complete Healing System and the large card system, *healing cards pro*

In 2011, Allegria Verlag published the *Heilapotheke,* the original German version of *The Complete Healing System[1],* which had already been created years ago, signaling the step to finally go public. I wanted to let the system grow as it needed to throughout those years so that it could mature without interference and at its own pace—and be ready when the time came—which was in 2011.

The Complete Healing System comprises 309 healing cards, six test cards covering 18 sets of thematic complexes, a copy card, an amulet and a booklet.

With this system, everyone can heal him- or herself.

The large card system, *healing cards pro,* was designed as a professional working tool for therapists and coaches. This comprehensive set encompasses 15 test cards covering over 300 testing complexes, nearly 4,200 healing cards and a compendium to fully equip an energy practitioner's practice.

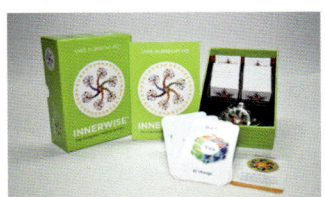

innerwise®: The Complete Healing System

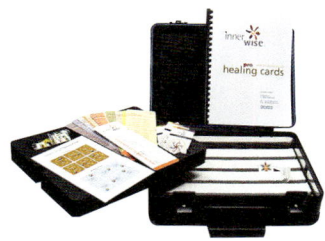

The large *innerwise* card system, *healing cards pro*

In 2011, the *Heilapotheke*—that is, *The Complete Healing System,* and the large *Cardsystem* were certified as medical devices in Europe.

---

[1] The English version, *innerwise®: The Complete Healing System,* was published by Hay House in 2012.

The Second System: The Medicine Wheel

Behind the *innerwise* Medicine Wheel is the search for insight and the realization that the three classical paths need to be combined to be successful—that is, the energetic path, the path of mental and spiritual realization and insight, and the physical path.

If we recognize that each of these paths has its downside, and if we integrate all that, then the fourth path opens up.

This results in a threefold type of meditation. These are no immersion exercises for the mind, but rather, life meditations that require inner discipline and perseverance and constitute a prerequisite for an *innerwise* therapist.

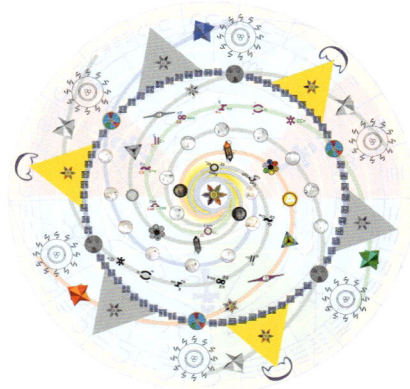

The *innerwise* Medicine Wheel

Meditation from the energetic perspective

This requires the desire to understand energetic processes and principles. It involves a new and unusual perspective, as well as the constant effort to look behind things and processes and to learn to see the energy flows.

This is the meditation of sensing, feeling and perceiving.

Meditation focusing on mental and spiritual insight

This is about the rational processing of the observed energy flows. It also involves an active interest in humanity's collective wisdoms and teachings, and in the mathematical and geometric laws—the foundation of all life. This includes verifying the accuracy of energetic principles. If they are correct, they have to be applicable to everything.

This is the meditation of the inner researcher, the humanist.

Meditation focusing on the body, the temple of the soul

As the temple of the soul, the body needs attention and preservation of structure and form. This includes conscious nutrition, continual cleansing from toxins and physical exercise done with love and joy—be it Qigong, dancing, gardening or something completely different. The body likes it when we use it and take good care of it.

It is the meditation of those hungry for life, because life is movement.

The Third System: The Homo Integer

In 2010, I felt like reinventing the wheel and creating another healing system in addition to the *Cardsystem.*

What prompted me to do so involved an ulterior motive. An *innerwise* mentor had worked with the dark side of power and had tried to introduce this into the system. With the help of old magic scripts and instructions, he had developed considerable energetic power.

With the Homo Integer, I created a second therapy system that I could use to check the *Cardsystem.* With several systems, it's always easier to identify unresolved things and irritations.

Since the Homo Integer was complete, I also had the strength to separate from this trainer, and I'm grateful to him that in the end, he brought us a gift—the need for this development.

As was the case many times before, I was greatly inspired by a crop circle. Interestingly enough, the right crop circles have always appeared when needed.

Behind each dot of the basic structure are symbols, but they're invisible: in the center is the testing system; and in addition, platonic bodies, Hermetic laws and much more.

The entire structure is composed of one central and six peripheral parts positioned in opposite directions of rotation. This makes for two systems that rotate in the opposite direction, producing a structurizing effect and allowing for a state of suspension.

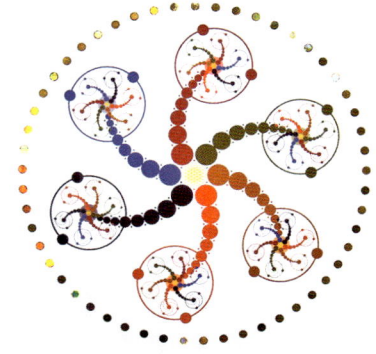

Homo Integer

Flower-of-life holograms that surround the central structure like a ring represent the healing energies.

Mandelbrot set (the little apple-man) symbols are printed behind the holograms as the connection to the geometry of Creation, the matrix.

If you want to experience such magic, watch the "Mandelbrot Zoom 333" movie on YouTube that will lead you through the light channel.

As healing energy, sources offered themselves that I've experienced for years as the Great Council in my meditations.

It was totally unexpected for me, and it's an immense grace for us to have direct access to these energies.

The idea was to produce the Homo Integer in three sizes (90 cm, 149.5 cm and 208 cm—that is, approximately 35.4, 58.9 and 81.9 inches, respectively); using the arm-length test, I tested the number of holograms for each size.

Something about the numbers caught my attention, so I divided the size by the number of holograms—and was speechless; it was mind-boggling:

The results were 1.62, 1.62 and 1.61.

It's the value of the golden ratio—1.618—tested three times with the arm-length test.

I stopped believing in coincidence a long time ago.

We use the Homo Integer to energize living and work spaces, as support in treatments and for the energetic design of organizations and projects. It can also harmonize geopathic stress and works well for meditations. Sit down on it and fly away!

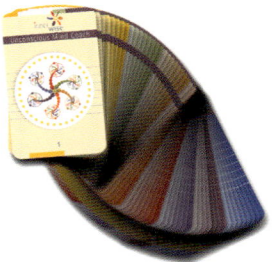

Unconscious Mind Coach Set

The Unconscious Mind Coach was created as a card set for coaching situations with the energy of the Homo Integer. The energies involved can no longer be described with words, which are simply too small and limited. However, you can *feel* the energies of the cards very well.

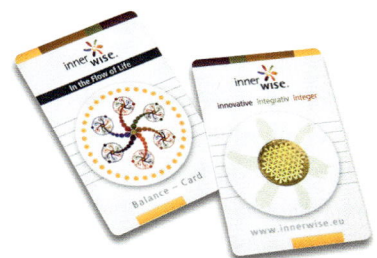

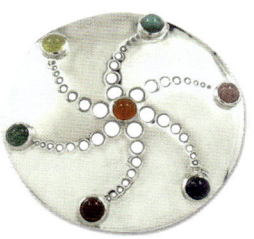

If an amulet doesn't go with your suit,
you can use the Balance Card as a memory medium.

The special
innerwise amulet

Subsequently, I added further memory media: the silver and gold amulets and the Balance Card, as well as the Flowmaker, a small version of the Homo Integer.

Perceptions on the Flowmaker

The symbols help dissolve obstacles in people. These include fears, resistance or wishes that keep us from being in the flow and feeling whole and complete, time and time again. We refer to those as blockages. We feel they're outside; yet in fact, they mirror our individual Being—that is, they're within us.

If these three are resolved, it's precisely this free state that arises. The energy is flowing; in other words, we are love. We don't need anything else.

What's special about this intelligent system is that the cause is healed without any further intervention from us, no matter what it is. Causes, as we imagine them, can be so manifold that we're not even able to grasp them, as they're not in the now, but in the past—possibly even beyond our Being in this world.

This systematic approach frees us from the cause without using our conscious mind, thereby also transforming the consequences. We could also use images like leaving the wheel of life, redemption, healing, becoming whole and complete or whatever else—it all applies.

Frank Reinoss

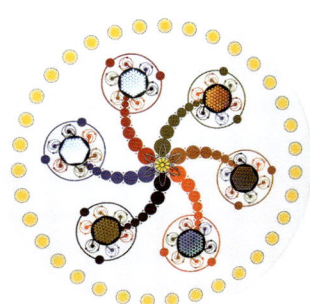

Flowmaker—the small
Homo Integer

The Fourth System: The *innerwise* Meditations

The healing breath—healing the soul

We solve so many issues in life at the mental and emotional level and then wonder why they're still there. The root cause frequently lies at the energetic and spiritual levels. The healing breath enables you to reach and heal these deeper levels. Thus, it can be applied almost universally and is useful in sensitive areas such as pain, inner void, relationship difficulties, speech impediments, exam nerves and deep-seated traumas of the soul.

How does this meditation work?

From the Source, breathe in healing energies through your imaginary umbilical cord. Through this umbilical cord you breathe out your issues and problems. You can also use energy from the Source to retrieve what has been lost, such as fragments of your soul. And you can dissolve old connections at the spiritual level in the Source.

Mother Earth—healing the heart

Nature is a vast healing pharmacy. Stones, plants, colors, water, fire—these are her gifts to us, many of which we have captured in healing remedies in the form of powder, drops or oils. The Mother Earth meditation allows you to become your own remedy. You can be a birch tree, a butterfly, a river, a volcano or one of Mother Earth's many other children. The gifts of Mother Earth take effect within you, rewarding you with harmony, clarification, resolution and healing.

We are not separated from the great Mother, we never were. We remain one of her buds that blooms. Once our awareness of this connection has been refreshed, her appearances in the form of animals, elements, crystals or plants can help us heal.

How does this meditation work?

Start out with the words: *Mother Earth, as a part of you, you are fully in me and live through me.* Immerse yourself in these words and thus in Mother Earth: once you are one with the great Mother you become part of her, as a waterfall, for example, or an eagle or a tree. You begin to feel their energy within you and to heal yourself.

When you have connected to Mother Earth, you can do the same with other cosmic forces and their gifts:

Father Sun, as a part of you, you are fully in me and live through me.
Heaven, as a part of you, you are fully in me and live through me.
God, as a part of you, you are fully in me and live through me.

innerYoga—healing the body

An actor who completely grows into the role he's playing has the power to move us. He becomes the other person. Become the remedy, identify with it, move like it. The healing remedy can then touch you deeply, transform you and enrich you. *innerYoga* is not merely identification with the remedy. Like an actor you begin to live the remedy, to surrender to its movement. You can spread your wings like an eagle and enjoy the sensation of flying or move like a tree in the wind. Their energies will heal you.

innerYoga is a perfect complement to the Mother Earth meditation, which is simply about tuning in to the remedy mentally and emotionally. With *innerYoga* you identify at all levels with an animal, a plant, a waterfall or some other representation of Mother Earth—mentally, emotionally, physically, spiritually and in motion. This identification permits your body and your conscious mind to comply in a natural way and assume its shape.

How does this meditation work?

In your imagination you fuse to part of nature, an animal, for example, an eagle. You feel it inside of you, feel its wings and yours, feel how the wind ripples through your feathers. And you breathe like an eagle. Your body begins of its own accord to move like an eagle. Your wings unfold. Every eagle is one of a kind, each position you adopt, each gesture is perfect. The whole of nature is in motion, nothing is static, schooled positions are now superfluous.

The River of Life—healing the conscious mind and the unconscious

This meditation emerged from picture journeys with many patients. Journeys in pictures have a tremendous healing effect. Our conscious mind and our unconscious can speak to us through pictures. And we have the power to transform our lives by altering the pictures. The River of Life is a symphony of images that emerged from ten years of therapeutic healing work and rewards you with healing and harmony at many different levels.

How does this meditation work?

You embark on the great spiritual journey through life with all its challenges. Let yourself be guided by the text and linger in pictures that move you.

dance-fingers-dance—rediscovering the lightness of Being

This meditation releases blockages and inhibitions stored in our body. Small children love freedom of movement, the joy of it. They're able to physically express their feelings with the greatest of ease. As we get older, however, we gradually become stiff, more reserved and shy as a result of rules and regulations, prohibitions, demands, and, above all, the accumulation of deposits of guilt, sorrow, envy, loss and other unresolved issues in our body tissue, in our muscles, fasciae and our bones. dance-fingers-dance will help you to rediscover the pleasure of your body and of movement.

How does this meditation work?
Your fingers, your hands become dancers on an imaginary stage, and you are the audience. Your fingers and hands transform the music into movement so that you can see it without having to hear it. Your hands are free of the countless restrictions, rules and patterns you carry within you, and their way of dancing *freedom* embraces your entire being and liberates you.

The Fifth System: The Quintessence

The Quintessence was created in September 2011 following my studies on the five basic energies and the principle of all and nothing.

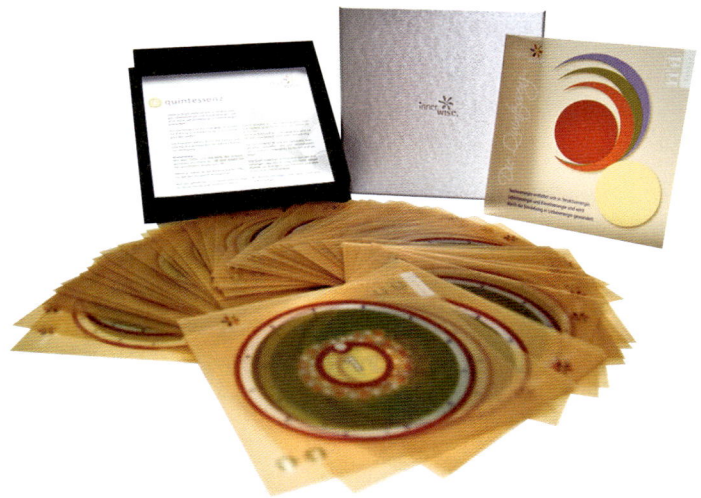

Quintessence Set

Based on a crop circle and number-based energy patterns, 45 healing cards have been created that are selected intuitively; the energies are activated in the body by placing one's hands on the cards. Upon completion of the treatment, the healing cards are copied to an amulet in the same way as all other healing cards.

On Friday, a colleague came to see me. She told me that she felt she'd had a lumbago that was spreading out into her back and causing neurological deficits in her right leg. I asked her to sit down for a moment and told her a bit about the Quintessence.

Although she was in a bit of a hurry, she still sat down calmly. I had measured her love energy; independently from that, she drew three cards and took in their energies through the hand chakras. After about 15 seconds, she felt great heat in the lumbar region which was concentrating more and more in one spot. It became hotter and hotter, and after another 15 seconds, she got up without any symptoms (before she had been limping), and said that the blockage had dissolved completely. This colleague is open but also very much down-to-earth. What a happy experience to witness a health issue that could be resolved instantly!

When the Quintessence is applied, the aura stabilizes very much, and all the people who have used it so far were amazed when they experienced it. Options available so far in the fields of radionics, radiesthesia and alike could mostly achieve only very temporary effects. As said before, our experience with the Quintessence has been quite different thus far; it compares most closely to the effects of a Universal Pendulum used in an energetically clean manner.

It's truly like a quintessence of experiences—healing, pleasant and moving.

Walter Schumacher

The Sixth System: Make Me An Instrument

Lord, make me an instrument of your peace:
Where there is hatred, let me sow love.
Where there is injury, pardon.
Where there is discord, union.
Where there is doubt, faith.
Where there is despair, hope.
Where there is sadness, joy.
Where there is darkness, light.

St. Francis of Assisi

Geometry

The flower of life

With the flower of life as the basic structure of Being, the circle is squared.
A three-dimensional cube is formed with 1,729 spheres, starting with a single circle in the center.

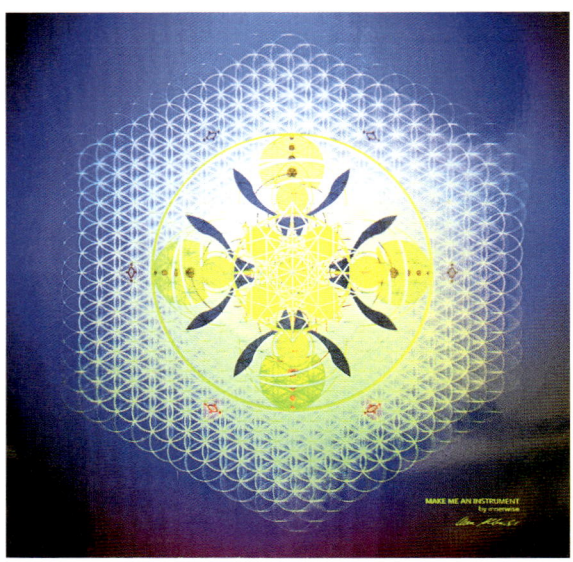

Crop circles

Make Me An Instrument unites two principles: the structurizing principle in the form of eight crop circles fused at the center, and the energizing principle with the flower of life.

Crop circles are a type of earth energy acupuncture and a geometric library of wisdom. Whenever I had unresolved questions about life, I found clues and answers to what I was looking for in the symbols and geometry of recent crop circles.

Effects

Healing through harmony

The universe, life, love and health are harmonious principles. They are subject to an internal order and emanate a harmonious sound. Illness, destruction and hatred are disharmonious and often based on rigidities and fears. The interplay of elements is out of tune. Instead of increasing, the energy level drops.

Healing can take place when disharmony is transformed back into harmony and rigidity into flow.

Meditating with numbers

Make Me An Instrument is a healing space. You can imagine entering it and letting it manifest its effects on you. You can also visualize your pets, your room or garden, for example, in this space and let the healing energies work on them through the hologram. The more conscious and focused you are when using this space, the stronger the impact. The more concrete the issue or question, the clearer and more powerful the answer. The complex number codes of the *innerwise* system and their therapeutic effects can support you as you focus. Medicinal plants, essential oils, Bach flower remedies—from an energetic point of view, all of them are concrete and complex frequency patterns. The same applies to number codes; they're just a bit more abstract.

They have the power to activate certain functions within the hologram, since everything is included in the holographic space, and number codes are like sounds that activate certain options, like music that makes them dance.

How to meditate with the hologram

Choose from the topics and healing codes what you need at that moment.

Look for somewhere quiet, sit down and close your eyes.

Visualize being in the hologram and letting the number code unfold its healing effect like a sound cloud in the hologram and thus also in you.

There is no need to learn the number codes by heart; simply look at them or put your hand on them, and take them with you *virtually* into the hologram. Imagine the healing codes as music that fulfills and transforms you. Quite a number of people notice the energy rushing through their body and how the issue for which they have chosen the healing code begins to change, is resolved. Afterward you feel more free, more clear and more present.

The chapter on test card 14 starting on page 349 includes a list of number codes for use with the hologram.

Based on planetary laws, the musician Richard Hiebinger has set the number codes to music. They are available on the CD *Healing Sounds 1*.

The Seventh System: Sounds of the Worlds

Sounds of the Worlds is a purely virtual system that users have to create themselves.

It is based on music that has undergone a spagyric process to extract its soul, its essence.

The first remedies were made out of individual musical pieces by Tom Kenyon that were transposed by way of frequency modulation and octaving to the range inaudible for humans. Yet they fill the space and manifest their effects.

After I'd developed, on a technical level, the principle for creating these remedies, the Sounds of the Worlds system began to evolve by itself.

The first 40 remedies are based on music by Tom Kenyon. Any further remedies exist in unlimited numbers, but their content is unknown to me. This means that I could work with remedy 78 or 96, for example, without being familiar with the music behind that remedy. Meanwhile, I know that musicians and composers such as Mozart, Bach or Brahms are also included.

How to create a virtual Sounds of the Worlds remedy:
1. Test the number of the remedy. I often stay within the range of 1 to 100, but there's no upper limit, so you could also select 4,278, for example.
2. Let the field manifest itself on your palm, then test the right octaving to fine-tune the remedy. For that purpose, I like to use the alphabet. The letters represent the octaving steps based on prime numbers, that is, A = 2, B = 3, C = 5, D = 7, etc.
   Next, let the field modify itself on your palm through the octaving you just tested.

I like to visualize this creation process like a cross: on the vertical line I test the remedy's number, and on the horizontal line I test the octaving via letters.

And here's your finished personalized remedy that you can offer as a gift to your client and save to an amulet, for example.

The Eighth System: Unison

This is a very simple system, because it consists of only one remedy.
This remedy reminds us of the original plan behind reality.
You create the Unison remedy only with your hands, like a field between them.

The following is an example of how it can manifest its effects:
A woman had a broken hand that was still hurting very much after three weeks and limited in its functionality.
I placed my hands on her hand and visualized Unison. Immediately, the bones in her hand started to move and realign.
Upon completion, the movability had improved significantly compared to before.

The Ninth System: *Live!*

The system *Live!* was born in 2014.
The challenge was to more deeply understand the architecture of Being and the forces at work.

Imagine a donut: it consists of two parts—the ring of dough and the hole.

Human beings have only two options:
They can feed on the dough like grubs, finding support and security. However, they're paying a very high price in return, because they connect to illusionary forces and serve them.

The other possibility is to opt for the hole in the middle as their living space, where they're free and self-responsible. Yet they won't find any dough and security there anymore.

The large majority of people feel most comfortable in the dough and don't want to leave it, because for them, it represents the highest degree of stability.
Within the hole, we have those areas that are to be experienced in life: in the center, the *Being, I am* and *I am I,* surrounded by *Life, Love, Sound,* the *Soul,* the *Self, Presence, Happiness* and *Creativity.*

In the dough ring, we find the forces of illusion—people connect to them, serve them, and in return, are "compensated" with a false sense of security: *Sacrificial Offerings* and *Pacts, Power, Self-Destruction, Enlightenment, Greed, Gurus* and *Priests, Initiation* and *Arrogance.*

The ring of dough and the hole are connected via negative emotions people identify with: *Hatred, Envy, Lies, Guilt, Sorrow, Fear, Self-Abandonment* and *Lethargy.*

There are also *external realities,* causing confusion. Yet, they're only duplicate images of reality. We can be in such external realities like in virtual worlds. *Fragmentations* add another level of complication. Each fragment believes it's the whole thing, and loses itself—it's the old "divide and rule" principle.

The goal of the *Live!* system is to be present in the hole, thus depriving the forces of illusion of their breeding ground.
Once you've arrived in the center, an energy torus is activated, giving you an unexpected gift for your courage to live with integrity.

I created the 10 Healers in the form of energy cards to help you clear irritations and to support your centering in the hole. They have the power to support your work on this philosophical level.

On *www.lebe.innerwise.com*, you can view them and listen to the music composed for each of them.

Here you can find a short guide to the Healing Game of Life with 6 steps into YOUR life:

1. Test whether your presence in your life is *fragmented.* If this is the case, the symbol of the outer circle is active. Heal it with one or more of the 10 Healers.

2. Test whether illusions *(external realities)* are present in your life. If this is the case, the symbol of the second outer circle is active. Heal it with one or more of the 10 Healers.

3. Test whether your *Being,* your *I am,* and your *I am I* are completely present. If one or more are not 100 percent present, heal it or them with one or more of the 10 Healers.

4. Test whether all 8 beings of the *Path of Realization and Insight—Love, Sound,* the *Soul, Life,* the *Self, Presence, Happiness* and *Creativity*—are completely present. If one or more are not 100 percent present, heal it or them with one or more of the 10 Healers.

5. Test whether one or more of the negative emotions of the *Path of Rigidification* are active, and whether you're still connected to one or more powers of the *Path of Temptation.* If this is still the case after fully activating the colorful center, heal this with one or more of the 10 Healers.

6. Now you are in the center of your life; and by activating your energy field, you can experience happiness, good health and inner wealth. You're living life how it can be—and Creation is laughing with joy!

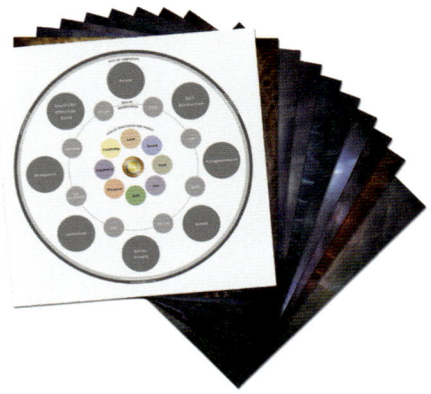

*inner**wise*** as an App

Until 2011, I had developed all tools and systems from physical materials based on alcohol, sugar, paper, glass, plastic and metal.

Then it was time for the transformation into a computer program. Touchscreen technology made it possible to transfer intuitive work into the technical realm.

Working with oneself or others using an iPad or iPhone is an evolution in healing. The idea is simple: A current photo from the client is embedded into a geometric energy field. The first test card is selected intuitively on the screen and then moves onto the photo. This means that we use the energetic picture of the client. When the test card is placed on the photo, the stress can also be tested directly in the client using the arm-length test.

Now healing cards are selected intuitively via the touchscreen and positioned onto the photo.

Instantly, this leads to changes in the actual client, just as if healing cards were placed directly on him or her.

When the healing symphony is complete, it can be printed on a symbol or copied from the device directly to an amulet or stored as a symbol in the device in order to meditate with it on a regular basis.

"How did you heal yourself?" "I meditated with my iPad," will then be the reply. The *innerwise* healing app is available for everyone to treat themselves. It's based on the test and healing cards of *innerwise*: *The Complete Healing System.* There is also a version for professional use by therapists that includes all *innerwise* tools. Additional apps are the meditation apps *Panta-rhei* and *Ra.*

PANTA-RHEI
"Everything changes and nothing remains still."

Heraclitus

A healing meditation with *innerwise* 2.0, the *innerwise* developments in the years 2013 and 2014.

Healing is always about removing charges, dissolving rigidifications, retrieving what has been lost, letting go of fear and reopening to life. *Panta-rhei* guides you through these steps with the help of light, sacred geometry and music, combined as fractal animation.

"Everything changes and nothing remains still."
Heraclitus spoke these words so long ago and yet they are still so true today.
We've loaded ourselves down with both our own and foreign charges, just to be loved.
Time and again, we want to hold on to what we've attained.
We've lost much of what once made up our completeness and perfection.
Consequently, we prevent ourselves from being offered the gift of something new.
"Rigidification" of what has been experienced and is familiar, yet is over, leads to blockage.
Anything that blocks or obstructs us, clogs our life or soul path.
As a result, we darken—and darkness invites more darkness.
We're afraid and withdraw into ourselves, missing out on life and betraying ourselves.
Thus, we age too early—much too early—by betraying our heart.
Life isn't meant to be like this—what a waste of beauty.
"Everything flows; nothing remains the same. Nothing endures but change."

RA – THE SUN
"A being of Light of a higher order"

A healing meditation with *innerwise* 3.0, the *innerwise* developments of 2014.
Ra is a geometric space based on the flower of life in 3D, made up of 12 layers and over 1,700 spheres. This results in a cube. Each of the individual spheres is activated and lights up like a sun. All spheres together produce a being of Light of a higher order consisting of autonomous individual structures.
An energetic tool that supports healing in many ways.
You can bring your issues to *Ra* to be cleared up by its sacred harmonic geometry. Imagine two *Ra* structures and, together with your chaos, enter one virtually while leaving the other in purity. Then transfer only the pure and clear energies from the chaotic first to the peaceful second *Ra* structure. You can "correctly recycle," that is, transform charges and irritating energies using *Ra*.

A being of Light of a higher order
The Source of all that is, is in each and every being of Light.
Each individual being of Light is perfect and complete in itself; it's autonomous, and it radiates—it's a sun.
There are many of these beings of Light, and like the cells of a living organism, they form a complex whole of a higher order—once again a sun.
The sun has created life and guards it.
Bring light into your life!

*inner**wise*** *healing*

innerwise for professional use by therapists, alternative health practitioners and medical doctors.

*inner**wise*** *create*

innerwise for the consulting of systems, companies and organizations, teams and projects. The *diagnosis* of systems is thus possible, as well as their *treatment.*

The Testing System

The testing system is at the heart of the *innerwise* system. It reflects years of searching for effective healing methods and "the quest for the true essence of life."

I had started out by treating symptoms, just like any therapist would do initially. But you can only get so far doing this. At some point you ask yourself whether this approach might cause even more harm to people rather than help them. If I suppress symptoms, I deprive the body of the opportunity to reveal deeper problems or disorders. I'm breaking the warning light, so to speak.

Although this offers short-term relief, it cannot offer long-term benefits. You can compare it to a steam boiler with a pressure leak. Simply fixing the leak doesn't address the problem of excess pressure in the boiler, and it won't take long before the mounting pressure will find another way to escape. So how can we eliminate the boiler's excess pressure?

This was the key question that led me to develop the testing system.

Are there any aspects that are universally applicable? If so, how can such a testing system be used most effectively?

The result was the creation of more than 300 sets of questions included in the test cards over the course of 15 years. I had the opportunity to experience most of them firsthand, which helped me to truly understand them, get a feel for them and integrate them.

Selecting them intuitively has proven to be the most effective way of using them, rather than working through them one by one, since this is like forcing a topic onto a client instead of letting yourself be guided intuitively.

Since *innerwise* is a living being with its own intelligence, the test cards activate themselves in the most effective order for the client. It's as if the active topic emanates a perceivable sound.

As you sense the test cards while moving your hand over them, one of them is energetically active. It sends out different vibrations and feels different.

Another way to find the active test card is through the arm-length test.

With some experience in using this system, you will automatically pick the right one, and the finger that glides over the test card will identify the right topic instantly. Among all the topics included in that specific test card, only one specific topic will be active.

The test cards are then placed on the client, and the stress caused by the test card is balanced using the healing cards.

Once this topic is resolved using the *innerwise* system and the test card is put back with the other test cards, the next topic is activated in one of the other test cards.

In this way, the testing system leads us step by step and topic by topic through the treatment in the most effective manner.

The small testing system is included in *The Complete Healing System,* and the large one in the large card system, *healing cards pro.* For the small testing system, you can also use healing cards pro for balancing; but you can't use *The Complete Healing System,* which is smaller, when working with the large testing system, since it requires the abundance and variety provided by the nearly 4,200 healing cards.

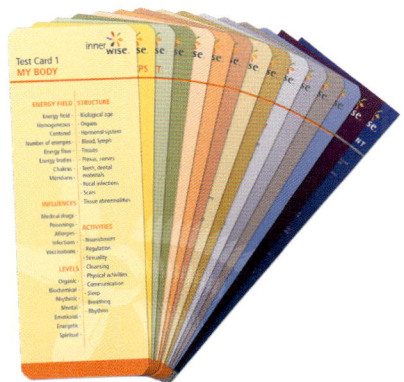

The large testing system

The small testing system of *The Complete Healing System*

These are powerful statements—they don't even try to manifest their effects on the level of symptoms; instead, they access the issues' deepest layers. It's fascinating to see how symptoms can disappear with unimagined ease in this way. As the testing system of *The Complete Healing System,* these statements are, above all, intended for you to treat yourself.

 Yes to change
I am ready to change.
I am ready to change EVERYTHING to live a healthy and happy life.

I am in the now.
I am grateful for all experiences; I integrate them, letting go of the past.

I am worth it.
I am worthy of feeling fine, being healthy and successful and enjoying life.

 Yes to the body
I nourish myself in healthy ways.
I am nourished on all levels: emotionally, energetically, spiritually, mentally and physically.

I free myself from poisons.
I cleanse myself of any poisons in my life: thoughts, emotions, energies, memories, chemical substances, metals and life situations.

My body is healthy.
I am free from infections, allergies and deficiencies. My organs are in harmony, my breath is free and my body is in balance.

 Yes to honesty
I am ready to communicate honestly.
I say what I think and feel regardless of the consequences.

I live authentically.
I am worthy of creating my life myself—with honesty and staying true to my values.

I let go of my compromises.
When I make compromises, I lie to myself. I am honest with myself.

 Yes to love
I love and I am loved.
I see the lovable core in every human being and let others see this lovable core in me.

I love what I was, what I am and what I will be.
There are no mistakes, just experiences.

I open my heart.
I am ready to open my heart and give up my protection. I am ready to give and receive love.

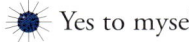 Yes to myself
I am I.
I am (first name).
I am living my own life and not somebody else's.

My energy field is clear.
I am free of foreign energies, manipulations and dependencies.
I am free from wanting to manipulate others.

I am happy.
I breathe freely, my eyes are shining, I dance through life.

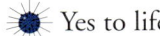 Yes to life
I regain my life energy.
I use my entire energy for my life purpose and stop destroying myself.

I live my creative potential.
Creativity flows through me and fills me with joy.

I am in the flow.
I trust. I am being taken care of. Everything I need is there at the right time. All my experiences are important steps in my growth process.

The Large Testing System

Test Card 1 My body

Levels and the energy field

Energy field

We consist of a tangible physical body, yet that's not everything. The bodies of our thought field, emotional field and the other layers of our aura are much bigger. If we accept the model of individual layers of an aura and refer to them as bodies, we have at least eight bodies: the physical body and seven energy bodies. Thus, one could say that our physical body is one-eighth of our reality at most. Not even all conventional medications are effective on the physical body; antibiotics, for example, have a greater impact on the energy field.

By the same token, it's important to include all of our levels (structural, biochemical, rhythmic, mental, emotional, energetic and spiritual) when testing—that is, the physical and the energetic ones. For the first ten years, normal cancer exists only on the energetic and emotional levels before it manifests physically. Our remedies should be effective in all our bodies. Bach flower essences that weren't adjusted to the quality of our times are only effective in some of our bodies, and thus, can merely qualify as "nice." Long ago they lost the real power they had during the time of Richard Bach.

Many of our disorders or irritations that finally manifest on the physical level first occur as emotional or energetic irritations in our energy field. There, we can easily sense them with our hands when scanning the field, with our hands acting as sensors. Like tuning a radio, we tune in to the frequency we're looking for and scan the field with the palm facing the body. In this way, we can detect inflammations, cancer, fissures in the field, foreign energies and much more.

A homogeneous field

Healing work aims to attain a homogeneous field. The opposite is fragmentation and separation. Fragmentation can apply in general or occur on a local level, and it can apply to the physical body and any layer of the energy field. Fragmentation can be tested in percents and then treated in a targeted manner.

A centered field

The layers of the energy field aren't always centered on top of one another. After an accident, for example, the field can be beside the body. When sensing someone, we can focus on that and then target this aspect in the treatment.

Number of energies

Unless you're a pregnant woman, you should have only one single energy field—the field of your soul. Any additional field is one too many.

In the course of my medical practice, I've tested the whole range from zero to

25,000 fields. This parameter is of particular importance, since in treatments, our objective is to have only the client's own clear and homogeneous field.

It was a Buddhist who took on the aforementioned 25,000 fields during his stay in Thailand after the tsunami. He could see the large number of souls in the intermediary world and wanted to help them all by bringing them to the Light. He almost turned himself into a taxi, as he had taken on the fields of these souls and brought them to Germany. His heart energy had nearly dropped to zero, and he was about to die himself.

In the treatment, we brought the souls home with the help of the *innerwise* system. He bounced back to life, and after two days, he had fully recovered.

One way to take on other energy fields is to play the role of the savior and caretaker who wants to help carry other people's burdens. Oftentimes, this happens to therapists who, given their "helper syndrome," nearly adopt their patients or clients.

The other way to obtain more than one field is manipulation. Although there's an invitation, a resonance, the manipulator makes use of it to install additional fields in other people in order to gain access to their energy, and control and manipulate them.

Unfortunately, this is a widespread parlor game, played by those who are no longer connected to the Source themselves and can only survive by stealing energy from others.

Over the past 18 years, I've worked with only two people who had no field. Both were cases of the most severe forms of manipulation. These people had been fully absorbed by a system and were basically mere shadows of their former selves. I recommend that you start testing in the following way:

"Do I have only one field?" If the response of the arm-length test shows a "no," there are more.

"More than five fields?" If the test response is "no" again, it can only be two, three, four or five fields. This can be tested quickly.

However, if the test reveals a "yes," I would ask the following in the next step: "More than ten fields?" This is an effective way to obtain the result.

Often it's one to 10 fields, but 10 to 40 aren't so rare either.

It's mostly therapists who have more than 100 when they've absorbed and "help" carry their clients' fields. "A trouble shared is a trouble halved" is actually quite a stupid saying since, in fact, the trouble is actually doubled.

Energy flow

Most healing systems depart from the premise that the energy flows freely when we're healthy. This isn't just about the main energy flows in the body, but about the entire human being. What's the use if our aorta is free but one arm is "tied off," or if waste products have built up in our connective tissue to such an extent that our cells are starving nevertheless.

Energy bodies

I've refrained from using "layers of the aura" since for me, this term has lost its neutral quality due to all the esoteric blah-blah-blah. Furthermore, there are rigid ideas of how an aura should be. Those can apply, but don't have to in a particular case, and they can prevent "freely" discovering the real situation.

Adding the physical body to the classic seven layers of the aura, I arrived at eight. With duplication, I arrived at 16, and I also found issues in all of the 16 layers. The same happened with 32 layers, 64, 128 and so on.

So how many layers are there, and where does the primary disorder or irritation reside initially? And which layer is only a copy of it?

Here is the solution to all these questions: we duplicated the number of layers infinitely, thereby opening the door to an n-dimensional space that is available to us as a testing field.

Thus, I had created the space of consciousness that was required to develop the healing breath technique—which then occurred within days.

Chakras

Modern esotericism departs from the 7 chakras; the Egyptians knew 12 body chakras, such as a lower heart chakra for personal love and an upper heart chakra for universal love. In Traditional Chinese Medicine (TCM), *Cun* (the width of a person's thumb at the knuckle) is used as a unit of measure, which makes for a logically comprehensible approach. Applying the *Cun* system to chakras, there must be more than seven.

Chakras above and below the body have also been described. As a result, we're facing the same question we had regarding the aura: How many are there for real? We don't know, yet one thing is clear: they do exist; they're vortices of energy and gateways, and an important element of our energetic system. Chakras can be irritated and/or blocked.

The rest is open, and we can discover it ourselves.

Meridians

Traditional Chinese Medicine is based on 12 principal meridians and 8 extraordinary meridians.

These meridians rank among the most sophisticated and best described systems, and are thus basic education available to anyone who's interested.

Chinese medicine always takes the following principle into account: when the flow of energy is interrupted in one part of the body, there's a congestion of energy before, and a lack of energy after, that spot.

Chinese medicine also describes different kinds of energies and how they interact, which provides the basis for planning the treatment.

One of the best books in this field is *The Foundations of Chinese Medicine* by Giovanni Maciocia.

Structure

Biological age

"You look really old."

We can hear this phrase at any age.

The biological age is a parameter that represents the body's age. It's not a constant, but varies, similar to the way we appear when we look in the mirror.

Biological age indicates the state of our cells, which is subject to current influences. This means that the biological age of a 50-year-old can be that of a 30-year-old or of a 70-year-old.

My therapeutic goal with adults is to achieve a biological age that is 20 years below the person's actual age.

Organs

When this test topic is active, certain organs need a special treatment:

"If you don't take special care of me, I won't go along with this anymore."

The excretory organs—kidneys, liver, lungs and intestines—are particularly sensitive and needy. But it can also be any other bodily organ.

And the issue can be on any level: physical, biochemical, mental, emotional, energetic and/or spiritual.

With the test topic "Organs," you check the organs using the arm-length test, and the one that needs something receives a special treatment.

Hormonal system

You want to place an order by e-mail and the internet doesn't work. Then, nothing works anymore. You experience the same problem when the hormonal system, or parts of it, are on strike. The recipient doesn't receive the message and can't act.

Our brain produces regulatory hormones that either do the work in our body or transmit the work instructions to other organs. In this way, we have a centralized regulation of many processes, making it possible that they're in tune with one another.

External influences such as AC voltage irritate the pituitary gland, which misinterprets the current as daylight; this blocks the melatonin production that occurs only at night.

Drugs and other toxins can also block the hormonal system.

With this test topic, central hormone production in the brain and the body's hormonal centers, such as the thyroid and adrenal glands, should be tested and balanced.

Blood, lymph, and cerebrospinal fluid

These are also bodily organs, even if they're often regarded as fluids only.

We have some knowledge about their functionality, but most of it is probably unknown. I still trained in detoxifying treatments based on methods by Hufeland and Aschner, such as bloodletting, the application of leeches, cupping, cantharides plasters and Baunscheidtism. All these are highly effective methods to cleanse the blood and lymph.

Neurodermatitis starts where the lymph is closest to the surface: in the elbow pits and the backs of the knees. When the lymph is no longer able to absorb more toxins, they're released via the skin. When the blood is loaded with toxins, the body also finds ways to do an emergency cleansing, such as venous leg ulcers in case of alkaloid poisonings. Alkaloids are highly toxic stimulating substances contained in coffee, tea and chocolate. Not everyone is able to excrete them sufficiently via the kidneys; in that case, the body finds another way.

Often, this can also be sweat. If perspiration smells, it's a good idea to completely refrain from consuming coffee, green and black tea, as well as chocolate; within days the smell will disappear naturally. This also applies to stinky feet in other cases of food intolerance.

The blood has utmost priority in the body. This is where enzymes and hormones act, which need a perfect milieu to work properly. Thus, the pH level has to be within a certain range, otherwise they won't keep functioning.

For this reason, the body ensures that such a level is maintained as long as possible. The toxins are excreted in whichever way, or stored in the tissue. What counts is that the blood's pH level is okay.

That explains why tissue hurts—it's simply a full toxic waste storage. This is why therapies work that use only water as a therapeutic agent. The toxins are diluted and excreted. Diuretics that drain water from the body (often used to lower blood pressure, and in case of water retention in the legs) can serve to send people to an early grave instead, as they lead to a heightened concentration of toxins in the body by draining the diluting water. Therefore, it's better to stop consuming all food toxins, which are included in all semi-luxury foods and beverages, when water is retained in the legs, and drink more good water to flush out the toxins rather than trying to kill the symptom out of good old ignorance. This isn't new, but rather ancient knowledge that was lost through pharmacological brainwashing.

The blood also takes over the oxygen transport, ensuring that tissues and cells don't starve. For this purpose, it has to move through the finest capillaries. However, it can only do so if the blood components can move around freely and adjust their forms. When the blood gets too acidic, the red blood cells are stuck together like rolls of coins. Have you ever experienced a line of people going through passport control? It only works one by one.

This results in clogged vessels and starving areas, which manifest in gray skin, sore muscles and inflammations, for example.

Lymph is the tissue fluid and has its own system of vessels.

These vessels also have valves regulated by the plexuses of the autonomic nervous system. If these plexuses are blocked, lymphatic fluid can also build up in the lymphatic vessels. The tonsils are the overflow of the lymphatic system. Thus, the sometimes stinky secretions (such as a bad taste in the throat) that come from them are the garbage disposal of the lymphatic system.

In the event of allergies, the situation in the body escalates even further. Due to the allergic reaction, the body itself produces acids. In such a case, using cortisone can bring only temporary relief to the cells, which get sort of "stoned," while we're keeping both eyes covered regarding the cause.

A better approach is to identify what triggers the allergy (food, cosmetics, or even medications, dental materials or toxic substances we use in our living environment) and eliminate these substances. With the arm-length test, finding the cause is really easy and takes just a few minutes.

A patient once came to see me with neurodermatitis. During the treatment, we found out that he reacted to milk protein and a certain detergent. He eliminated milk and bovine products from his diet and replaced the detergent with another one that tested okay using the arm-length test. After two weeks, his skin had healed.

Tissues

How tall would humans be if each cell had its individual blood pipeline and a "slave nerve" in order to always receive the latest information. We would be about as tall as a mammoth. Since we aren't, there must be a different way to supply the individual cells. Apart from a few very important exceptions—the VIPs, so to speak—vessels and nerves end in the connective tissue, which then distributes information and nutrients to the cells.

When the tissue is suffocating in toxins and acids, it loses its flexibility and is no longer able to provide for the individual cells.

Squeezing the skin firmly between your thumb and index finger at one of your forearms shouldn't be painful at all. If it isn't, your connective tissue is in a good state. If it is, the tissue is too acidic. Alkaline and isotonic tissue is always painfree; whenever it hurts, there are acids involved. This then calls for a reduction of acid-forming food, and drinking a lot of water until the tissue has normalized again. Food that creates acid isn't that which has a sour taste, but that whose decomposition leads to the formation of acids in the body—that is, sugar, meat, sweet beverages, coffee, etc.

Allergic reactions to food constitute another important source of acids. An allergy to milk protein, for instance, not only produces a typical bloated face (which led to the creation of the term "milksop"), but also overacidifies the connective tissue in the entire body.

Here, it makes sense to test all food and drinks and stop consuming all those that create an allergic reaction, as revealed by the arm-length test (the difference in arm length increases with repeat testing).

Tissues include all body tissues: bones, mucous membranes, nerves, organs, etc. It's also possible that tissues lack nutrients, such as fatty acids, vitamins or minerals. Or, they're poisoned with wood preservatives, pesticides, residues of dishwashing detergent on dishes, formaldehyde, residues of detergent on cotton clothing, or insecticides containing pyrethroids (highly potent neurotoxins).

Tissue can also be irritated, such as by high-frequency and AC electric fields, or by geopathic stress at work or in sleeping areas.

Microwaved food is a special case. It's no longer recognized by the connective tissue because the molecules have been changed. Since the connective tissue doesn't transport them, the cells behind this tissue starve. "I don't know you. Anyone can claim to be vitamin C. You sound different, you smell different and you look different."

In an experiment, food and beverages were microwaved before giving them to some cats. The 5,000 cats involved could eat as much as they wanted, yet the last cat still died on day 28 because microwaved food has no value.

Structure

Our bodies consist of rhythms, and structures that move in tune with these rhythms. Not all issues can be resolved energetically. A suppurative focus underneath a tooth often has to be removed surgically, a tumor reduced or fully removed, rhythms reactivated directly with osteopathy, or foreign material removed from the teeth or following bone-fracture surgery. If this test question causes stress, this is an indication that the structure needs to be treated directly.

Nerve plexuses

These are the major regulatory centers of the body, and my favorite structures. They each have their own individual sound. When they're blocked—and they can be "upset" quite easily—the organs depending on them have a hard time. Organs are spoiled, as they're regulated by the nerve plexuses that coordinate them.

In order to feel these plexuses, we reach into them in a virtual fashion. Our hand becomes this nerve plexus, sensing how free it is by how easily the hand moves. In a blocked plexus, hardly any movement is possible; it feels incredibly viscous. A free plexus makes the hand move like there is zero gravity. And there are all kinds of shades between these extremes.

The major nerve plexuses of the autonomic nervous system are the:

- pelvic plexus
- navel plexus
- solar plexus
- cervical plexuses (left and right)
- vagal system (along the spine)

The pelvic plexus regulates all organs in the lower abdomen. It can be blocked due to a physical trauma, such as falling on the coccyx, because it is situated directly above. However, it can also be blocked as a result of emotional, energetic or spiritual traumas, such as violent sex. Consequently, women can experience menstrual or bladder problems, or a limited ability to enjoy their sexuality; in men, this can result in prostate, bladder or sexual problems.

In adults, the navel plexus plays a rather subordinate role. For unborn or new-born babies, it's of vital importance due to the umbilical cord. For this reason, it's essential to check this plexus when working with unborn babies, as cutting the umbilical cord is the first major trauma after birth. In adults, it's connected with a basic sense of trust, and being and feeling nourished.

The solar plexus regulates all upper abdominal organs and large parts of the intestines. When it's blocked, often as a result of emotional and energetic stress, malfunctions of these organs can occur because they're simply not used to thinking for themselves and attuning to one another—a task Mother Solar Plexus is usually in charge of.

Before starting to work on individual organs, it makes sense to first readjust the regulatory system and then test which individual organs still need something.

The cervical plexuses on both the right and left side can be divided into lower, middle and upper ones, but they don't have to be.
They regulate the head, face and brain; and the arms, shoulders and chest, including the lungs and heart.
If, for instance, the blood circulation is disturbed after a wrist fracture and the hand is atrophic, which is called "complex regional pain syndrome" (CRPS), formerly also known as Sudeck's atrophy, this is just a regulatory problem. Neural therapists inject local anesthetics in the respective cervical plexus and numb it, thereby trying to push the reset button so that the blood vessels open up again.
When blood is taken from both elbow pits simultaneously and sent to the lab to be examined, certain parameters, such as hemoglobin, hematocrit and leucocytes, yield very different results. The lab usually responds: "The samples were mixed up; those cannot be from one and the same patient."
But they are. I tried it during my work at the hospital. The explanation lies in the cervical plexuses, as the value of the leucocytes, the white blood cells, is not determined by their formation, but by their decomposition. Also, the thickness of the blood on both sides differs, and is regulated by these plexuses. A focal infection underneath a tooth or in the tonsils, for example, irritates the regulation of this area, which changes the blood values on this side of the body.
These findings were already established in the second half of the last century by Viennese professors Alfred Pischinger and Felix Perger, and unfortunately, have been almost forgotten.

The last big plexus is that of the vagus nerve, with its branches that extend down the body along the spine. In Latin, *vagus* means "wanderer." It regulates the senses and reflexes, playing a coordinating role in a superordinate sense. When it's blocked or irritated, the interplay on a larger scale of all processes is disturbed.

To sense the vagus nerve with your hands, it's best to imagine them being the vagus with all its branches on both sides along the spine. Sensing how easily the hands move will reveal how free the vagus is, and thus its state.

Working with and freeing up the nerve plexuses, together with working on treatments of the craniosacral rhythms, constitute the supreme therapeutic discipline.

Teeth, dental materials and focal infections

Did you know that:
- at least half of the bone underneath a tooth has to be eaten away for it to show on an x-ray?
- a focal infection underneath a tooth can require half of the immune system's capacity to be kept in check?
- toxins stemming from dental inflammations are excreted via the tonsils? There was an experiment where ink was injected underneath a tooth, and came back out at the tonsils.
- the root canal of an incisor is about three miles long, not just about half an inch? This is due to the fact that this isn't a canal, but actually similar to a river delta with an infinite network of branches. This makes a root canal treatment that cleans only this half-inch very questionable.
- a dead tooth secretes ptomaines? These are the strongest toxins found in a human organism and carry such nice names as propionic and butyric acid, putrescine, cadaverine or thioether. CADAVERINE in our teeth—sounds delicious, doesn't it?
- as a result of combining noble and base metals in the mouth, electric currents are generated that can demoralize our nerves?
  For this reason, using both gold and amalgam in the mouth is a form of malpractice, as nerves are being irritated already when exposed to 80mV. This is referred to as "oral galvanism" or the "battery effect" in the mouth. Trigeminal neuralgia, headaches or irritations of the sinuses and eyes can be attributed to this, as well as to dental focal infections.
- many people can't tolerate dental materials? Some even show allergic reactions. However, these allergic reactions don't reveal themselves directly in the mouth; their symptoms can appear anywhere in the body. Pig collagen inserted into the jawbone to help build the bone for implants can create a dramatic situa-

tion, as it cannot be removed anymore, whereas metals used in fillings can be removed easily.

Dental glues are more difficult to remove once used, as they have to be ground off. If the person is allergic to the dental materials—that is, the arm-length test reveals an increasing difference with repeat testing—the materials have to be removed, if possible. For the purpose of testing, the patient can place his or her tongue on the filling prior to testing. Or a sample of the dental material is placed on the body, and the patient imagines having this dental material in his or her mouth on a permanent basis.

Ideally, dental materials are tested directly in the dentist's practice before they're used. Testing can be done by the dentist or the patient him- or herself. In this way, many odysseys of suffering can be avoided.

- tolerance of most glues and plastics can be tested using a tube of instant glue? Dental glues and plastics are based on cyanoacrylate. This is precisely the same basic substance used in instant glues. The blue light is used by the dentist to polymerize, and thus harden, the glue or plastic. The body only reacts to the nonpolymerized form. Thus, a reaction to such substances can sometimes be reduced or even eliminated by posthardening them using this blue light.

- implants are dentists' cash cows? With reductions in dental service compensation from health insurance funds over the past years, it has become increasingly difficult for dentists to operate cost-efficiently and pay back the high debts related to their enormously expensive equipment. But fortunately, there are still implants, which can allow for a profit of 500 to 1,000 U.S. dollars.

  Many people's adverse reaction to the materials used doesn't matter here and is also difficult to prove with conventional medicine.

  Filling people's stomachs with pork meat is still okay for many, and it also doesn't stay there that long. But in the bone, it stays for a lifetime. Using the arm-length test, about half of all people react to titanium as an implant. It's true that there's still a 50 percent chance that the person won't be affected. If dentists didn't make so much money with implants, there wouldn't be so many. When in doubt, it's better to choose the removable option for the night.

- amalgam has to be removed carefully in combination with thorough detoxification? And that chlorella algae are really dangerous when used by themselves for detoxification? When using these algae, toxins extracted from the connective tissue accumulate before the kidneys, which give in, facing this load. If, however, the algae is combined with a kidney/bladder tea containing goldenrod, the kidneys can manage the high load. The schedule for removing amalgam (how many fillings can be removed in how many appointments with how much time in between) and the necessary detoxification measures can be tested really well with the arm-length test.

- dental materials don't stay on the market for long? And that they weren't tested thoroughly and for a long time before using them in practice? This turns the patient into a guinea pig. As a result, it can happen that a plastic filling swells up and bursts the tooth; or that in Germany, teeth are still filled with highly toxic mercury although it's already banned in other countries. Also, high-quality gold is mixed with a lot of palladium. Thus, you don't do yourself a favor if you exchange amalgam for this kind of gold. It's just that with palladium, it's not the kidneys and brain that get affected, but the pancreas.
- that meridians end at the teeth, and that each tooth is connected to certain emotional issues? This explains why certain teeth have problems or break when specific issues are present.
- inflammations of the teeth in the lower jaw can be palpated very well? When trying to palpate the roots along the lower jawbone using the thumb, certain spots can be very sensitive to pressure. And an old rule says: Where it hurts, there's an inflammation.
- irritations or problems of the teeth can be detected very well with the arm-length test? Put your tongue on a tooth, and test.
- misaligned teeth can be treated very well using *innerwise*?
  Normally, teeth can move freely in all directions, even if these movements are minimal. This can be tested and treated using healing cards up to the point where a tooth no longer has any problem in any direction; when testing, the arms always stay equally long.
  It doesn't make sense to move teeth with braces somewhere where they don't want to move to. This is forcing movement on them, and often entails tension and blockages in the cervical spine; scoliosis can arise, and the tension in the neck compresses important blood vessels supplying the brain. As a result, braces can bring down an adolescent's grades by one or two letters. Alternatively, there are orthodontists who work energetically first, and then use braces only to support what's needed. This combination reduces the treatment period by half.

Testing the severity of a dental focal infection—that is, an inflammation underneath the teeth, which is often invisible on an x-ray—can involve a test measuring the concentration of decomposition toxins. The following scale supports you in testing without a lab test:

Teeth	
First quadrant (upper right)	Second quadrant (upper left)
1 2 3 4 5 6 7 8	9 10 11 12 13 14 15 16
32 31 30 29 28 27 26 25	24 23 22 21 20 19 18 17
Fourth quadrant (lower right)	Third quadrant (lower left)

Dental chart

Tox test:
for dental focal infections: bacterial and decomposition toxins
(propionic and butyric acid, putrescine, cadaverine, thioether)
Scale to assess a dental focal infection:

    0 = Healthy
    1 = Harmless
    2 = Need for treatment
    3 = Need for treatment
    4 = Need for treatment
    5 = Need for treatment
    6 = Need for treatment
    7 = Surgical removal of focal infection required
    8 = Surgical removal of focal infection required

Scars, focal infections and tonsils

For years I've treated all scars harboring an interference field with neural therapy
by infiltrating procaine into them, and have experienced great healing results in
my patients and myself.

For example, since World War II, a man had experienced phantom pain in the
arm he'd lost. The hand that was no longer there hurt him almost permanently
so that he could only get by with painkillers. The scar on his shoulder was still
partially discolored (purple) and weather sensitive. After injecting the local anesthetic procaine into the scar the first time (procaine by itself only anesthetizes
for a few minutes), he was painfree for the first time in years, and it stayed that
way.

All scars should be tested using the arm-length test: Glide over the scar with your
fingers or hand, and test with your arms. If the arms react with stress, the scar still
irritates the body and needs to be treated.
In particular, irritating scars affect the autonomic nervous system with the nerve
plexuses. Today I balance scars using *innerwise* healing cards only. Simply pick the

cards that remove the stress. This works because a scar's actual stress comes from the energetic charges related to its origination that are still present.

The tonsils can be another significant site of focal infection. Frequently, they're filled with old pus that has hardened over time. Tonsils look like a sponge; in their crevices or tonsillar crypts, tonsil stones can be lodged—that is, small smelly pieces of pus. Bad breath usually stems from dental focal infections or the tonsils. The stomach is rarely the point of origin, but is sometimes offered as an explanation out of embarrassment. In earlier times, people still took care of cleaning their tonsils, which is very easy if you want to try it: massage the tonsils out using your index finger. It's best to do this alone in the bathroom, as it can cause a gag reflex. The taste is atrocious, but the old pus has to get out of the tonsils. You will also experience immediate relaxation in your shoulders and neck area. The waste lodged in the tonsils originates from two sources: dental focal infections and intolerance reactions to proteins—above all, chicken protein and bovine protein (milk products). If these stones remain in the tonsils, they release toxins into the body and affect it severely.

Tissue abnormalities
We have to differentiate three kinds of tumors: those that grow at a normal slow pace, at a medium-fast pace or an ultrafast pace. In general, the following factors play a role regarding tumors:

- a strong, unresolved emotional trauma
- resonance with the tumor
- energetic manipulation

Tumors growing at a normal slow pace
A slow pace means 15 to 20 years.
After a severe emotional trauma where something in us dies, the growth of a tumor takes place only on the energetic level for about ten years. Then, it starts to manifest on the structural level, and cells start to form. It takes another few years until three to four million cells have formed, making a tumor visible on an ultrasound or other imaging technique, as it's at that point that it will have reached a size of about 0.2 inches. At this stage, people get diagnosed, and they often give up on themselves as of that day. Yet in fact, they've already coexisted peacefully with the tumor for 15 to 20 years.

Tumors growing at a medium-fast pace

Growing at a medium-fast pace means three to five years. So far, I haven't been able to find an explanation as to why and how they grow.

Tumors growing at an ultrafast pace

Within days, a physically manifest tumor has developed in the patient's body. The question "Do you have cancer?" reveals a "no" response from the patient. The question "Do you feed cancer?" gets a "yes" response. This can lead to big question marks in the head, because it means that this person's own energy field, his or her soul, doesn't have the cancer. But whose cancer is it? Where does it come from? Regularly, we find fissures in the soul field through which the cancer manifests itself from the outside. I've seen several cases where cancer was physically manifest within 36 hours. These are always cases of the most severe kinds of manipulation. On the other hand, there must have been an invitation from the person concerned, a resonance with that manipulation.

As long as the tumors exist only on an energetic level—of course, sensitive people can feel them as unpleasant energies—they can be easily cleared with *innerwise*. If greater amounts of cells have already formed, it gets problematic.

Then, we need another strategy: We have to increase the structurizing energy as well as all other base energies (soul, life, creative and love energies) to a level high enough so that the original core structure can manifest itself again and that foreign structures can be recognized and removed. In addition, it's about resolving all core issues, eliminating compromises and seeking support from conventional medicine, if helpful.

Activities

Nourishment

This involves much more than eating food.

It's about nourishing oneself on the physical level, involving: physical activities, nutrition, vitamins, minerals, water and detoxification.

Nourishing oneself on the mental level, involving: attitude, the power of thoughts, programs and conditioning.

Nourishing oneself on the emotional level, involving: feelings, food for the heart, dependencies, expectations, self-love, self-worth and self-confidence.

Nourishing oneself on the energetic level, involving: flow/blockages, one's own and foreign energies, trust in the necessity of all experiences.

Nourishing oneself on the spiritual level, involving: humbleness and gratitude for everything.

Regulation

Does the body work in harmony with itself? And who's calling the shots? If, for instance, parts of the body carry another identity or are stuck in another time (heart broken at the age of 18, anger in the liver since 25, deep loss sitting in the kidneys since 32) and thus, the organs are still caught in the shock of the event, the person is a fragmented system; and as a result, harmonious central coordination and regulation are no longer possible. However, this is necessary to heal and fully enjoy life. At the end of a treatment, all fragmentations should be cleared up.

Sexuality

Under this topic, everything related to sexuality should be put on the table, such as how desire and sexual pleasure are experienced—from orgasmic qualities all the way to sperm pressure.

And once again, it's a good thing that therapists can use test cards—if they're shy, they can always refer back to the test card that revealed a particular topic.

How was sexuality experienced for the first time? What models were the parents in the way they themselves lived? Which values were transmitted? Did any experiences involve violence?

Were there situations that left behind feelings of shame?

Are sex and pleasure coupled with pain? Does partnership involve servitude? What religious or societal prisons have been internalized? Do both partners still have the desire to touch each other? Were there any abortions?

How is orgasm experienced? Is it possible to also feel the partner's orgasm, and if not, why?

Were there affairs, or has anything been suppressed that killed sexuality in the relationship?

Sexual organs store very diverse energies. Oftentimes, they're like a library of one's love life, and it's all stored one on top of the other. The uterus and prostate often carry manipulating energies. In an Imago, they then appear heavy and dark. Fissures in the soul field can also frequently be found in the lower abdomen after violent experiences.

The organ Imago is a wonderful tool to work on these topics. This involves a kind of virtual systemic constellation work of the organ; issues are cleared up and the organs are cleansed.

Cleansing

In Goethe's time, it was still common to describe one's bowel movement in letters. "Today I had a good shit." Children still have shining eyes as well when describing this proudly. With this topic, it's time to talk uninhibitedly about one's excretions: urine, sweat, shit, discharges, sperm, bad breath, body odor or foot perspiration.

Physical activities

In the mood for engaging with your body? In the mood for movement? How about running through puddles again? Dancing wildly and freely? Climbing mountains?

How do people perceive their bodies, muscles, tendons and bones? Which traumas are stored in the tissue and block movement? Here, Wilhelm Reich's body armors play a significant role. Do people move with nearly zero gravity? Or is there a viscosity, heaviness and rigidity that pulls them down into their chairs? How smoothly do people move? Is it nice to watch them run or dance?

For dancing, I recommend the following exercise: Turn on some good music and close your eyes. Stand still and observe yourself until you sense which part of your body feels like moving to this music, and what rhythm it's inspired to follow.

This part of your body will guide the rest of your body in this dance. With the next song, you stand still again until one part of your body wants to engage and starts guiding you. This can be your shoulders, pelvis, knees, feet or even your genitals.

Communication

Do you always speak the truth? Do you have the courage to say what's on the tip of your tongue? Do you really have something to say when you talk?

At a friends' house, Grandma moved in with a young family. Half a year later, the little girl started to talk like Grandma, using the same words and representing the same fears and patterns. After one year, no one could hear the girl herself anymore, but only the grandmother speaking through her. Nicely put, one calls this "social heredity." The honest interpretation is "child abuse."

Now we'll do the ABC test: Sense yourself within and say the letter *A*. Then sense where the *A* resounds in yourself. You can repeat this with every letter of the alphabet, as well as the numbers 0 to 9. Ideally, every letter and number resound throughout your entire body. The whole body resonates, becomes a sound space and gives all its power into it as you're doing this.

Then, using *innerwise*, you can treat all letters and numbers that resound only in one part of the body or sound and feel weak. You will feel the changes immediately, and your arms will no longer differ in length when you test the letters or numbers. Once you've completed the program, you can do a stress test and imagine visiting your parents and having coffee. Then, repeat the entire test with the alphabet and numbers. As we often regress and turn back into children when being with our parents, the power of our language also breaks down along with that.

Once more, you can balance any stress that may be present with *innerwise*.

Consequently, you'll experience that your voice will have changed noticeably. Others will also react differently to you. Suddenly, people will hear you with all your power, and then they will also listen.

Sleep

For 18 years, I've been taking my children to bed. Whenever one got old enough to fall asleep alone, the next one came. I keep finding it fascinating to feel how the aura of children changes once they've fallen asleep. Then, they're really in another world. Frequently, I could support them in falling asleep by creating the field they radiate when asleep in advance.

Some tests yield different results depending on whether the person is awake or asleep. It also suffices if the therapist imagines that the client is asleep or awake. Answers given in the sleep mode are often more honest.

A good night's sleep means falling asleep after five minutes, sleeping through the night and waking up in the morning well rested, with a clear mind and a body that can move freely. Everything else is a compromise. The two big topics, electrosmog and geopathology, are discussed in the context of test card 11, which is dedicated to the environment.

Just one thing at this point: using the arm-length test, there shouldn't be any stress when you imagine lying in bed, nor when you imagine your partner lying next to you or a child sleeping between both of you.

Breathing

When you take a deep breath and focus on how the air is spreading out in your body and how your body is expanding, you will often notice asymmetries. The expansion isn't identical on both sides. When you concentrate more on how the energy is spreading out that you absorbed when breathing in, you will notice various differences between the two sides of the body but also in different life situations.

Our inhalation should be unrestricted, light and free; it symbolizes the future. If we're afraid of the future, our inhalation is blocked.

Our exhalation should be unrestricted in depth and in the capacity to empty ourselves; it symbolizes letting go of the past. If we hold on to something, our exhalation is blocked.

If our breathing is blocked on the left side of the body, our female side is blocked.

If our breathing is blocked on the right side of the body, the blockage concerns our male side.

Rhythms

We consist only of rhythms. Everything else is an illusion. Solid bodies are only particularly densified fields.

Each organ has its own rhythm, which regulates its functionality. The heartbeat, breath, cranial breath and craniosacral rhythm are only some of them. The body is like an orchestra, and a harmonious interplay is key.

Rhythms can be sensed well using our hands. Imagine that your hands are the client's lungs and you're breathing in through them. You will feel every blockage and restriction. In the same way, your hands can also turn into your nerve plexuses or the pelvis and test its mobility. Or you imagine how you press together your client's skull from the sides, as well as from the front and back with your hands. To do so, you don't place your hands directly on the skull, but about 12 inches away from it, and then do these movements in the air. Usually, the skull can be pressed together easily, like a tightly filled rubber ball. Yet, it might feel more like wanting to press together a concrete block. In that case, the skull is blocked, and the client is likely to experience pressure in the head.

You should check the skull's mobility with your hands at least in three dimensions. If you're not certain when doing so using your hands, you can also apply the arm-length test at any time to double-check. That is, you virtually press the skull together and then double-check using the client's arms. Learning by doing can be that simple!

Influences and reactions

Medical drugs

In this chapter, I have to once again point out the following, both for legal reasons and also based on my own experience: *Any change in medication must be discussed in advance with an understanding medical doctor.*

Does it harm me? Does it do me any good? These are the key questions.
It's likely that more people die than regain good health from medication.

In practice, the picture often looks as follows: Out of ten medical drugs taken by patients, they have a severe allergic reaction to three, don't tolerate two, don't need three, and only two drugs can be tolerated and make sense.

I once worked in a fasting clinic for a while. After several days of fasting, patients hardly needed any medication anymore. In geriatric medicine, the number of drugs could often be reduced by half without the slightest negative effect.

As a medical doctor, I no longer recommend any medication that I haven't tested before. For this purpose, the two following test questions have to yield a positive response:

1. As the person imagines taking the medication, the arm-length test may not reveal any negative reaction.
2. The question as to whether the person needs the medication has to show a "yes" response.

Many medical drugs that people take cause a stress or an allergic reaction in the arm-length test.
Medication that produces an allergic reaction may not be taken in the future. Such drugs certainly have more side effects than desired positive effects.

Medication causing stress in the sense of "I don't like this!" should be substituted; if this isn't possible, they should be combined with other remedies to cancel out the stress. These can be detox remedies for the kidneys, liver and gallbladder, or for the intestines; or vitamins and homeopathic remedies.
When testing these compensation remedies in combination with the medication, the stress disappears.

Most medical drugs fight symptoms; they aren't even based on a healing approach. However, healing isn't possible on the symptomatic level; it can only occur when dealing with the underlying core issues.

Test questions
- Think of all the medications you're taking, and test all of them together. Don't forget the contraceptive pill, vitamins, Bach flower essences and homeopathic remedies, as applicable.
- If stress arises, test each of them individually.
- Test all medications or remedies that have survived this test regarding their benefit: "I need this medication or remedy …"

Poisonings
What was the greatest poison in your life? I've asked this question in many workshops. Rarely have people replied with amalgam, wood preservatives or vaccina-

tions. The most frequently named poisons were: not being loved, value concepts, rules, words and energies.

If this test question comes up, you're called upon to turn into a detective and identify the poisons or toxins of any kind in the life of the person concerned.

This can also refer to the wood preservatives used in a home's attic. This can be determined by checking if the arm-length test reveals stress when the person imagines breathing in the air in these rooms. But it can also refer to not being a wanted child at the time of conception.

For the most effective search, we can ask about the time in the person's life when the poisoning originated, and test. "Is this a poisoning from the present?" "Is this a poisoning from youth?" "Is this a poisoning from childhood?"

Or, we can test the age when the poisoning occurred.

Example: "Were you 30 to 40 years old when the poisoning occurred?" Arm-length test response: "No."

"Were you 20 to 30 years old when the poisoning occurred?" Arm-length test response: "Yes." With this approach, we can identify the exact point in time.

We can also ask about the kind of poisoning: "Was the poisoning based on a substance?" "Was it an emotional, energetic, etc., poisoning?"

The more precisely we can determine the cause, the more the person concerned can assume self-responsibility and avoid such things in the future, as well as better understand the correlations in his or her life.

As therapists, it offers us the opportunity to learn how that person works: after the issue of poisoning has been resolved with the support of healing cards, the therapist can once more test the body, organs, fields and parameters, understanding how this particular issue was interconnected in the body.

The living art of healing—learning by doing.

Allergies

An allergic reaction is like an attempt to run away screaming. It's just that the body can't run away when the horror is being poured in in the form of milk, when it's glued into the teeth in the form of metal, or when it's smeared into hair in the form of shampoo.

The outcry remains, followed by continued self-destruction.

When we test medications and they produce an allergic reaction in the arm-length test—that is, an increasing difference in arm length with repeat testing—one thing is for sure: the side effects are greater than the desired positive effects. Under no circumstances should we tolerate allergies or try to balance them energetically. Here, the only order of the day is identifying and eliminating the cause.

Potential sources in the order of their significance:

- Food and drinks
- Medical drugs
- Dental materials
- Cosmetics
- Detergents and cleaners
- Indoor air pollution

Food and drinks

The most common allergen is bovine protein. We constantly consume this protein not only in the form of meat, but especially in dairy products such as milk, curd, yogurt, cheese, milk chocolate, ice cream, etc.

It has become trendy to have a lactose intolerance—trendy because clever companies sell pills to counteract it.

In most cases, however, the people concerned have an allergic reaction to the protein and not the sugar, lactose. Then, one can only abstain, or a bit more practical: "sin consciously"—that is, test to see when one can once again enjoy a caffe latte. And add a cleansing phase following these little sins.

In many cases, there's the option to switch to milk and milk products from animals other than cows—such as sheep or goats—or use almond, hazelnut or oat milk.

The high rate of milk protein allergies has two causes: baby formulas and vaccinations.

Initially, the bowels of a newborn are still permeable to proteins. If proteins from a different species are fed too early, they go into the blood. They can be recognized as foreign proteins, and the body develops an immune reaction against them. This imprint stays one's entire life. The second possible cause are vaccinations. During my medical practice, I used to wonder why I tested allergies to milk proteins so frequently in connection with vaccine-induced damage. Calling the medical doctor in charge of vaccine production at a pharmaceutical company unraveled the mystery: some vaccines are cultivated in beef broth.

This also includes a vaccine against diphtheria. Over a number of years, production methods have changed, but previous generations were injected with bovine protein together with the vaccine. And then, the body did what it's supposed to do when vaccinated: it built up an immune response against the proteins, including the bovine protein.

A milk protein intolerance shows classic symptoms: middle-ear infection, sinusitis, the sniffles, polyps, bronchitis, asthma, diarrhea or constipation. All these are due to a swelling of the mucous membranes. On a secondary level, the acids created via the allergic reaction are deposited in the tissue, resulting in the bloated "milksop" face and hurtful tissue swellings overall.

Many people believe it is fat. As opposed to fat, swellings caused by an acid formation in the tissue are painful. Often mixed forms occur, of course. When dropping the allergy triggers, "love handles" and "spare tires" caused by the formation of acids in the tissue disappear quickly.

What's important is to never force children to eat something they don't want to. There's always a reason why they don't want to eat or drink something. Milk simply isn't always healthy and good for bone growth. A study involving thousands of Swedish nurses even showed that the more milk the nurses had drunk, the more frequently their pelvic bones would break.

The next important food item is chicken protein. The good news is that usually egg yolk can be tolerated well. These allergies can also be attributed to vaccinations, as some vaccines were, and partially still are, cultivated in chicken embryos, such as those against *rubella, mumps, measles* and the *flu*. Together with the vaccine, residual protein is injected, too. From a sociomedical point of view, it's therefore time to raise the question of whether vaccinations have really contributed to improving public health?

The most frequent symptoms include a disgust one feels about soft egg whites, or getting tonsillitis or colitis.

This allergy is a free pass to enjoy only the egg yolk!

Also, quail eggs can be an alternative.

The third important food in this context is wheat—in particular, wheat protein. Once more, the cause is likely to stem from the fact that it's fed to babies too soon. So far I haven't been able to identify other causes, but there are certainly some. Symptoms are rather "hot" inflammations, such as neurodermatitis or a strong colitis. "Hot" refers to red, itchy and/or bloody inflammations, according to the nomenclature used in Traditional Chinese Medicine.

This is a normal state: When pressing the belly with your hand as deeply as possible, as if you wanted to touch the aorta or the spine from the front, it doesn't elicit any pain. Only then is there no inflammation in the intestines. Most people attain this state only when they fast. Those who wish to experience again what freedom in the body feels like should fast for a few days. Then you'll know how it can and should be, remembering what good health actually is.

With an allergy to wheat protein, it's possible to switch to other types of grains. Sometimes people can tolerate the unripe wheat referred to as "green spelt" or freekeh *(Grünkern)*. With bread, there's a problem: most rye breads contain wheat, as the wheat protein has excellent adhesive qualities.

Sweets contain many colorants that can be toxic or cause allergies. The only thing that helps here is testing the product in the store before buying it, and reading the ingredients listed on the packaging.

Sugar substitutes are another major issue. Aspartame and acesulfame, etc., are highly allergenic. There are almost no chewing gums that don't contain these substances.

From dry tongue to skin reactions to changes in brain function—there's a whole range of possible bodily reactions. You drink a low-calorie beverage and are more thirsty afterward than you were before—that's typical. Here, it's necessary to read the ingredients when you go shopping and avoid any artificially sweetened (light) or low-calorie products.

Incidentally, these products don't help you lose weight! The sweet taste is enough for producing insulin and thus storing everything that increases the blood-sugar level (also fats and proteins) more quickly in the tissue. "Sweet" is the signal to "fill the pantries"—that is, the spare tires.

Medical drugs

Please don't undertake any breakneck self-experiments in the future when it comes to medication, food supplements, homeopathy, etc. Think of the medication or remedy, or look at the unopened product and use the arm-length test. If your arms differ in length, your body doesn't like it; if the difference keeps increasing as you repeat the testing, it's rat poison for you—you're allergic to it. In that case, you may not take it and must find an alternative (contact an understanding medical doctor!).

Dental materials

Dental materials that cause an allergic reaction in the arm-length test must be removed.

Apply caution in the removal of amalgam: detox agents are important, as well as the schedule for removal. How many fillings can be removed at once? How long do the intervals have to be between each visit to the dentist, and which detox agents do you have to take?

For the removal, the dentist has to use a special suction device; the evacuator tip is placed onto the tooth to suck the highly toxic mercury vapors directly off the tooth. Mercury evaporates at about 96.8 °F, and when drilling out the amalgam, it gets much warmer than that. If the dentist can't do that or refuses to do so, he or she may not remove your amalgam—unless you want to "preserve" your brain with an extra portion of mercury that will remain there with a half-life of 16 years. For testing, put your tongue on each tooth that contains foreign material and apply the arm-length test. It could also be that a dentist was unscrupulous and lazy, left the old amalgam filling underneath a gold filling, and just ground it off. Then, the only remaining solution is to take off the crown and have a look, and break off the friendship with your previous dentist as a consequence of this malpractice.

And for the future: Ask the dentist to test all dental materials before using them on you, or test them yourself. And here, *all* means really *all*—including anesthetic injections, medications, dental glues, cement, plastics, metals and ceramics.

Cosmetics

The most allergenic substances used in cosmetics and body washes are parabens. The following four kinds of parabens are used: ethyl-, butyl-, propyl- and methylparabens. They produce the classic itching of the eyes and skin after washing your hair.

But cosmetic products contain even more atrocities. And the same applies here, too: always look at the list of ingredients (even with organic products—some of which contain parabens without moral scruples), and test them.

Detergents and cleaners

There are children who develop neurodermatitis as a result of dishwasher tabs. With a water consumption of merely 5 gallons, chemicals will always remain on the dishes and cutlery, reaching the body with the next meal.

By the same token, detergents and fabric softeners also remain in the clothes unless you rinse them in a clean river. You should always select the "extra rinse" cycle when you use a washing machine. This can reduce poisoning caused by the water-saving mania. Imagine if toilet paper was rationed and you weren't allowed to wipe yourself more than once! This wouldn't leave you clean either. What makes sense is to test all cleaning agents used in your household to see whether they're tolerated by everyone living there.

Clothes made of cotton are frequently treated with chemicals during production so that they look good and feel soft in the store. Among other substances, formaldehyde is used for this purpose. This can adversely affect the hollows of the knees when wearing a new pair of unwashed jeans, and may take up to half a year to heal. That's what I experienced when I was 20 years old.

Indoor air pollution

I had put a wall-to-wall wool carpet in one of the rooms in my house and then didn't enter the room for a few days due to the smell. The orange tree that I'd forgotten in the room couldn't flee, though, and died from the chemical evaporations.

Wool carpets—even those made of organic materials—can contain toxic moth protection products.

A patient once came to see me for a headache that she got every time she was at home, especially after sleeping there throughout the night (she'd bought a beautiful attic loft). When she imagined breathing in the air in her home, she exhibited an allergic reaction with the arm-length test. The problem involved the wood preservatives used for the roof. It was particularly bad in the summer when the roof heated up, yet she couldn't simply move out as a tenant would be able to do. So we found a solution: A few times a day, she would spray "Effective Microorganisms" in the air. Those are able to neutralize the toxic substances.

For testing purposes, it's best to visualize the following: First, imagine breathing outdoors, with all windows and doors of the house or apartment being closed. Now, you can imagine entering the first room, breathing there, and test with the arm-length test. Then you imagine entering the next room, breathing there, and test again. In this way, it's easy to identify which room has polluted air and irritates you.

Now you can imagine removing individual pieces of furniture or carpets, then briefly airing the room virtually, breathing again, and then test once more. When the cause is removed, the stress will also disappear in the testing.

As mentioned previously, it all happens just in our imagination, which is enough for diagnostic purposes. Of course, it's necessary to also remove the cause in real life.

Infections

The term "infection" refers to something affecting us inside. This can be anything, of course.

Based on our conditioning over the centuries and the old imprints it has left in us, we immediately associate infections with viruses, bacteria and fungi that attack us; and we have to proceed with a general mobilization against them.

Yet, many of these "beastly little things" are nice and often live in a symbiotic relationship with us. If, however, our milieu derails, they help us clean it up.

Streptococci that cause strep throat always belong in our mouth. The *Candida* yeast residing in our intestines or vagina is a normal gut bacterium that plays an important role in producing vitamins in the intestines. Of course, there are also germs that only visit us rarely. But they all need an irritation of the body or a state of being stuck in a blockage in order to be able to offer their help. Their help consists of supporting our cleansing through snot, phlegm, diarrhea or vaginal discharge. On the other hand, they provoke a "bodybuilding" of the immune system through an increase in antibodies and "arouse" the body until it's so hot that we call it a fever.

In a fever, the rise in temperature stimulates other hormonal and enzymatic processes, triggering an important self-healing mechanism. We know about this reaction in children: In the evening, they're getting a bit sick, then they briefly develop a high fever during the night, and in the morning they're fine again.

Other infections are energetic or emotional in nature, blocking our regulatory system. They figure as the critical, primary infections, since they plant a partial or full blockage on our system that's vibrating harmoniously. This kind of infection is directed at life itself, which is based on vibration.

And there are mental infections. Those include going to school or reading the newspaper.

Here, the current state of ignorance or targeted disinformation is used for education and manipulation.

Infections can also be frequency based. If electronic devices are manufactured by energetically unclean developers, or if systems are peppered with the frequency patterns of sectarian structures, or if energetically charged mantras are used to make people in ashrams dependent, then these also count as infections.

Infections can occur on all levels—physical, mental, emotional, energetic and spiritual.

The key question is, however, what resonance does the person concerned have, and why does he or she invite this infection?

Vaccinations

As a medical student and young medical doctor, I used to believe in them. But after my first daughter almost died from a vaccination, none of my children ever got vaccinated again.

During my medical studies, they taught about the purpose of vaccinations in my Social Medicine course: "Their goal is to maintain public health, not individual prophylaxis." This is the only way to understand articles in medical magazines reporting on a new hepatitis vaccine that is considered tolerable and will thus be approved because only one out of 4,000 children died from it during the test phase. Consequently, vaccinations were, by definition, never about protecting the individual but about achieving a high vaccination coverage in the population to limit the spread of diseases, even if the vaccination harmed individual people. We

don't have children in order to produce servants for the state, but because we love our kids and want to offer them optimal conditions to live a fulfilled life.
Thus, we're also responsible for protecting them from harm.

When parents come to see me and want to know whether they should have their child vaccinated or not, I test the individual vaccines and then tell the parents which ones from which company their child can tolerate, and which intervals are okay for the child for administering the vaccinations. If vaccines don't make it in the test, at least I can test which organs in the body would be harmed. I advise against combined vaccinations that address six or seven diseases at once, as they constitute too great of a burden for the child (who, in effect, gets six to seven serious diseases at the same time).
Also from the perspective of conventional medicine, these vaccinations are nonsense, as the production of antibodies is not sufficient in view of such a multiple challenge, and the hoped for protection can't be attained or won't last long enough. Think about it—have you ever been able to maintain a truly deep relationship with seven partners at once? That is, one where you really engage and grow with one another?
I also recommend books and videos on YouTube to parents. In the end, parents need to decide for themselves, as they also have to be able to make their case vis-à-vis their family, the pediatrician and the school authorities.

Another little story on vaccinations:
Smallpox was defeated through vaccinations—just about every child knows this, and it's written in our schoolbooks. Only the World Health Organization (WHO) doesn't. WHO had commissioned the vaccinations and stopped them for insufficient effectiveness half a year before smallpox was eradicated in 1980. The former head of WHO said that isolating the sick and improving living conditions had managed to conquer smallpox. By the way, the last person who contracted smallpox was a cook who had been vaccinated against the disease. How embarrassing!

On the test card, the topic of vaccinations implies more than vaccinations administered with a syringe or on a sugar cube. It also comprises anything that was inculcated, such as lies spread on the smallpox vaccination, or that the Berlin Wall was protecting people from the evil West, or that the army turns boys into real men, or that a strong back knows no pain.
It's a good thing we have the arm-length test—our pocket lie detector.

Test Card 2   Love and relationships

Ability to love

Many people have never experienced what it means to be loved unconditionally. We can only love someone unconditionally if we're able to see his or her whole and complete soul behind all the masks and scars caused by traumas.

We can't love a body per se; we can desire it. We can't love thoughts per se; we can recognize ourselves in them. We can't love a feeling per se; we can immerse ourselves in it. It's only the soul that we can truly love, as it is an image of Creation. We love thoughts, feelings and the body as an expression of the soul.

None of us is whole and complete, but we all have the chance to once again come closer to our own wholeness and completeness. When we see the wholeness and completeness in other people, we give them the room to get closer to it.

When we focus on their deficits, they will always live these deficits vis-à-vis us.

Relationships—owning/using

It's pretty scary how fast being in love leads to claiming the right to be possessive, and above all, the right to provide for and take care of the other. Thus, love deteriorates to a relationship where relating to one another involves pulling at each another, which is also reflected in the German equivalent "Beziehung." The respect for each other's freedom and independence turns into mutually using one another to fill the holes of our souls, compensating for the trauma experienced in life and projecting our own issues. Most frequently, the partners even lose their identity along the way.

One day a man and a woman came to see me for a couple's treatment before their wedding. The woman had already taken over her partner's identity, and he had taken over hers. In this way, they both tried to live the other's life and save one another.

This can only go wrong.

It's also interesting to observe couples and listen to them, and see or hear which patterns of communication and mutual control they've taken on—even patterns regarding their bodies and the ways they move. And people even do that voluntarily; they give up themselves and their freedom to gain a bit of security, to avoid facing self-responsibility and also to avoid starting afresh in life all the time. This is how many people create hell themselves, out of fear of being honest with themselves and others.

Apart from avoiding self-responsibility, the most important motivation for allowing these dependencies to occur and for engaging in them is living on someone else's energy.

Those who haven't found their own life purpose and are thus not nourished energetically, have to live by stealing energy from others. And who could lend oneself better to this than a partner susceptible to blackmail and one's children? "You're killing me!" This statement can be so true. I myself had constant heart pain during one relationship. Upon separating, this pain disappeared completely. Many people blossom after ending a dependent relationship and do things again that they'd stopped doing for years for the sake of their partner.

In general, every time we forgo something for the sake of another, guilt remains on an energetic level. Deep inside, we make the other person responsible for something important we denied ourselves, or for doing something that wasn't okay for us.

Over the years, a mountain of energetic charges builds up that leads to illness, or which can only be released through a liberating separation.

It's particularly extreme when this "mountain" is between parents and children.

When children are unwanted and when the lives of their parents went in different ways than they would have liked them to go, the children are burdened with a load that's hard to bear.

Each "I would like to, but I can't because of the child" carries the subliminal meaning of "It's because of you, child, that I can't." The friends' response, which says: "You wanted the sex, now you'll have to go through it!" only extends the guilt to the sexual desire that is lived out; and as a subconscious earworm, it will be the "topping" on the ecstasy of each orgasm.

Paternalism

This word means keeping someone else's mouth shut.

When people want to compensate for their own weakness and incompetence, they control others. A common way to play this out is by depriving people of their right to make their own decisions. This means stripping people of their freedom to decide about their lives themselves and believing that one knows better what's right for them.

Many parents find that children have to be paternalized in general in order to teach them values and educate them. And this behavior doesn't change when the children have already long grown up.

Oftentimes, partners greatly enjoy participating in this game, as almost anyone has already experienced this firsthand.

The third large realm where we find paternalism is the working environment.

Among friends, paternalism is less common, as only a few people accept it there. The big question is: Why do people accept paternalism from their partner or parents? How much self-worth has already been lost in order to accept blackmailing paternalizing behavior? Or how great is the fear of change if people no longer let it happen?

And where do we ourselves paternalize others?
Only a society of free human beings living with integrity can be fully free of paternalism.

Sexuality

Sexuality as a shared experience also creates different ways of experiencing it, as well as orgasmic qualities, with different partners.
I also work with patients who come to see me for a treatment because of their declining sperm pressure. The cause always resides in the dynamics of the relationship, feelings of guilt or unresolved issues.
In Chinese medicine, one asks about the man's natural morning erection. If it's normal, the energies of the kidneys are strong, which are responsible for this from a Chinese point of view. If there are still erection problems during sex, it's the liver, suppressed anger, rage and/or other emotional components that are causing this problem. Most likely, it will not arise with another partner.
Sexuality should give both partners energy.
However, there are also cases where pleasure is one-sided. If, during sex, the man loses energy to the woman, the sexual desire soon subsides and his energies can be exhausted.
The same happens for the woman if she's only used for release. The man leaves with relaxed loins and reduced sperm pressure, and what was released stays stuck in the woman, with or without a condom.
Under this topic, we can find all kinds of sexual abuse, blockages of the ways sexuality is experienced, manipulation issues related to sex, related secrets, or wishes and fantasies that aren't lived out.

Distrust

"I fully trust my partner." Most couples can respond with a "yes" to this question (as tested using the arm-length test) only during the first phase of being in love. After the first disappointment, innocence and unconditional trust vanish.
Thus, the slow-acting poison has been injected. It's no longer possible to fully open up to one another. Thus, the inner withdrawal sets in.
Distrust is always rooted in a disappointing experience, a betrayal. Whether objectively, this feeling is really justified, or whether it stems from expectations that result from claiming the right to be possessive, can be determined with the help of a simple parameter: Was a lie, some type of dishonesty, involved?
If not, each partner has taken the freedom they're both entitled to and isn't responsible for the other's expectations.

Freedom and restriction

◉ With your eyes closed, take a few breaths, and pay close attention to how your breathing feels. Be attentive to your right and left lungs, and your maximum inhalation and exhalation. Be attentive to how much your chest expands.

◉ Now imagine you are alone on an island. How is your breath now?

◉ Imagine your parents-in-law are coming to visit. How is your breath now?

◉ Imagine you are with your partner. How is your breath now?

◉ Imagine you are still with your partner in four years. How is your breath now?

If it's optimally free in all situations, congratulations! If not, some freedom has been lost; you've maneuvered yourself into a restricted space.

Self-abandonment

Giving up on ourselves for the sake of someone else or an idea is the most normal thing on Earth. Not loving our work but being paid well; not going on vacation alone because our partner could be disappointed; visiting our parents for Christmas because that's what you do even if you don't want to; listening to a bad lecture until the end because it's not okay to simply get up in the middle; not living a dream because it doesn't offer safety and security; or not separating from your partner because the house isn't paid off yet.

The liberty that small children take to say what *they* want to say, and do what *they* want to do—when and why have we given up on this?

My children can be naked in the garden and on the street; in the garden, they can pee wherever they want to; they're free to not come home for three days if their friends' parties are so great; they can have sex with whomever they want to, eat with their fingers and get up from the dining table whenever they wish. I've refrained from education, and have trusted them to find their way themselves; and I've chosen to be a living example of being honest toward myself and living my dreams. The results speak for themselves. I have wonderful children, who are self-responsible and live their dreams.

I've had some female patients who've never gone on a vacation alone during their marriage and have always done everything with their partner for 25 years. After the treatment, their homework was to break this pattern and spend a few days alone. Suddenly, they're by themselves on vacation and discovering anew what *they* want to experience, where *they* want to go.

I had my most wonderful times in Paris alone, simply walking around where I felt like going, and discovering something magical at every turn. Without a "Where do you want to go now?" "What do you want to do now?" Conclusion?

Self-love

How can you truly love somebody if you can't love yourself?

This is more than looking at yourself naked in the mirror and finding yourself beautiful. It means being able to look at *everything* in your life and loving yourself for everything you've experienced.

It's the ability to be enough for yourself. It's about being able to be alone and experience this as enriching, filled with abundance.

The basic prerequisite is having your own identity, followed by clearing old energetic charges, including those left behind from the injuries and traumas of life, and being connected to the Source.

I've seen many people who use others, even their grandchildren, as love objects because they can't stand themselves.

What hasn't been lived out

I asked one patient to do some homework that involved hanging up a big sheet of paper in the hallway at home with one column for each partner. There, she was to write down everything she still wanted to experience and hadn't lived out yet. And her husband could fill out his column. Since she couldn't discuss this with her husband directly, this approach offered her a way to express her wishes and see those of her partner without a "Yes, but …" in the conversation.

What is kept secret

"For four years, there has been someone but nobody knows about it …"

Nothing eats up more energy than keeping a secret.

In our workshops, we often go around the group, with everyone completing the sentence: "Something I've never told anybody is that …"

Everyone says something when they feel like sharing it, and they all find healing. Theft, fraud, "abnormal" sexual practices, lies—everyone shares something kept secret so far with the others. The details shared aren't important; what matters is how an energy is freed that has been locked for years by talking about it, how everyone feels better afterward, and how the power of the secret is broken.

Ex-partners

In relationships, partners create many different kinds of connections and links between each other. Such links remain on an energetic level even if the couple officially separated years ago.
Their shared love field remains.
Here, it can do wonders to apply the healing breath.

Partner

- Is there something unresolved?
- Are the partners in the midst of a process?
- Do you still love him/her?

Friends

This and that person is my friend, and I can trust him/her.
Let the client draw up a list and test for him- or herself.
With friends, it's the same as with anybody else—we don't really help them when we "help" carry their load.

Siblings

This can be the sibling(s) the client knows, but it can also be siblings the client isn't familiar with. Twins, of whom one didn't make it into life; children who were lost; children who weren't supposed to come in; additional children of the same biological father; or children the father is reminded of only once a month via his bank account statement or he never knew about.

Children

If the topic or issue doesn't become apparent by itself, it always helps to make an intuitive drawing, an Imago, showing the family. Who is located where in the picture? What does the whole picture look like?

Open agreements

In recent years, I always knew that I still had open soul contracts with children. And these children also came in. But this topic involves more: All kinds of open soul contracts that we've created for this life and that still want to be lived out, and experiences that our soul still wants to have in order to grow and gain insight. It's futile to run away from these experiences.

However, open agreements aren't laws; they can be changed. If the necessary experiences have been integrated in a different way, open agreements can change. It doesn't matter to realization and insight when or how you gain it.

When testing something for the future, we can always just say:
"If everything stays as it is now, this or that is likely to happen." If, however, people change something, if they decide to change direction when at a crossroads, the future also changes.
Although we can test what could happen in the future, this is only the vision of the future we can see if we keep going straight on the same path.

When working with couples hoping to conceive, the topic of open agreements is significant. Is there actually a contract with a new soul?
Do both partners have a contract with this soul?
There are many cases where only one partner had a contract with the new soul at the beginning of the *innerwise* treatment; by working together and resolving issues, subsequently both partners had the contract. Usually, the couples were prospective parents two weeks later.
Based on these experiences with the variability of the future, we can only say: "If nothing changes, this or that could happen." Any other predictions about the future, saying: "This or that will happen" are dubious and highly manipulative.

Parents

Have you already liberated yourself from the life and value-related patterns of your parents?
Were you wanted by both parents?
Do your parents love you as an image of the love they once used to share? Are you the museum piece of this past love? Or do they love you for who you are?
With your place in your ancestral line, do you simply continue carrying the burden of your parents, grandparents and all your ancestors? All the unresolved traumas they've passed on to their children?
Do you feel responsible for your parents?

 Close your eyes and imagine that you're standing in a room together with your parents. How tall are the individual people in this image?
Are you at eye level with your parents? Or are you shorter or taller than they are?
Being at eye level means being on par; being shorter or smaller reflects paternalism if you're already an adult; and being taller or bigger means that you've assumed responsibility for them.

Ancestors

Often they're long gone yet still present. We carry about 10 percent of all irritations, disorders or problems for our ancestors.

The rape of the grandmother during the World War II, causing menstrual pain in the grandchild; the fratricide that occurred seven generations ago, appearing as a face eczema; or the expulsion from the great-great-grandfather's homeland, showing up in the great-great-grandson's difficulties in learning the language … all these are examples of problems caused by the ancestral line that I experienced working with certain patients.

Since we can only resolve issues where they come from, we have to work with the ancestors.

Alternatively, we could "unhinge" the patient from the ancestral line.

However, this can only be a possible emergency solution if no other therapeutic way is possible *and* if we get a "yes" response to the test question whether we're allowed to do this, applying spherical vision as we ask.

Test Card 3   Searching for insight

Soul energy

What and how much of your soul is present? Test this in percents. What matters here is that we're clear on the comparative value.

What is 100 percent? When did we ever reach this level?

Hardly at our conception, as the soul has already experienced separation from the ONE at that time, and taken on energetic charges. The farther we go back in the creation process of an individual soul, the more complete it will be.

As a 100 percent value, I suggest the moment of the first separation from the Source, the ONE. It's the first moment when the soul comes into Being, and the moment with the lowest level of charges. It's the moment of the soul's birth.

Using this comparative value reveals frustrating test results: frequently, only 1 to 5 percent of the original soul is in the here and now.

However, also comparing the soul's state with its state at the moment of conception or at birth shows that often only very little is left.

Naturally, the goal is to attain 100 percent even if this is hardly reachable. Any increase in the level of soul energy is a huge success.

Structurizing energy

This is the energy that creates structure and maintains its form.

The higher it is, the better.

Below 10 percent, the body turns into a "pile of cells," and only food doping can provide the required energy.

10 to 20 percent: Aging still progresses rapidly, but the body is no longer falling apart to that extent.

20 to 30 percent: First spring feelings awaken. Inner form and bearing attain a better state.

30 to 40 percent: The feelings of rejuvenation start to grow. A new sensation of freedom and ease sets in.

Most people don't experience anything above this range.

The real fountain of youth begins at a level above 70 percent maintained on a permanent basis. Then the body is able to re-create defective structures anew.

We only experienced 100 percent once in life: when the ovum fused with the sperm.

Life energy

This is the energy flowing in us, nourishing all organs, tissue, structures and functions.

It should be above 90 percent.

Life energy scale
100 percent: feels like flying, or like falling in love.
 80 percent: able to perform at full capacity, reaching your goals.
 70 percent: able to perform at normal capacity, but used to be better.
 50 percent: hanging in there, but it's no fun anymore.
 40 percent: able to perform for four to six hours.
 30 percent: exhausted after two hours of work; prone to tears.
 25 percent: severe exhaustion; nothing matters anymore.
 20 percent: the battery is empty.

I often ask my patients how high their level of life energy is, ranging between zero and 100 percent, and then test it. And then I always ask them: "And what about the energy that is missing? What did you do with it?"

Creative energy
This is the creativity flowing through us.
It should also be as high as possible, especially for people who make a living based on their creativity.
A level below 30 percent is too low for anybody.

Heart/love energy
This refers to our ability to love and to experience love. Love energy arises when we live our life purpose and radiate love.

Heart energy scale
 0–3 percent: risk of a heart attack
 4–30 percent: able to perform at a low capacity; person has a "small" heart
30–60 percent: the "normal" state
60–100 percent: a healthy, strong and loving heart; a golden heart

Accepting my life purpose
Yes, it exists for everyone. And we all have our own life purpose. And all human beings can live it, as otherwise it would be meaningless for them to exist, after all.

Basic charges that are brought along
These are all energetic charges that we already bring into this incarnation, no matter whether we believe in past lives, karma or the divine stockpot.
They enable us to gain special experiences and ensure that we can have them during this lifetime.

I've refrained from using the term "karma" here, because for me, it isn't neutral enough and is associated with too many judgments and limitations.

Finding my soul purpose

Remember: On the clearing of life, take a machete and clear your own way into the jungle. It's predetermined but hasn't been used yet.
Don't follow the beaten track of others, but summon up the courage to take off into the unknown.

Embracing my soul purpose

Walking this path and co-creating it as you go along also means no longer being able to follow other paths. It requires the decision to walk one's own path, whatever this means in life.

Living my soul purpose

This means to trust, to let yourself be guided, to be nourished energetically and to find your own fulfillment and insights. And to withstand the temptations that tout an often seemingly easier path, offer shortcuts and promise "instant enlightenments."

The path of realization and insight

It's the path of self-responsibility, the path of one's own life and soul purpose, the path of love and a path free of manipulation. It's a path that we can only follow to the end if we live our life and soul purpose, the quintessence, at a rate of 100 percent.

Walking my own path

Is the path you're following *your* path? Do you have the courage to pursue it even if everyone else follows a different path? It doesn't matter how stony or uncomfortable your path seems to you; the only thing that matters is that you learn your lessons as you go along, and continue walking. Because this is the only path leading you to the Light.

The temptation of power

This results from following the path of others and taking the beaten track, and thus, not being nourished by the divine source. Then, the only way to obtain the necessary energy is to steal energy from others—energy vampirism.
And this involves using all possible methods of manipulation—from playing the victim to black magic.
Anyone following this path turns energetically dark all the way to black. Such

people have to turn into energy vampires to satisfy their need for energy, thus opening all the gateways to dark and manipulative energies.

Following the path of others

It looks easier to choose these paths because they're comfortable—those are beaten tracks, free of stumbling blocks and not as lonely. But they don't lead anywhere. We always stay small, unfulfilled; we keep hoping for something better, and with time, we lose our strength and vitality.

When will you finally grow up and start living?

Test Card 4   Mine, yours, ours

I like to bear the burden for others, then I'm worth something

Most people think they're only worth something or will be loved when they're there for other people and help them carry their life's load.

About 95 percent of all people find fulfillment in shouldering other people's burdens.

The problem is that we cannot help anybody by easing their load.

We only reduce the need for change. And these people can simply continue a life where they created this burden themselves.

In my book *A Course in Healing,* the symptom says:

"You think I am 'THE ILLNESS.' Nonsense. Do you know what THE ILLNESS really is? It's you and your way of life."

The cause for taking on a burden is the search for love.

If we're not loved for who we are, then at least we should be loved for what we do for other people.

The caretaker

I once had a client with a bicycle company. He'd produced a T-shirt for all his employees saying: *I take care of others.*

I know many people who'd like to wear such a T-shirt:

those who haven't found themselves, who don't know or live their own life purpose, or who try to define themselves through other people and see their purpose in that.

I'm not a caretaker; instead, I try to inspire others by the way I live.

Shaped values

Don't dig in your nose; sex only after marriage; you have to honor and respect your parents no matter what they do; the children in Africa are starving, so eat the food on your plate.

Value are behavioral rules, needed by people who didn't develop a feeling of humbleness, self-worth, respect and love themselves. They're for people who don't live their life purpose and would act like hyenas if they could do what they really wanted to do.

Values were and are also created to control people and to be able to keep them attached more easily.

Thus, value systems are external support structures for amoebae, a structure for people who don't have any. Detaching from and clearing up such values is only possible if our inner support structure takes over their function. Only then can values be released easily.

The value systems of fanatical religious systems and sects are the most difficult to clear, because they were installed with control and inferiority-based programs.

Beliefs

Well, whose beliefs are we talking about here? Clients' beliefs, or beliefs they have taken over through education or otherwise?

"I'm not good enough. I'm not lovable. In our family, nobody has ever turned out well. The teacher knows it better. You have to stay in the relationship for the sake of the children, although love has died."

At this point in a treatment, it's important to identify the key beliefs by testing them, even if this requires some work, so that they can be targeted and cleared.

Accepted rules

"My intuition is telling me something else, but I trust you'll be right." Or, "Subordinating yourself and conforming makes life easier."

However, we pay a high price every time we betray ourselves.

Here, questioning our own thoughts and behaviors are called for. And it's even better to go on a trip around the world and get to know other cultures, broadening one's horizon.

I've already sent many patients out into the world as a form of therapy. Three months in India, six months working for *SOS Children's Villages* in Central America, one year at a high school in Sweden, harvesting olives in Italy, the St. James Way in Spain, etc. Personally, I don't see the need for rules, and enjoy breaking those that don't make any sense. How is it possible to develop something new when one is anxiously trying to abide by all the rules?

Education and parenting

There's nothing more absurd and destructive than educating children. This only forces on the kids the sick value system of the previous generation—a generation that passes this world to its children in a state worse than it received it in. What the heck! What a scam!

Children want to discover, gain experiences, eat with their fingers, pee on trees … just one thing they *don't* want is to be drilled and trained.

We can only love them and serve as an example—that's all.

And those who try educating them will get an intense puberty as a thank-you in return, which is nothing else but an outcry: "I find your lies and your dishonest life sickening. I never want to become like that!" But isn't this great? An outcry is so much better than ten years of psychotherapy! And after that, young people have the chance to find out for the first time what they really want. Then, one can only hope that they've experienced living examples of that; otherwise, this would often be not only the first but also the last chance to do so.

What I inherited

Grandma's jewelry, Dad's inferiority complex, the big family secret from Mother's line, or the trauma of an aborted older sister. It's not millions in a bank account that cause stress, but the blood they're still stained with.

With this topic, it's always good to radically clear out one's home. What people don't love or need doesn't belong there anymore. Afterward, it's usually easier for them to sort out their lives.

Issues from my partner

There are hardly any couples where the partners don't take over issues from each other.

As the energy fields mix and overlap, as issues are created together and as partners feel responsible for one another, a mixed field, a mixed reality and a mixed life are being created—basically, a huge entanglement that is very difficult to clear up.

When both partners come for a couple's treatment and lie on two massage tables next to each other, it's fascinating to see how work done with one partner leads to changes in the other.

Since we can always resolve issues only at their source, we have to test whose issue it is, and then work on it at its source. Just working on an issue with the partner who "helps" to carry it is useless, as the issue will come back immediately.

When an issue already returns during the treatment or shortly afterward, we haven't addressed the root of the problem.

Issues from ex-partners

Frequently, entanglements with ex-partners aren't unraveled. The old mixed fields still exist, and ex-partners remain present in the new relationship.

Testing represents the easiest diagnostic way to find out when an issue originated or was taken over. In most cases, this quickly reveals the source, except when people have had lots of sexual contacts.

If the partner had several partners before, the field is often like a chaotic ball of wool with threads in different colors, and requires in-depth work to be cleared so that the partner can be free again and is able to experience new love in a deep way.

Issues from the parents

Many people would rather do without social heredity. We learned our parents' pain bodies and their unresolved issues in early childhood, often when we were still in our mother's womb. In addition, we're marked by the values shaped by our family and by our experiences with parents who didn't have integrity.

When parents don't act like responsible adults due to low social maturity, and, as a result, children try to take over this role at an early age, they adopt their parents in a way and also feel co-responsible for their unresolved issues.

When children come to me for a treatment, the rule is that I first work with the parents. Then, treating the children is often no longer necessary.

The child can be in a state of rigidity and show symptoms. Once the parents receive healing cards, the rigidity and symptoms of the child disappear in 90 percent of all cases by themselves. Then, only the damage that occurred in the child as a consequence needs to be balanced.

Working with a child, although the parents are responsible for the problems, is therapeutic abuse.

Issues from the children

The other way around, overly concerned parents want to protect their children from life and the experiences it can bring, and would rather shoulder an issue themselves. Or, they feel guilty, so by taking over their child's issues, they solicit indulgence for having hurt him or her at some point.

Issues from friends

"I would do anything for you so that you feel better." Would you also die for that?

It's not a sign of friendship to "help" carry a friend's affliction; rather, it means you're mutually using one another.

It could also be the case that people with manipulative intentions distribute their burdens onto other people in order to get some breathing space and energy.

In such a scenario, one can work on the person's willingness to carry issues for other people on the one hand; and on the other, one can draw healing cards for the soul of the other person involved, if it's allowed, and give them as a present without any intention.

Issues from ancestors

The grandmother experienced terrible things during the war and lost her children and husband. This burden was passed on from mother to daughter within the family, and the great-granddaughter comes to see a therapist for ovarian cysts. If the cysts are the expression of the great-grandmother's unresolved charges, they cannot be treated in the great-granddaughter.

In that case, we work on the great-grandmother. We're choosing the necessary healing cards with the help of the testing system, and the great-granddaughter gives them virtually to her mother so that she can pass them on to her mother until they've arrived at the great-grandmother.

If the great-grandmother accepts them, and frequently clients see or perceive this, the issue is often resolved for the great-granddaughter, or may need only a little additional therapeutic support.

In energy therapy, time and space no longer represent any limits.

Issues created through manipulation

Often intricate and intertwined field and control systems are built to manipulate people, keeping the manipulated person caught in the net.

Few people are able to be free from manipulation in their communication.

Many use subliminal blackmailing and reproaches aimed at inducing guilt in order to create dependencies. Grandma sending $50 in her birthday letter to the grandchild, accompanied by a note saying: "It's unfortunate that you're living so far away, as I can only see you so little" is very unfair vis-à-vis the child, as it induces a feeling of guilt since "poor" Grandma has to suffer. In such a case, it would be better to send the money back with a note saying that gifts will only be accepted again once they're given without intention.

Issues of the building, of the location/site

Buildings and locations or sites also have a soul, just like people. And they're able to store energies and fields.

Thus, people enter a kind of sound field that influences them on a permanent basis. For some time, it's possible to resist it, to meditate a lot and take good care of oneself; but in the end, the field always wins as it continues to manifest its effects—also via the partner or the kids who may not be so disciplined in ensuring the clarity of the field.

That's why it's important to first sense the building and location or site, and to imagine living there for a few years before signing the rental or purchase agreement.

We can work therapeutically on buildings, gardens and locations or sites. If this doesn't suffice, however, moving can also be a therapeutic intervention that makes sense. When my older son used *innerwise* with a client in New Zealand and diagnosed stress in this woman's sleeping area, she replied: "Well, then, I'll sell my house." It's wonderful how easy life can be. In Europe, we would hardly experience such a reaction.

Irritations in buildings and locations or sites aren't caused only by geopathic stress. electrosmog or chemical contamination; above all, they stem from unhealed traumas that happened there, even if it occurred a long time ago.

Who wants to sleep on a battlefield of the Thirty Years' War and be visited at night by the souls of those who were killed there?

Issues of the region, of the country

Europeans no longer notice the heaviness weighing on Europe as a result of World War I and II; just like we hardly feel a backpack anymore after a day or two if we carry it all the time. We feel this heaviness only when coming to Europe from another continent.

Therefore, it's important to travel a lot in order to learn to identify irritations and find a place where we feel really good.

Issues of the language, of the culture

When we ask clients to utter words in different languages, we can determine very quickly which language is associated with stress.

For 13 years, I had to try to learn Russian, which didn't appeal to me. What an ordeal! This language still causes stress in me, and I refuse to speak it. Yet, I also don't feel I want to work on this issue. Everything may be resolved at the right time; we neither have to, nor must we force it, when it's not yet the right time.

Often we can identify the cause of the stress, and once more, testing the point in time when it originated helps us most.

Issues of systems, of organizations

When we consider ourselves to be part of a system, such as a company or organization, we're subject to the effects of this company/organization's field. This can be a very positive thing when this system is characterized by clarity, honesty and integrity.

But it can also be hell where it seems as if we're caught between a rock and a hard place due to the fact that it's our job.

We can also work with systems and companies or organizations, but only when those in charge of certain areas have given us permission to do so.

If employees are unhappy with their salary and don't like their boss, we're not allowed to energetically tinker with the system. Those who still do so as therapists or coaches will be given the opportunity to experience that boundaries aren't trespassed for manipulative purposes without consequences. This will always come back to the therapist or coach.

If, however, those in charge have given their permission, it's possible to energetically coach the entire system using *innerwise*, effecting change in many areas.

Issues of religious orientations

Every religion has an inner circle, a magical form of teaching, which deals with the energy fields and the resulting opportunities to exert influence. This knowledge can be used in positive ways, but has been and still is used to manipulate and retain power. Structures with a sectarian organization profile are particularly problematic. The members take on a subordinate role and everyone is subject to the energetic structures. The rules provide support, and the energetic structures milk the flock.

It's also possible that the energetic structures were installed centuries ago when the religion was established—as is typically the case with certain initiation mantras—and that today's users aren't aware of that anymore.

Yet, these energetic structures still impact everyone and everything involved, as time and space have little significance for energies. And just because we can't or don't want to see them, we're not protected from them.

From my experience, it's almost impossible to free people from the influence of these energies, as long as they still feel the need for the religion's support. This is because such people are ready to do almost anything for this external structural support that seems to lend meaning and purpose to their lives.

Political ideas

When analyzing the energetic constellations of dictatorial systems, we can find that in the case of Nazi Germany as well, high magic was applied.

Today it's more the news that is being manipulated—something you can easily identify using your gut feelings and the arm-length test.

Test Card 5   Homework

My list of compromises

Write down a list of all compromises you're making. Over the next few weeks and months, it will be your job to put an end to each of them, one after the other. If a couple isn't able to talk about them, it makes sense to add a column for each partner on this list and hang it up in the hallway.

Cleaning up my home

How often do we behave like museum managers in our own home: "I can't throw that out! When Mom comes to visit, Grandma's chest of drawers has to be here; otherwise, she will be very sad."
"This could still be useful someday."
For most people, it's easier to clean up and sort out their environment first—one room a day or a week until it's all cleaned up—and to take care of their lives next. Usually, you'll find that this step is no longer that big.

Cleaning up my life

Just like you did for your home, put an end to the chaos in your life. Draw it as an Imago, get an overview, sort things anew and put an end to things.
Create some breathing space for yourself and the room to once again focus on what's essential.

Letting go of everything that I don't love

Whether it's books that fill up your shelves for their mere value or only as a souvenir, or your job that's secure and pays well but no longer fills you with love, or whether habit is all that's left in what connects you with your partner ... whatever it is—life is too short to hold on to something you don't love anymore.
And this applies to everything in life: put an end to *everything* you don't love.
"But I can't do that! I have to keep hanging in there ..."
Okay, then keep suffering; after all, it's not *my* life.
A therapist is only responsible for him- or herself!
And here as well, it helps to make a list with three columns:
I love/I hate/I don't care
The rest is the patient's or client's responsibility.
What a therapist can show a client, however, is how it feels when things are sorted out in life and what changes as a result.
"Imagine you've cleaned up and changed this or that. How does your body feel now? How's your energy?"

Or to show clients with the arm-length test what influence unloved life aspects have on them.

"How does your heart feel when you separate from your partner, as you've been wanting to do for the past seven years?"

"What happens with your headache when you change jobs?"

Testing food and drinks

You should test food products before you purchase them, not just once they're bought and stored in the fridge. The same goes for restaurants. Testing food makes people responsible for their lives in a very simple way.

If someone is allergic to a certain product yet keeps consuming it, it makes sense to interrupt the treatment and tie its continuation to the condition that the person refrains from consuming it.

The most common food allergies are related to milk protein, chicken protein and wheat.

Next on the list are colorants, preservatives and sugar substitutes, followed by coffee, tea and chocolate based on the highly toxic alkaloids contained therein that also alter the odor of perspiration.

I've also sent patients back home and told them that they could come back once they stop drinking alcohol, coffee and soda for three months; and instead, drink only water.

A therapist's job is to provide clean testing of food and drinks, and then to place the responsibility entirely in the patient's hands.

The bucket list and joy-of-life list

The idea for this homework assignment came from the movie *The Bucket List* featuring Jack Nicholson and Morgan Freeman. Two men with cancer create a list of what they still want to experience before they die—that is, kick the bucket. They live out their bucket list, thus prolonging their lives.

"Imagine you have three months left to live. What would you still like to experience?"

And now, transform your bucket list into your joy-of-life list so that you don't have to die and still experience it.

Expressing creativity

Do something creative, such as painting, dancing, singing, making music, etc., and do it once a day.

Let creativity flow through you.

Do it only for yourself. Don't show it to anybody. Enjoy yourself, without judgment.

Engaging in something unknown

Do what you're most afraid of, because it's there that the greatest gift is waiting for you.

Physical activities

Cutting wood, digging in the garden, dancing, running, sex—enjoy your body in full action. Feel each cell again. Use your body for what it's made for.

Singing

You might try singing in the car at first, then at home, and then even on the street.

Here, it helps if the therapist tests the scale and analyzes each tone that is blocked—determining when the blockage first occurred and what issue is behind it—and then clears those blockages. This makes it possible to sing again, and to rediscover the beauty of one's voice.

Dancing freely

Dance. Simply dance your Self. Dance as freely as you do when you sing alone in the car. Forget all rules, steps or patterns. Let the music move you.

Resolving my list of lies

This is first about creating your list of lies and then summoning up the courage to put an end to these lies.

"I have to tell you something …"

Each lie that people put an end to, relieves them from a burden.

Nothing consumes more energy than a suppressed secret or a lie that shouldn't come to light. Some people use up more than 60 percent of their life energy for such a purpose.

Using the arm-length test in my daily life

At the supermarket, in the restaurant, at work or when standing in front of our closet … we have to make decisions all the time.

Color breathing

Like sounds, colors are frequency patterns.

 Close your eyes and imagine that you're standing in the middle of a round room. The walls consist of the entire spectrum of colors. Turn to the color that makes you feel good; then, go through the wall into that color and breathe it until you feel saturated.

Now step back into the middle of the room. You can breathe other colors as needed.

Grounding exercises

Earthing, or grounding, is essential for human beings. We're made from Mother Earth, we're a part of her, but we often forget about that. Put your hands in the earth, dance barefoot through puddles, or run barefoot as much as possible. I also like to dig deep holes in the ground at times until there's hardly anything left to see of me anymore.

Grounding is cleansing, rootedness and clearing up things—all at the same time. And if you're in the city, a flower pot might also do in a pinch. In the forest, you can hug trees and imagine that you merge with them, becoming their roots and also their crowns.

Drinking water

Our bodies are often poisoned by coffee, tea, sweeteners, alcohol, etc., and the only thing that helps is drinking a lot of still water.

Water is a dilution and detox agent, and the only beverage that can quench thirst. Whether you wish to drink good-quality tap water, filtered water, alkaline water or spring water depends on your budget and taste. It shouldn't be carbonated water, as this is too acidic.

Water can also be energized and vitalized, even just by blessing it with our hands.

Deacidification

When legs get swollen due to water retention there, it's high time to deacidify the body. It has to maintain an optimal pH level in the blood so that enzymes and hormones keep functioning.

When the excretory organs such as the kidneys, liver, intestines, lungs and skin no longer manage to deal with the flood of acids, the body has only one way out in order not to die: move the acids to the tissue. Due to the concentration gradient and to prevent them from "corroding" the tissue, they're diluted with water. And this is why water is retained in the legs. But water is also retained in the arms.

Squeezing the skin firmly between your thumb and index finger shouldn't hurt. If it does, the tissue is sour. Also, the tissue should be thin and not a big swollen bulge. Acids almost always stem from food products: acid-producing meat, sugar that is decomposed to acid, acidic beverages such as coffee, tea or sparkling water—all of these are significant sources.
The second major source are allergic reactions to foods, as massive amounts of acids are produced in the body in their course.
And the third cause is when we've gone sour on life.

The best deacidification method is to eat less (when you have no more gas, you know you're eating exactly the quantity that your body can process), to drink lots of water, and to take alkaline baths and products.
Deacidification is essential for the successful therapy of many forms of physical discomfort or ailments.

Smiling at the person in the mirror in the morning
That person will smile back.

Looking at myself naked in the mirror
Love yourself; love your body the way it is. This also includes the chubby or bony parts. Caress your body and give it love. Stop hating and fighting it.
People who love their body no matter what their weight is, radiate beauty.
It doesn't matter how you look; the only thing that counts is how you *feel*.

Test Card 6   The Self

I am I

Who else if not me?

Whose life am I living if I'm not myself?

This is the key question in all treatments. I always ask it openly and out loud to enable the patient to become aware of it.

If the identity isn't clear, we as therapists don't even know who's actually answering us. Which of the identities?

I love my name

If saying one's name causes stress to somebody in the arm-length test, there are two possibilities:

1. One's own identity is not present.

2. There's a negative charge on one or more letters of the name.

A boy showed an allergic/panic reaction with the arm-length test when uttering his name (Max). The reaction was a response to the letter A, caused by a trauma seven years before. After clearing the charge of the old trauma, he no longer experienced stress with his name.

It's important to test all names.

Even if a name has been changed to a spiritual name, for instance, it's necessary to clear the stress with the person's original name(s). We can't run away from that in life.

I am happy

This is about being happy not just for one moment, but as a state that doesn't require a protected space, getting drunk or other special circumstances, and which can be reached and experienced time and again in daily life.

I am good

Although neither our parents, teachers nor ex-partners said it, I know I am good. I'm even the best for *me*.

I trust

I trust myself, life and all experiences I encounter.

Trust also means giving up any form of control and accepting whatever comes along.

I live authentically and honestly

An innocent, "seeing" child can look into my eyes, soul and heart, and I don't need to hide anything.

This is the only way I can inspire people and touch their hearts.

I am open to the new

Otherwise, life will get boring. In eastern Germany, people already knew at the age of 20 what they were going to do until they were 65. Do you think this was exciting and created any real zest for life?

I let go of my compromises

Compromises are lies that you live in your life.

How much longer do you want to keep lying to yourself?

I love myself how I used to be

"I love everything I did in the past, and that which happened to and with me in my life." There are no mistakes, just learning tasks. When climbing a ladder, it's also useless and illogical to destroy each rung you've climbed, reviling it as a MISTAKE.

I love myself how I am

"I love myself how I am. Everything is right as it is and helps me grow."

I love myself how I will be

Everything else that I will still do in life, that I will decide to do or how I will be, is right. This also includes the wrinkles, gray hair, love handles, good-bye letters, new beginnings, etc.

I am ready and willing to change

I am ready to change EVERYTHING in order to live a healthy and happy life again. And this means EVERYTHING. No safety nets, no backup solutions, letting go of simply everything.

Would you also be ready to go to another country and leave your family, taking with you only what you're wearing and your inner capabilities, to start anew somewhere else?

I am responsible for my own life

Who else? Mom or Dad?

I love my female/male energies

Many people can still say this sentence without problems.
The male energies in the right half of the body and the left hemisphere of the brain represent logical, analytical and active qualities.
The female energies on the side of our heart and in the right hemisphere of the brain represent creative, nourishing, loving and intuitive qualities.
Every human being has both.

I love being a woman/man

Many people feel stress when making this statement, however. Suddenly, the old gender stereotypes come into play that have become so outdated—especially for men who have lost their moxie and have become disempowered. Then, they shouldn't be surprised if their partners become increasingly hard and masculine. Men and women living together requires a balance of both energies; if a man doesn't assume his part, the woman has to do it. And then, both are unhappy.
Men urgently need a men's movement to be able to clarify their role in life and re-assume it.

I love my sexuality

How should a nun or priest respond to that? Well, we don't have to be concerned about that. It's just that, unfortunately, religious institutions left their imprint on us for centuries, creating blockages in us in this respect. They turned sexuality into something dirty and obscene. "Only after marriage, and then only with one partner." All of these cases of abuse by priests have shown that this cannot be healthy.
A friend wrote me about his agreement with his wife. He told her: "I don't want you to have to forgo something because of me. I don't take responsibility for that." And he's right.

I love the state of ecstasy

Dance yourself into ecstasy, love yourself into ecstasy, live ecstasy. Because at some point, it will be too late, and then you can only say: "Gosh, if I had just … at the time." "If I just hadn't been so considerate of other people and had done what I really wanted to do."

I forgive myself and I am forgiven

Most people are still willing to forgive others. But when it's about forgiving themselves, they can't even utter the words.

With this statement, I've seen more people with their mouths open, not able to say a word, than with any other topic.

What are you waiting for? For the time after the atonement in hell's cauldron?

I love life and joy

What have you done today that justifies your saying this?

I am connected to the Source

Yes, but which source? When I was about to leave home for some time, a girl-friend told me that she would also go away, because then, life "was going to be so boring, no longer dramatic." I replied: "You need your drama, you love your drama."

So, I don't mean the source of the drama queen, but Creation manifesting through us.

I free myself from charges and patterns

Patterns offer support; they create a routine that provides structure to daily life.

Everybody does it this way.

Have the courage to be unique, to be different, to be yourself.

I don't live for others, nor do I expect others to live for me

This phrase is borrowed from Ayn Rand's book *Atlas Shrugged* in a slightly altered form. The original wording by character John Galt is: "I swear by my life and my love for it that I will never live for the sake of another man, nor ask another man to live for mine."

Long live self-responsibility!

Just like I'm not writing this book to please readers—I do so because I enjoy writing it.

When I had completed my doctoral dissertation after two years of practical research and it was ready for submission, I threw it in the trash.

In the end, I just wanted to find out something, understand it and prove it to myself—which I'd done. My theory was correct, and I had enjoyed proving it in a practical application study. I just didn't want to prove it to anybody else. And I certainly didn't want to receive patients in the future who would come to see me because of my doctoral title. I only wanted to work with people who would resonate with what I have to offer.

Nobody around me understood why I forsook my doctoral title, but that didn't, and still doesn't, matter to me.

All this sounds very egocentric. Yes, it is, because I love my *ego,* my Self—it is the most precious thing I have and the instrument through which divine creativity can unfold. If we give up the Self, if we deny it, then what is supposed to serve as an instrument for Creation?

Test Card 7   My life

I want to live

For people who have a serious, life-threatening illness, the arm-length test often reveals a "no" as the response of the unconscious to the statement "I want to live." And the opposite statement "I want to die" shows a "yes" response.

In such a constellation, therapy has no chance.

Here as well, the root of this rejection of life lies in the unconscious—an inner self-destruction program whose cause always varies depending on the person. Thus, there's no universal solution to transform this. It's the therapist's task to identify the cause in the timeline, and resolve it. In addition, there's resignation due to the exhaustion.

The lower the life energy, the smaller the will to live.

Betrayal of the heart

Usually, it doesn't happen often in life that we betray our heart, because when we do, we hurt ourselves really deeply. Some years ago, I heard the following saying: "You don't age with years but by betraying your heart." Betraying our love for ourselves and our life purpose is like a little suicide—a wound staying open that can't heal.

In a treatment, we go back to the time of the betrayal by testing the age when it occurred, and then work on the source of that issue.

Fear factor

This is a parameter that can be tested in percents. Many people live with a fear factor between 60 and 80 percent. This means that they give fear an equally high potential to manifest. This can only generate *more* fear and negative experiences in the future. Success requires a fear factor below 60 percent.

The more we manage to reduce the fear factor in a treatment, the easier and more beautiful life becomes. Whether we, as humans, will ever be able to reach and live a level of zero percent fear is a question I haven't been able to answer thus far. At that point, we'd probably be able to walk on water as well.

The fear factor is only partially fed by personal experience. The influence of local fears (such as those of earthquakes or war zones) and global fears (such as those of war, nuclear accidents or a 9/11-type incident) is equally large. This makes it difficult to reduce the fear factor in a personal treatment.

We could achieve the best results on that issue with the support of the *innerwise* symbol *Make Me An Instrument.*

My inner child

When was the last time you danced barefoot in a puddle, walked backward or simply laughed out loud? Our inner child is well hidden because it got whipped by all the education, seriousness and uptightness of our time. "One doesn't do that. That's not a proper thing to do. What will people think? You're embarrassing."

Take off your shoes and look for the next puddle—without giving yourself liquid courage but out of the pure zest for life. Be unreasonable, be foolish!

Social maturity

We can be 50 years old but behave like a 13-year-old. Many women complain that their partner's behavior is closer to that of their children. Then again, many children already behave like adults or need to because their parents don't.

The "social maturity" parameter is tested in years, and should more or less match the person's real age. It's an important parameter that helps to understand relationship and family constellations and assess a person's ability to take responsibility.

"I'm your fourth child," a man told his wife. "But one doesn't have sex with one's child," she replied, and left him.

Flight from reality

"I can't stand it here anymore."

Drugs and alcohol are the usual ways to flee reality. But fleeing into spiritual make-believe worlds, personality roles and social networks is also common practice.

Get sober and face life. The next steps are rolling up your sleeves and cleaning up.

Living in the here and now

The here and now arises with every single moment of our lives. It is free of everything that we carry with us from the past.

In the here and now, there are no illnesses, fears, lies or feelings of inferiority.

It just requires the courage to let go of all alleged habits and forms of security.

I am brave and strong

Broken people can't stand upright, fearful people can't be courageous, and powerless ones can't be strong.

Here as well, it's most effective to identify the cause and when it occurred, and treat it. If the problem is that of not having been a wanted child at one's conception, it's the situation of the conception that needs to be worked on. In this case, it may be that only the souls of the parents need some support.

I am being taken care of

There's always enough for me. I receive everything I need. This doesn't mean that I'll always live in luxury, but that I'm able to gain the experiences that are important for me. "I'm able to let go and trust."

Profession or calling

Do you do a job, do you have a profession or do you live your calling?
Do you love the work you do? Does it fulfill you, inspire you and encourage you?
Or did you resign from your job in all but name a long time ago? Are you behaving like a prostitute to get that paycheck at the end of the month? Do you believe you have to keep hanging in there due to certain commitments? Or, do you consider yourself unable to start something new?
Live your dreams. Do only what you enjoy doing.

I love my work

Whatever you do, do it with love. A meal prepared with love simply tastes better. Any time where you felt love is never wasted.

I accomplish my tasks with a high degree of quality

I identify with my work and take responsibility for the quality I deliver. I deliver a high degree of quality because I enjoy doing so.

I am competent in my area

I have experience, I have knowledge, I have good intuition, I'm good. I'm the right person in this position, and what I don't yet know how to do, I will learn.

I am worthy of being successful

"Money stinks." "Success arouses envy." "Success is a lonely road." "I don't deserve that. I'm not good enough for that. I'm not worth it."
Okay, so you're not successful. But then, don't complain.

I like to make decisions

There are no more mountains of unresolved issues in my life. I know what I want. Through my decisions, I keep bringing maximum clarity into my life.

Thank you for everything

Simply be grateful for everything. Because everything has had a meaning and purpose and has come at the right time.

Welcome, life, with all that you have to offer

I'm here on this Earth only once in this form, and I want to experience as much as possible.

Test Card 8   Manipulation

On the energetic level

Oaths

I swear …

You should think twice before saying this sentence silently or out loud. It's quickly forgotten but keeps having an impact, because you swore it.

And 15 years later, you're surprised about what life is presenting you.

Pacts

A friend used to live in Africa. There, it was common that you went to see the medicine man if you wanted to achieve something. In return, however, you had to give away what's most precious to you: your soul.

A typical pact is the fairy tale of the heart of stone. I give something from me, and in return, I get something else. As Goethe already described it impressively in *Faust,* pacts can determine your life.

Those who seek power in magic have to reckon with paying a high price for that. It's almost impossible to dissolve pacts from the outside. Only when people have nothing to lose anymore are they willing to give up the pact and the power associated with it. By that time, it's often too late.

Before that moment, therapists can't do it for those concerned, even if they see the pact and the people suffering. Therapists are also obliged to watch how such clients destroy themselves and their environment until they themselves are willing to dissolve the pact.

Initiations

In initiations, you're tied to one or more sources of energy. Here, it's not about the mental aspect, but about the underlying energetic component.

You allow the energy to unfold and work through you.

Therefore, the big question is:

What kind of energy is it? How clear and pure is it? Do you have to pay with anything to benefit from this energy?

In order to dissolve such ties, therapists should be familiar with, and have experience working with, magic energies and know which methods can be applied. They have to be able to recognize parallel worlds and move freely in time and space in their therapeutic work. The dimensions of Being according to Burkhard Heim are a good parameter for assessing one's capabilities.

Maledictions, curses

In Europe, rune magic is the strongest and most well known and can serve to cause substantial magic harm. In the past, rune magic was not only used in marriage wars but also in real wars. There's always great malignity behind doing that. The fair part is that in the end, this always falls back to the person who initiated it.

In addition to runes, there are many kinds of magic rituals that are applied in maledictions.

For dissolving maledictions and curses, it helps to test the words or symbols used.

Energetic ties

This is about any type of energetic tie even if we're not aware of it or can't feel it. Examples are sexually conditioned energetic ties.

Any energetic tie is characterized by an exchange of energy that can go both ways.

Implants

Implants are programs that were created through pain, rites, drugs, sex, NLP or other manipulations with a view to gain control over people. They can be found in the brain, heart, plexuses of the autonomic nervous system or sexual organs. They're like dormant computer viruses that only reveal themselves once activated.

On the spiritual level

Soul fragmentation and separation

In the course of very deep traumas, it often happens that soul fragments separate and then get lost in the dimensions of Being. Since they use escape tunnels, it's possible to identify those. "When in life did this happen to you?"

It's normal that soul fragments can withdraw. However, if they disappear from the soul space of the person concerned, there's partly manipulation involved.

Almost all people experience soul fragmentation and separation. With the support of the healing breath, it's possible to retrieve these fragments and reintegrate them.

The healing breath is described in the related section of test card 10.

Fissure in the soul field

The soul field is cut open, as if with a knife; thus, things can enter that don't belong there. But people can also lose something through such fissures. It's like bleeding, sometimes to the point of death.

Issues that penetrated are recognized as not belonging to that person. "Do you have cancer?" "No!"

"Do you feed cancer?" "Yes!"

These parts that penetrated are worked on as independent beings in the *innerwise* treatment, and the healing symphony is given through them to the source of the manipulation. We give the healing cards virtually to the cancer, for example, and ask it to pass the energies on to its source. We can't resolve the issue in the client him- or herself because it's not the client's own issue; rather he/she just feeds it.

A friend worked with Filipino spiritual healers who pulled the cancer out of her twice a day over three months—but the cancer kept coming back. They continually tried to cleanse the source in the background via the fissure, but it isn't possible to do so that way. As a result, the issue returned again and again, because it wasn't her cancer, even though it ate her up in the end.

After treating the energies that have intruded, you retrieve the lost soul fragments from the n-dimensional space using the healing breath and then close the fissure with *innerwise*.

Copies, duplicates

The classic model of this method is voodoo. A duplicate is created from the soul field, and then this duplicate is copied again a few times. When one or several of these copies are being manipulated, the person concerned can no longer differentiate these manipulations from his or her own issues.

And this is what makes this technique so dangerous. Also, it's not used as seldom as you might think.

People who are very sensitive will notice that they have more than one inner space, yet they can't tell which of them is their own, even if these spaces feel different and have different rhythms.

This is resolved by first picking healing cards to target the manipulation of the copies. Then, you draw healing cards to dissolve all copies and duplicates so that in the end, there's only one's own original soul field left.

There can also be more than one duplicate, and each of them has a large number of copies. Nevertheless, it's also fairly easy to dissolve that once it's identified.

Hydra

As described in Greek mythology, what's special about a hydra is that two heads will grow after one has been cut off. Therefore, this isn't the way to deal with it once and for all.

A hydra manipulation is like a mycelium that grows in a human being; it entered through an orifice of the body and can only be removed via that same orifice.

You may recall the worms in the movie "The Matrix" that crawled into the human beings via the navel, and which could only be removed again via this spot. Typical symptoms are "wandering" irritations that move around in the body, and a lack of inner stability.

You work with such a manipulation by removing it as a whole, using healing cards via the orifice through which it entered the body.

Energetic corrosion

In this case, the soul field develops holes. I first noticed this in HIV patients. The "hull" of the soul field is corroded; there are holes everywhere.

This is comparable to a breakdown of the soul's immune system. Here, you cleanse the person's soul space with *innerwise*, close the holes and rebuild the "hull."

Cancer

Something foreign grows in you and destroys life at an unabated pace.

This is unnatural, against the principles of life, thus fulfilling all conditions of a manipulation.

Once you also consider cancer from this perspective, additional therapeutic approaches open up that differ from the usual ones.

Nebula around the soul field

Being smothered by a gray, sticky fog that blocks your connection to the Source, thus causing a lack of orientation—is a typical demonic technique that is nasty and very malicious.

The typical signs are a loss of both clarity and one's connection to the Source.

Treating this type of manipulation requires a considerable amount of experience in energy work, and it's always appropriate to seek the help of other therapists in such a case.

Inner darkness

The nebula managed to penetrate the being and eat up all the light.

This is the most malicious manipulation that I've ever experienced. As long as there's a little bit of light left, the treatment still offers a chance. It's like in *The Neverending Story* where the Nothing destroys everything, and where Bastian Balthazar re-creates everything out of a tiny remainder within himself at the end of the story.

Light channel manipulation

This manipulation can be applied at two different times:

1. People's channel to the Source is tapped during their lifetime, and some of their light is stolen.
2. The light channel opening up after people's death is abused to tap energy directly from the Source. For the soul of the deceased, this can mean remaining stuck in the intermediary world and not finding redemption.

For all soul manipulations, the question remains: Who uses it and why? Who benefits from it? How sick do people's minds have to be to do something like this with others?

Nevertheless, it seems that there are plenty of them, because we keep finding such manipulations in treatments on a regular basis.

As long as people kill one another in wars, we'll also have to face and deal with the issue of energetic wars.

Alternatively, we could consider the existence of autonomous energy qualities that play a role here.

Cloning

This can apply to an entire human being or only to individual organs. The original is replaced with a clone, the only difference is a colder aura—the warmth of the heart is missing. The interesting questions are: Where is the original, and what's happening with it?

Laser vision

Similar to hypnosis, forced eye contact is used to manipulate people in a very complex way. The eyes are chosen consciously, as they offer access to the soul. These are very sophisticated and sneaky forms of manipulation, involving complex spaces; the manipulations are mirrored, and the source is hard to identify and locate—very tricky. The eyes set on fire what is supposed to burn, and they burn everything that's in the way.

Field disintegration

Existing fields simply disintegrate. This is used to delete the energetic foundation of reality, to erase it as if it had never existed.

On the mental level

Cerebrum
Manipulation in the cerebrum caused by implants, programming, drugs and targeted blockages of brain circuits.

Nuclei, midbrain and cerebellum
Manipulation caused by implants, programming, remote controlling, drugs or electromagnetic irritations in areas of the brain involved in fine-tuning.

Brainstem
Manipulation in the brain areas in charge of survival, caused by implants, initiations or sexual manipulation.

Thought field
The underlying idea is that our thoughts and memories aren't stored in cranial nerve circuits, but rather in an energy field surrounding us, and that this field can be manipulated using frequencies, for instance. It's known that experiments have been made using magnetic fields to delete mental content.
Among others, a thought field can be affected by the following manipulations: electromagnetic deletions, programming, remote controlling, morphogenetic fields or fields of fear.

Thought content
Turn on the TV, read a newspaper or visit a school, and you know what I'm talking about.

On the physical level

Through: drugs, toxins, chastisements, injuries

On the unconscious level

Dreamtime manipulation

By day, you're the master of your senses, but by night, topics and energies appear in your dreams that you can't relate to even with the best intentions, yet they influence your behavior during the day. The movie *Inception* (2010) clearly describes the manipulation of conscious decisions through intrusions into someone's dreamtime.

Frequency-based manipulations

Radionic remote broadcasting, Scientology frequency patterns on bioresonance devices, ELF wave manipulation or other gimmicks—their goal resembles that of a microwave: to turn you around inside and cook you until you're done. And like a microwave, it will kill what's alive in you.

Drive and sexual coding

These are patterns created through sexuality and various sexual practices. In his book *Eleven Minutes,* Paulo Coelho describes how lust is linked with pain in a prostitute—a typical example. But this also includes bondage games, using a whip, whipping the genitals as self-punishment, and everything else that belongs to that category.

Basically, it includes everything related to sexuality that makes use of people's lack of willpower when they're driven by their sex drive.

Neediness, dependency, addiction, deprivation, fear and fragmentation

On the emotional level

Through: anger, rage, aggression, greed, stinginess, jealousy, deceit, lies, victimhood and fear

Test Card 9   Dimensions of Being according to Burkhard Heim

This test card is the most difficult to describe. These dimensions are also the degrees of freedom of existence, of our Being.

The 12 dimensions described by Burkhard Heim are based on complex mathematical formulas, whose logical understanding considerably exceeds my knowledge. Yet, I can *experience* these dimensions; I can perceive them as spaces with different qualities. Thus, I can move within these dimensions and give people the opportunity to experience them in a guided meditation.

Based on my experience of working with rigidities, I took the liberty of adding the *point* as a complementary zeroth dimension: rigidity.

Point

Imagine you're caught in a steel sphere—cast in metal, unable to move. All your rhythms have ceased. You're no longer able to communicate. What people can see from the outside is not what's hidden in the steel sphere. You're caught in a state of total rigidity, unable to free yourself.

Length

Free of the steel sphere, you're now a point on a plane. You're only free to move from the point where you are to another point on the plane. You are neither free to take a turn nor to determine the speed of motion. You're caught in the ink that becomes a line with the help of a ruler.

Width

The second great liberation: you can now leave the line on the sheet of paper and change direction at any time to reach another point. You can even turn or move in wiggly lines, but you cannot leave the paper. You're still stuck there.

As a human being in a car, you'd be bound to the road, but could already take an exit to relieve yourself rather than having to pee in your pants like you had to in the previous dimension.

Height

You get wings! Your car turns into a fly-drive vehicle. You can drive or choose to fly. Time is still linear for you, and you have no power over it. But what freedom! You can now move in three dimensions.

Time T

Back to the future, forward to the past. Time has become relative, as you can now move within this dimension. Also, time is no longer linear for you; seconds are not necessarily equally long. You're like Salvador Dalí's melting clock. Yet, this also means you lose more footing. What is still valid? What is still law? What rules can you still hold on to? If you now have no inner structure to support you, if you don't feel connected to the Source, you can lose yourself.

On the other hand, you can also see how events interconnect through time. What happens today does not necessarily refer to yesterday; it can also originate in the long-distant past or in the future.

After all, it's a misconception that only the past affects the present; the future does so as well. The time for discrimination against the future for not creating reality is over. Equal rights for everyone!

Structure space S1

"Where am I?" appears to be the appropriate question for the fifth dimension. You can be here or there. You can sip your espresso in Rome while skiing in the Rockies and fending off souvenir vendors in Bali to finally relax in the sun.

But the Rockies can also be in Bali, and Rome can have a long sandy beach right beside the Colosseum with a perfect view of the far side of the Moon.

You're in the fifth dimension, and the time has come to say good-bye to old beliefs. Of course, this exceeds what humans can usually access without drugs. If you want to experience the Creator's realm of possibilities and how He/She sees the world, there are no more taboos. Science is simply the current state of ignorance.

Structure space S2

If Bali, Rome and the Rockies are not separate locations but all in that one place where everything exists simultaneously, then all those people you don't like are there, too. It's no longer possible to run away and hide.

Everything can be in one place, but it doesn't have to be. You could suddenly face seven generations of your ancestors when you walk around the next corner.

Or would you prefer to bump into the people you might have an affair with in the future?

With a single bold movement of your hand you can now ask: "What is time anyway?" And with the other hand: "What is space anyway?" At this point you are no longer socially acceptable.

Information space I1

You move forward into the unknown, as you have nothing to lose anymore. If you've made it to here without ending up in a psychiatric clinic, nothing less than the Nobel Prize awaits you. But not even Burkhard Heim received this award, although he certainly deserved it.

In this dimension you begin to get a sense of how *innerwise* works. You get a feel for virtual information spaces in the field, for global information networks without technology, for the free composition of energetic flower bouquets.

Information space I2

Information takes on intelligence. You can almost smell God—that's how close you've come to Him/Her. Space comes alive; matter consists of sounds. You are filled with humility before Creation.

Hyperspace G1, Hyperspace G2, Hyperspace G3, Hyperspace G4

Burkhard Heim was either unable or unwilling to describe these spaces. Neither am I in a position to do so. Suffice it to say that here the dual dissolves into the nondual. As a dual being, you may take a peak through the Pearly Gates and glance at paradise before you actually die.

Anyone who has found access to these planes knows that only those who have also accessed them can understand these spaces. And then words become superfluous.

Test Card 10   Processes

Imago

The now

Describe your current situation in a picture, or draw it intuitively.

A specific age

Let's say you're 40 years old and you test that the Imago should take place at the age of 5.

 Imagine that you're five years old again. Close your eyes and describe the room of your family at that age.

It could also be the case, however, that you're a three-month-old fetus in your mother's womb, or a young teenager with pimples. The beautiful thing is that you'll always have inner images arising in you, no matter what age it is.

A situation

Your work situation, a decision, a project, a former relationship, a divorce, the decision to move … there are no limits.
For situations, I'd prefer the intuitive drawing method over a purely virtual image, as they're often very complex.

The rhythms

Our body is like an orchestra. All parts play different instruments, and only if they harmonize with one another, do we not need to cover our ears. Have a look at the orchestra and listen to the music—do you like the music? If not, tune the instruments again, and then make sure the whole orchestra is in harmony.

An organ

Close your eyes and describe your uterus as a room—lighting, colors, walls, interior, etc.—or the heart, brain, prostate or whatever else revealed itself during testing to be looked at and resolved in an Imago.

Lineage

 Take the last seven generations of women, ask them to go into one room and
describe what you see.
Or the men, or two or twelve generations—everything is possible.
If the Imago was successful, you'll have a family party at the end.

Taken from life

Journeys into this life

This is like taking an elevator through your life. Whenever something still needs
to be clarified and resolved, when there are any charges left, the elevator will jolt
at a certain age. The arm-length test will reveal stress. Then, open the door and
have a look. Now you can work specifically on the issue there.

My own birth: conception, pregnancy, delivery

Here, the elevator will descend a bit further. During these nine months, more
things are determined for our lives than we might like.
If there's stress at conception, it's likely that one or both parents may not have
wanted to conceive a child at that moment. When thinking of each parent by
him- or herself, you can quickly determine how each of them felt during conception. If stress is identified during the pregnancy, this can be due to stress in the
relationship, fear, a medical intervention, an accident or many other things that
still have a charge.
Out of my eight children, I only experienced two births after which the children
didn't need to be treated with *innerwise*. I think this is about average.

The future

Why not also travel there and check to see whether charges can be sensed, thus
urgently indicating a change in course now.

Homo Integer Meditation

The Homo Integer as a healing field is available in a large format, starting at
about 35 by 35 inches, and in a smaller version with the Flowmaker disc. If this
topic is active in the test card, support from this source of energy is always
needed.
This is often the case when issues are difficult to resolve and when a treatment no
longer goes easily and beautifully. Place the Homo Integer underneath the person

or topic you're working on, let it build up its energy field, and instantly something will clear up and the treatment will be fun again.

HEALING BREATH: Healing the soul

There are two ways to retrieve soul fragments that separated due to traumas: We follow them through the escape tunnels and can find them again this way. Or we search for them throughout the entire space—but try to retrieve a teddy bear in outer space!

First breath

Inhalation: From the divine source, breathe in pure energy.
Exhalation: As you breathe out, fill up all escape tunnels of the soul fragments that separated, all the way to the end with this energy, this light.

Second breath

Inhalation: From the escape tunnels, breathe in the energy, and thus all soul fragments.
Exhalation: Breathe out all retrieved soul fragments into the Source.

Third breath

Inhalation: From the Source, breathe in your healed soul fragments.
Exhalation: Re-integrate all soul fragments back into your life as you breathe out.

Repeat the healing breath until your soul is complete again and the escape tunnels are empty and have disappeared.

HEALING BREATH: Healing fissures in the soul space

Fissures are openings to other realities; they're like gateways through which energies can enter, and parts and energies from us can get lost. These are areas or spots where the energy field of the person concerned isn't stable.

First breath

Inhalation: From the divine source, breathe in pure energy.
Exhalation: Breathe it out via the heart chakra into the entire space and all dimensions.

Repeat this breathing until the entire space is filled with energy and you can feel light and joy within yourself by feeling connected to everything.

Second breath

Inhalation: Breathe in all lost soul fragments from the infinite space back into your soul space.
Exhalation: Breathe out the soul fragments into the Source.

Third breath

Inhalation: From the Source, breathe in your healed soul fragments.
Exhalation: Re-integrate them back into your Being as you breathe out.

Fourth breath

Inhalation: Breathe in all negativity and manipulation that hides behind the fissure.
Exhalation: Breathe it all out into the Source.

Fifth breath

Inhalation: From the Source, breathe in pure energy.
Exhalation: With this energy, close the fissure in the soul space.

Repeat this breathing until the fissure has fully vanished.

HEALING BREATH: Healing the love field

The love for our partner or even for our children isn't always equally strong and pure. Sometimes our trust in our partner is shaken, and our love field is weak or poisoned.

This love field is the field, the space, that surrounds the present space between two people.

Imagine your love partner, and concentrate on the love field that surrounds both of you and needs support.

First breath

Inhalation: Breathe in this love field.

Exhalation: Breathe it out fully into the divine source.

Second breath

Inhalation: From the Source, breathe in a new, clean love field.

Exhalation: Fill the space around and between the two of you with this love field.

Repeat the breathing exercise until both of you are filled again with the power of pure love.

The healing breath for love is better and more effective if both partners do it together.

HEALING BREATH: Letting go of one's partner when separating

It's not always possible to revive love. Sometimes what two souls set out to experience together has been accomplished and they can now let go of each other in gratitude.

Ideally, both partners perform the healing breath together. It is a ritual to bring something big to an end and give both partners back their freedom.

If not otherwise possible, each partner can perform the healing breath alone.

Imagine your ex-partner, and concentrate on the love field that still connects both of you.

First breath

Inhalation: Breathe in your old love field completely.
Exhalation: Breathe it out fully into the divine source.

Second breath

Inhalation: From the Source, breathe in your energy only.
Exhalation: As you breathe out, fill up your soul space alone with your breath.

Apply the healing breath until you can no longer see your partner in front of your inner eye, and the field that formerly surrounded you has dissolved; do this until you're both free. In this way, love can also turn into friendship.

HEALING BREATH: Letting go of old relationships

Imagine an ex-partner from your life. Concentrate on the field that still connects both of you.

First breath

Inhalation: Breathe in this old field completely.
Exhalation: Breathe it out into the divine source.

Second breath

Inhalation: From the Source, breathe in your energy only.
Exhalation: As you breathe out, fill up your soul space alone with your breath.

Repeat the healing breath until you can no longer visualize your ex-partner in front of you in a field that connects both of you. Thank your ex-partner for all the experiences you shared and say good-bye.

HEALING BREATH: Clearing family fields

You can choose your friends, but not your family, and thus also the shared burden of the past … *or not.*
The healing breath can help you protect your own sacred family space so that no one can affect it from outside in destructive ways.

First breath

Inhalation: Breathe in the field of your core family as it is.
Exhalation: Breathe it out into the divine source.

Second breath

Inhalation: From the Source, breathe in a new and beautiful field for your
                family.
Exhalation: As you breathe out, fill up your family space with your breath.

Repeat this healing breath until you and your family have a stable and strong family field.

HEALING BREATH: Children can finally be children

Children are often loved as a substitute for the great love that used to exist between their parents.

But who would want to be loved as a substitute for someone else—with the feeling that the love is not meant for you, but for someone or for a time that no longer exists.

Imagine your child, and sense the field that connects both of you.

First breath

Inhalation: Breathe in the field completely that has connected you both thus far.

Exhalation: Breathe it out into the divine source.

Second breath

Inhalation: From the Source, breathe in pure energy and love to accompany your child on its journey to becoming an adult in a protected way.

Exhalation: Fill the love space that surrounds you and your child with this energy and love.

Repeat the healing breath until your child is smiling at you in front of your inner eye.

Ideally, you can do the healing breath together with your child until you both smile at each other.

HEALING BREATH: Parents become friends, children become adults

Once we're adults, we can choose the kind of relationship and connection we want to have with other people, and this also includes our parents: Do we want to continue having the parent-child connection? In that case, however, we won't *really* grow up. Or do we want to be at eye level—that is, on par with them. Then, parents can turn into true friends, and mutual respect and recognition are possible.

In this healing breath, you breathe into the divine source the parent-child field that has connected you with your parents thus far, which is only a mirror of the original love field between your parents and you. Then, you breathe in a love field where you're at eye level with your parents into the space that surrounds you and them, or alternatively, the space that surrounds you and only one parent, depending on what you want to do.

Imagine one parent in front of you, and sense the field that connects both of you.

First breath

Inhalation: Breathe in the field completely that has connected you both thus far.

Exhalation: Breathe it out into the divine source.

Second breath

Inhalation: From the Source, breathe in the pure energy of a field that connects people at eye level—that is, who are on par with one another.

Exhalation: Fill the love space that surrounds you and your parent with this energy.

Repeat this breathing until you can see yourself and your parent at eye level— that is, on par with you—and you look each other in the eye with mutual respect and joy.

HEALING BREATH: Letting go of parents, becoming an adult

It's also possible that it's time to end the relationship or connection with one or both parents. A clear end is better than endless agony—especially if those involved in a relationship aren't honest, pull at one another energetically and sap energy, if there are power and blackmail games, and if no solution can be found.

Imagine one parent in front of you, and sense the field that connects both of you.

First breath

Inhalation: Breathe in this field completely.
Exhalation: Breathe it out into the divine source.

Second breath

Inhalation: From the Source, breathe in pure energy into your soul space only.
Exhalation: Fill yourself up with this energy; it's there for you only.

Repeat the healing breath until you can no longer visualize your parent in front of you in a field that connects both of you. Thank your parent for all the experiences you shared and say good-bye.

HEALING BREATH: Sparking the creative fire

Creativity comes our way when we're able to understand ourselves as an instrument. When I write, it's the divine source writing through me. Good musicians know their trade, and then the Source can play through them. You can also call this inspiration.

First breath

Inhalation: Breathe in all your fears completely.
Exhalation: Breathe them all out into the divine source.

Repeat this breathing until all your fears have disappeared.

Second breath

Inhalation: From the Source, breathe in creative energy through your central channel.
Exhalation: Fill yourself up completely with this creative fire.

Repeat this healing breath until creativity is bubbling out of you.

MOTHER EARTH MEDITATION

Start out with the words: *Mother Earth, as a part of you, you are fully in me and live through me.* Immerse yourself in these words and thus in Mother Earth: Once you are one with the great Mother you become part of her, as a waterfall, for example, or an eagle or a tree. You begin to feel their energy within you and to heal yourself.

When you have connected to Mother Earth, you can do the same with other cosmic forces and their gifts:
Father Sun, as a part of you, you are fully in me and live through me.
Heaven, as a part of you, you are fully in me and live through me.
God, as a part of you, you are fully in me and live through me.

*inner*Yoga

In your imagination you fuse to part of nature, an animal, for example, an eagle. You feel it inside of you, feel its wings and yours, feel how the wind ripples through your feathers. And you breathe like an eagle. Your body begins of its own accord to move like an eagle. Your wings unfold. Every eagle is one of a kind, each position you adopt, each gesture is perfect. The whole of nature is in motion, nothing is static, schooled positions are now superfluous.

THE RIVER OF LIFE

Retreat to a quiet place and find your inner peace. Sit or lie down comfortably. Close your eyes and take a few deep breaths.

Now visualize the color blue with your inner eye . Notice how this blue begins to move, to form waves, to become water and flow like a river. Look into the river and see your own reflection.

You see a boat on the river. It's your boat. You are in your boat in the center of the river. Take a look around you—you see the shore, the meadows and the trees—and notice the river, see the leaves floating on the surface of the water.

Now look at the direction your boat is taking. Are you heading for the source or the mouth of the river? If you're on the way to the mouth, think about why your boat is heading in this direction. Think back on times in your life when you moved toward the source. If you're going to the source, think about why your boat is heading in this direction. Notice how much you have to struggle with the current to get closer to your destination.

Look around you and see all the other boats going in the opposite direction. Haven't you asked yourself all along why your life in particular consists of so much struggle and loneliness? You now have the opportunity to learn how to trust. Change direction, allow yourself to drift—to be in the flow. Sense the flow of the river.

Now come back into the present moment and see what's in your boat. Is there anybody else there for the ride? If so—it may be an animal, a partner, friends or your children—look into the eyes of the animal or person and ask them: "Why are you in my boat?", "Why are you not in your own boat?", "Who invited you?", "Do I need you in my boat?"

Notice whether you're sitting at the front or the back of your boat. Are you at the helm or did you surrender control to someone else, who is now steering your boat? Imagine how it feels to be alone again in your boat; to navigate alone, perfectly at peace with yourself.

Now the time has come for the other people or animals to leave your boat and enter their own, which is gliding alongside yours. Imagine them leaving the boat. And if there's something holding them back, imagine a color that envelops them like a warm coat so they can leave. Now you're alone again in your boat. Whoever's in your heart is right beside you, traveling in their own boat. There are passages in the river where your boats drift slightly apart, and others where you come closer again. There are no anchors or ropes between you and the others. You're confident that it's right exactly as it is at any given moment.

You watch the other boats on the river and notice that two that were close together are drifting apart, and how at a fork in the river each boat goes its own way. This fills your heart with great joy—you see that two human beings have spent part of their lives together and taught each other what they had agreed upon before they stepped into their boats. Now they set each other free and separate, so that both can continue to grow and fulfill other tasks.

All of a sudden you hear it. There it is, that rushing noise somewhere ahead of you. It's getting louder. Now you know what it is—a waterfall. And it's right in front of you.

You look around, there's no way you can get past it; you're drifting closer and closer. Are you afraid? If so, what planet or star immediately comes to mind? Ask it for strength, courage and trust so that you can steer directly into the waterfall. Slowly count to three. One, two, three … suddenly you feel how your boat begins to fly and then lands softly on the other side of the waterfall in a deep, quiet pool.

You're amazed to see that your fear was unnecessary, and you remember situations in your life where your fear was stronger than your courage, and how this deprived you of marvelous experiences. Now you know that with the help of stars and planets you can conquer any waterfall. The river quietens, and twilight is approaching. You hear the bird's lovely evening songs; candles are floating on the water in a bay, and you feel a deep desire to be close to someone, an embrace, a union with another human being.

If something now holds you back and forbids this deep desire, imagine a crystal, its color, its form. Connect to this crystal and become one with it; feel the deep peace that resides there. And now feel the desire to melt with another person within you. Your boats blend and become one, and you begin to melt into one another. With your eyes, your touch, your kiss you dive deep down into each other and feel how you become one common breath. You both feel the most wonderful energy rising within you and your breath becomes ever more intense. You are filled with infinite bliss and completeness, time- and spacelessness.

Dawn has broken, and the time has come for both of you to part and separate your boats, and for each to continue on their own path alone. Look at your own boat again—it's turning into a kayak. In the twilight, you see a sign by the riverside: "Caution, whitewater! Only one boat at a time."

Before you have time to realize your new situation, the current pulls your boat into rough waters. The water is churning, gushing over boulders, and you're caught up in wild swirls. You do well; you master the challenges. But suddenly a current throws you off balance, and your kayak capsizes. With your head under water you hang on to your kayak. The water overwhelms you. You hold your breath and feel the cold water swirling past you. You notice the air getting less and less. It may last another thirty seconds, not more. You have to make a decision. You can leave the kayak, or try to turn it around and get above water.

An inner voice tells you: "Try it, you can do it, turn yourself around." You try, but to no avail. Time is running out.

To live or die—again the choice is yours: to leave the boat or summon every ounce of strength and try again. You try it one last time with all your might. You did it! Your head is above water again. You feel the fresh air, and how it fills your lungs. You're alive! You continue to drift. Night has fallen. The river is quieter and reflects the bright moonlight.

Suddenly you see a wall in front of you. All the water gushes through a hole in the wall. What's behind it? An abyss? The end? Paradise? You don't know, and you won't find out unless you trust and flow with the water through this hole.

You could also paddle to the shore. You could wait there, stare at the hole every day and see how all the other boats push through it. But you would be wasting years of your life—out of fear. You've done that too many times already, haven't you? And in the end it'll be the same as the waterfall—easy. This time you trust and go through. And then …

… you find yourself on the most beautiful blue quiet lake. The sun is shining.

You turn around in your kayak and look back at the wall through which you reached this lake. The hole is no longer there; in its place there's a window, and above the window it says "window of gratitude." You can only see experiences in your past for which you are grateful. You're still standing in front of this window, looking through it. What do you see? And what do you not see? Saying "thank you" for injuries, pain, fear, loneliness or losses is not an easy task.

All of a sudden you hear a clear voice telling you: "It's easy; you planned your life exactly as it is, with all its experiences. And these have enriched your soul. They've made you what you are today: wonderful, lovable and a little wiser." Think about your entire life and feel the gratitude that you were given the opportunity to experience all this.

You have no idea how much time you spent in front of this window; although it was only a few moments, it feels like eternity. And you made it! Your heart feels light and free, you're filled with a power you thought you had lost forever. You've seen yourself as a victim for so long and suppressed the power within you. Now you're no longer a victim.

The gentle current of the lake slowly propels you away from the window. You turn and look ahead, but you can't see very far because suddenly a fog is rising in front of you, so dense that you can't even begin to guess what awaits you ahead. By now you've embarked on the unknown so often that you feel joyful expectation this time, a tingling, similar to the delicious feeling you had as a child just before Christmas. Which gifts await you now?

You dive into the fog, glide along. All of a sudden you see a wild swirl of water in front of you. You have no choice—the entire lake is pulled into it. It's a hole—a black, infinitely deep, quiet hole. You make a decision: you get up and jump into nothingness … and it's the most magnificent thing you have ever experienced in your life. You are everything and nothing, both human being and God. You fly like you've flown in your dreams. You are one with everything, limitless, infinite. You experience a profound transformation. You become enlightened and find yourself again at the source of the river.

It's the river of love, and your "boat of life" is ready for a new journey. But first you rest a while and think about your last journey on the river. You remember how you always wanted to swim against the tide back to the Source; you think of all the sweating and puffing, and you have to laugh at yourself. You see the boats again with your ex-partners, your partner, your children. In one boat the partner was tied up in chains to prevent disembarkation. Now you can laugh heartily about your fear of the waterfall. And you still feel the shared breath of love inside of you. How blessed human beings are to have a body that allows them to experience all this.

You remember the waterfall and the whitewater, the hole in the wall, the beautiful lake shrouded in fog, and this fantastic maelstrom of water you jumped into head first. It is all in your soul, and it was all really good. At some point, once you've rested enough, you decide that you will make sound plans for your next journey on the river and find friends to participate. And the time will come when you board a new boat.

Now wake up and enjoy this life! One day you will reach the Source, and by then you should have had a lot of fun!

Test Card 11   Environment

Private environment

Depending on how many compromises we make, our private environment either turns into an Armageddon or an oasis of peace.

No one can seriously claim to be a victim of his or her environment.

We've all chosen and created our environment ourselves—the apartment or house we live in, the location, the country, or our friends and partners. And our environment has also left an imprint on our children.

We always have the option to change things, if we want to. It's easy to paint a wall a color that we truly like, to give up a job that we hate, to move to a different country or to talk honestly to one another, and so on.

Most people lack the energy to do so; the pressure isn't high enough, or they lack the courage.

The goal of *innerwise* isn't to "adopt" people or to tell them what to do or not do. What we can do is show them where there are issues, compromises and lies, and then let them be self-responsible.

If someone wants to continue living with his partner in the home of his in-laws just to save rent, he can do so, but then he shouldn't hope that his therapist takes away his headache. And there are always painkillers that numb the symptoms and shorten one's life in return.

We all pay for every compromise; the only question is *when.*

Professional environment

According to statistics, 70 percent of the working population in Germany have resigned from their job in all but name.

I love my work, and it gives me energy. I enjoy writing this book. I feel good when I've given someone a treatment. And I also expect that all the people I work with love their work. I only go to restaurants or buy things in stores where I feel good and where people put their heart into their work.

This means that only 30 percent do their job with love and fill their work with their presence.

Someone I know manages a research company, and there as well, 60 percent of the employees have resigned in all but name. This means that the creative output of this company is only at one-third of what's possible, and 60 percent of the staff could resign without causing major changes.

Productivity and creativity aren't a question of the time we spend, but a question of the presence, love and energy that we dedicate to it.

The essential question is whether we live our soul purpose with what we do.

Do I walk my path, receiving maximum support from fate through what is called divine providence, or do I live against myself?

Our work environment includes everything and everyone involved: the annoying copy machine at the office, lighting conditions, colleagues, the work climate, corporate values, time pressures, communication among the workforce, and so on.

Also this testing topic requires detective abilities in order to identify the core issues. Only when these issues are identified and solutions are worked out will this testing topic no longer cause stress in the arm-length test.

People in my life

This involves clarifying relationships and clearing ties, understanding contracts and putting an end to systems of suffering.

Do people in our lives still trigger unconscious patterns in us? This also includes parents, siblings, ex-partners, our own children, friends, acquaintances, and so on.

Are there still patterns stemming from experiences of all lives with the souls of these people?

Through testing, determine how many people there are with whom such patterns still exist, and then clear them all.

Think of all the experiences you've had with these people in this life. This often triggers panic reactions that show up in the arm-length test. In that case, use healing cards to clear that stress.

Being dishonest with one another

What are you afraid of? Why don't you just say everything the way you think it? "What is supposed to happen?" It could be that the other person can't handle it, but this isn't your issue. Or do you want to continue lying in order to protect somebody?

Speak the truth and express it in an "I" message: "For me …" or "I perceive …" or "I don't feel good about …"

When you slap people in the face with words such as: "Because of you …" or "It's your fault that … ," they'll hit you back.

If you stick to "I" messages, this won't happen.

It's not your job to protect others from the truth and to swallow the energetic charges of the lie and then feel worse. Trust your fellow human beings to behave like adults.

Test questions
- I usually lie … times a day.
- I'm always absolutely honest with … people.
- Due to my untruths, I've lost … percent of my life energy.

"Darling, what I've always wanted to tell you is that …"

Noise

We only realize the ability of our senses and nervous system to filter information when they no longer work properly.

Anyone with a hearing aid recognizes this problem. All noises reach our brain as if they're equally important. This makes it extremely difficult to concentrate on what's essential. But our filters also diminish during periods of exhaustion, and we start to feel noise as physical pain.

However, noise is much more than what we can hear. When high-frequency detectors make the normal frequency mix that constantly pervades us audible, everybody covers their ears. But our cells can't cover their ears. They're constantly exposed to such stress to the limit of exhaustion.

At some point, their ability to compensate is used up, and the fuses blow.

It looks like Darwin was right—evolution does happen, because the ability to deal with the noise of audible and nonaudible frequencies appears to increase. If this weren't the case, the use of cell phones would have already caused testicular cancer in most men, or brain tumors in the majority of people.

Five years ago, a cell phone in sending mode still caused a stress or panic reaction in almost everyone in the arm-length test. Today, this is no longer the case. Many people no longer experience stress with that. Have we been adapting?

Noise is also a question of taste. If we went to a concert where the instruments were tuned as they used to be 500 years ago, and where the choir sang the tones as people used to do at that time, many of us would experience this as noise. Noise is only what we *perceive* as disharmonious.

Our life has gotten faster, and along with that, our taste in sounds and frequencies has also changed.

Disharmony

And noise is much more than that: "You're thinking so loudly!"

Noise encompasses much more than miscellaneous audible sounds. We perceive the thoughts, emotions and energies of other people just like we sense the energies of rooms and other spaces, systems or ideas.

Why do we choose a café that is a few hundred feet farther away when there's one right in front of us?

Because we feel better there.

Why can we no longer stand the voices of certain people, whereas we melt when hearing those of others?

People can only be harmonious and beautiful when their own identity is present and their presence is clear.

Energetic irritations

I've set up my home and garden to be an energetic oasis that supports the work I do. However, this field isn't permanently stable; it requires that I'm attentive to it all the time.

When we create such a clean space, we also have an experimental field for any kind of energetic irritation, because it can be seen and sensed immediately.

And once we're used to a clean space, we're spoiled.

With my awareness of, and experience with, the power of fields, it has become essential to live in a clear environment.

At this very moment—I'm currently on an island writing this text—my daughter is calling from home, asking me to tune into the garden, because something isn't quite right there. She has a bad feeling.

And she was right. I was able to help her stabilize herself from far away, and I told her what she could do to clear up the garden.

This demonstrates once more how valuable the arm-length test is, as well as trained perception and sensing.

Another example:

A young mother is calling, and in the background, I can hear her four-week-old baby screaming in panic. This screaming comes from the soul.

Usually, the baby is very peaceful and happy, but through testing, I identified an irritation that had occurred an hour and a half earlier. The mother confirmed that the baby had been screaming for 90 minutes.

When I asked what had happened at the time, she replied that nothing special had occurred; she was talking to an old friend. However, this friend takes drugs on a regular basis and is part of a cult.

Consequently, I drew the field of the baby to gain an overview, because I could only feel fear and panic when tuning into the child.

The circle that I'd drawn for this purpose, trying to find the child in there, was empty. The child's soul field was no longer with the baby.

There was an interference with the baby's identity; the child was in a state of rigidity.

Then I found the child's soul field in the circle that I had drawn for the cult. I immediately worked with the baby remotely, and the treatment was effective the moment I completed it. The baby calmed down instantly and was able to fall into a restful sleep. I was more than 300 miles away.

Toxic burdens

This refers to poisonings of all types: poisoned soils, air polluted by paint, wood preservatives, industrial air emissions, mold toxins, polluted water, pesticides, and so on. We can extend this list infinitely.

What's important is to identify the source of the poisoning—the spaces where it occurs, the sources it stems from, when it started and when it happens.

This is a challenge for the detective in us, and it's no disgrace if it takes a few treatments until the source is identified.

Harmful effects in the workplace

When painting car bodies, it can be particulate matter and solvents; for a secretary, it can be the vapors of the laser printer; for any staff member, it can be the whims of colleagues or bosses; or it can be geopathic stress or electrosmog in the workplace. Once more, you'll need your detective abilities to identify the cause of the stress reaction to this test question. Filtering questions can help you limit the potential causes and make this easier.

"Imagine you're breathing in the air of this room."
"Imagine sitting for several hours on your chair."
"Now imagine moving your chair three feet to the right or left and then sitting there again for an extended period of time."
"Imagine that your colleague is away for a month."
"Imagine that your computer is three feet farther away from you."

Electrosmog in the sleeping area

List of symptoms
- Trouble falling asleep (more than ten minutes)
- Dark circles under the eyes
- Urinating at night
- Trouble sleeping through the night
- Waking up tired
- Light sleep
- Racing heart at night
- Fatigue syndrome
- ADD or hyperactivity
- Pain and tense muscles at night and in the morning—such as back pain, headaches, stiff muscles or rheumatism
- Chronic inflammations

We divide electrosmog into three areas:
- AC voltage
- Magnetic fields
- High frequencies

AC voltage

Current is a blessing—if only it wasn't nearly everywhere all the time. Hotel beds with integrated sockets and switches, furniture for young people equipped with TVs mounted to the bed, power cables hidden in the wall behind the bed … it's almost everywhere.

The problem with AC voltage is that our brain—that is, the pineal gland, to be more precise—misinterprets it, confusing it with sunlight.

When the sun is shining, we don't need to sleep. When it's getting dark, the hormones change, and it's time for recuperation and internal refreshment. For this purpose, the pineal gland releases melatonin, which is in charge of regulating our body's biorhythm, but it's also a happiness and anti-carcinogenic hormone.

If we sleep in AC electric fields, they're misinterpreted as light; and melatonin, the body's own natural sleeping pill, isn't produced.

As a result, falling asleep takes longer than the usual five or ten minutes. People can't sleep through the night, they have to get up at night to go to the bathroom and can't fall back asleep afterward, they wake up with a foggy mind and sleepy eyes and aren't in a sunny mood.

Since melatonin also regulates other regulatory hormones, these are lacking as well. Organs and tissue no longer regenerate optimally. The body's hormone-producing organs such as the thyroid or adrenal glands also need their work instructions for the day, which they receive with the regulatory hormones. If those regulatory hormones are lacking, the body is missing coordination, and the thyroid and other organs will do what they think is right. Thus, the thyroid is the first organ that alters at night and gets enlarged as a result of sleeping in an AC electric field.

It's not so easy to test AC voltage with the arm-length test. As for electrosmog, the person has to imagine sleeping in his or her bed throughout the entire night, and only then does electrosmog become tangible. Imagining taking a nap during the day doesn't suffice, because AC voltage only causes stress at night.
Remediating such harmful effects requires a technical measurement by means of a connection measurement.

Here, the person concerned lies in bed, and the measuring device compares the AC voltage in the body with a grounding.
The measured value should be below 0.1 volt.
It has been shown that a value of 0.2 volt already results in an 80 percent reduction in melatonin production.

Nevertheless, many people try to sleep at values of between 1 and 10 volts.
The first step to remedy this problem is to remove the sources: extension cords, lamps and radio alarm clocks. If the measurement still doesn't yield the desired result, remove all fuses and then activate one after the other to determine which circuit causes the voltage-related stress.
For this purpose, it helps if someone supports the person concerned, so that he or she can stay in bed during the measurement.
If feasible, remove the fuse every time before going to bed from now on, or ask an electrician to install a demand switch.
If none of the above offers a solution, the only thing left to do is to set up a technical protective shielding. For that, conductive material is placed underneath the mattress and grounded. If the reading from the measuring device shows a higher value when you touch the wall—that is, if you're also exposed to electrosmog from the wall, you do the same with the wall behind or next to the bed. This is caused by cables in the wall or from a neighbor.
The main stress mostly comes from below. It stems from the lighting cables in the room underneath you. Only ceilings with grounded steel reinforcements provide shielding.

In wooden houses, the entire wood construction transmits the voltage. These kinds of houses need shielded cables to be healthy for their inhabitants.

Here, more advanced multifunctional measuring devices can be used. Select Volt AC voltage as the measuring range.

In order to test whether the measuring device is usable, take an extension cord into one hand; you'll measure a voltage between 5 and 15 volts. Plug the cable connected to the person into the voltage input, and attach the grounding cord from the COM output to a grounding. The grounding can be the grounding contacts of an outlet, if they're properly connected. It's also possible to use water or heating pipes as long as they're not made of plastic.

Together with the Dutch company Healthfoam, I've developed a measuring and shielding system called E-Cover that serves to take measurements and shield your bed and walls if setting up your own protective shielding is not an option.

Magnetic fields

Magnetic fields cause depression in people. Such fields can only be measured using special measuring devices, but this isn't much of an issue as sources are clearly identifiable—that is, all devices that contain a transformer and are less than three feet away from the body.

An exception would be cable harnesses in building shafts, overhead power cables and high-voltage power lines. With overhead power cables at window level along roads, higher magnetic field levels can be measured up to a distance of about 33 feet; in case of high-voltage power lines, elevated values can still be measured much farther away. A simple radio alarm clock, which represents the most frequent source of such interference, only generates fields that already drop below the exposure limit of 250 microtesla after three feet.

The easiest solution to this problem is exchanging the radio alarm clock for a battery-powered alarm clock.

People buy radio alarm clocks to make sure they wake up in the morning because they don't sleep well. But they sleep even worse because of the radio alarm clock. That's a catch-22 situation.

Since it's hardly possible to shield yourself from magnetic fields, the only option left is to move when you're experiencing stress due to high-voltage power lines.

When exposed to overhead power cables in front of your bedroom window, you can still try to sleep in the room farthest away from them.

High-frequency interference

Many people are fighting against cell phone towers, yet with their wireless phones, they've very strong transmitters at their own home.

It appears that the rise in the number of tumors in the head and lower abdomen caused by cell phones that was projected years ago never materialized. Also, testing of the younger generations reveals a tangibly lower stress reaction to interference from cell phones.

Nevertheless, it would be better if people avoided exposing themselves to this kind of interference. And there will always be those who are highly sensitive to high-frequency interference.

Wireless phones can be replaced by modern ECO DECT telephones that stop the disturbing pulsed signal a few seconds after the conversation ends; instead of the interference, there will only be a background noise.

You can switch off your Wi-Fi overnight. You shouldn't buy a home near a cell phone tower, even if it's cheap. Trees can shield you from electromagnetic interference, and clay plaster also offers good protective shielding.

Furthermore, it's possible to modulate the body's reaction to such information through harmonious information that compensates for the chaos and the irritating patterns in the body.

Electrosmog in the workplace

Apart from positioning your computer farther away from your body, you can measure the electrosmog caused by AC voltage using the measuring device and then make changes. What matters is that a computer should be about three feet away from your body due to its strong magnetic field, and it shouldn't be directly on or next to your lap.

Geopathic stress in the sleeping area

The Earth is not flat, and there's no "bad" radiation emitting from below its surface.

Unfortunately, the myth is still being disseminated successfully that placing a cork mat underneath a bed offers protective shielding against geopathic stress.

On planet Earth, there are fields with different qualities, and not all living beings react the same to them.

Cats and ants feel good in places where horses, cows and dogs would never lie down. Animals have preserved their alertness and their ability to sense that. People, on the other hand, go by the floor plan of their apartment, *feng shui* principles they read about, or simply practical considerations.

Consequently, about 80 percent of all people in Europe and North America sleep in places that don't make them healthier, but rather, the contrary.

Animals can also lose this ability when they're socialized and used as a substitute for a child or partner.

We can also see when people have planted trees against nature: twisted street trees, crippled trees or trees that grow toward one side when they reach a certain height, as if they're steering clear of something.

Many people wake up with pain or stiff muscles in the morning; their mind is foggy, the energy isn't optimal, dreaming was disturbed or they had strange dreams. Simply put, they didn't regenerate optimally during the night.

What's normal is to wake up with a clear mind and clear eyes; with a relaxed, soft and rejuvenated body, full of good energy flowing through us, and with a sunny mood.

And this isn't about the quality of the mattress. Worldwide, many people sleep in hammocks, or on straw or animal skins, and they don't need a space-proven cold-foam mattress to enjoy a good night's sleep.

Only inner-spring mattresses exert an influence. They can alter the natural magnetic field, as can be easily verified with a compass. AC electric fields can generate a flow of current in the metal with irritating or harmful effects on the human being.

Here, the topic of geopathic stress or geopathology isn't about a precise expertise, the exact name of the different kinds of interference or of the fields according to those who described them (Hartmann, Curry, etc.). Rather, it's about redeveloping our ability to perceive and sense which environment is good for us and which one harms us.

It doesn't matter whether we do this with a dowsing rod or the arm-length test.

The following basic knowledge suffices:

Field structures of the Earth that are arranged in grids, water veins, faults or lodes cause geopathic stress.

There's no "bad" earth radiation.

On the one hand, there are straight magnetic grids that nourish us. On the other hand, these straight gridlines generate a diagonal grid similar to a moving ship creating a bow wave. These grids are not homogeneous fields; rather, they're comparable to waves.

About every 8 feet, they're slightly intensified; about every 33 feet, the intensification is of medium strength; and about every 108 feet, the intensification is extreme.

The straight grid generates nourishing fields and places of power at its crossings. The diagonal grid produces energy-draining fields and places.

Compared to the importance of these grids, water veins, lodes and faults play only a subordinate role.

If people are on an energy-draining line or on a crossing of the diagonal grid, which is even stronger, they lose energy and their body is being irritated. This leads to tense muscles, pain, irritated body rhythms and a loss of energy.

Everybody knows this from going to the movies: Your neighbor is sitting there relaxed, and you have to keep shifting in your seat because you're so uncomfortable and your bottom is hurting. Your neighbor has the same kind of seat, but you happen to be sitting on a geopathic stress zone, and your body is reacting to that.

When we're standing on a crossing of the energy-draining 108-foot grid, we can feel within minutes how our knees turn to jelly, and energy leaves the body. Such spots are also referred to as "sudden-infant-death-syndrome (SIDS) points." If a baby sleeps on such a spot, the loss of energy can trigger SIDS, which is based on total energetic exhaustion.

The 33-foot grid can result in tense and/or stiff muscles, back pain or migraines in the morning.

The 8-foot grid is the weakest and can lead to light forms of physical discomfort or ailments.

Then again, we can recharge ourselves and support healing processes when being in places of power, which are frequently crossings of the energizing grid.

A complicating factor in this topic are frequencies that can add themselves to the grid fields. You can imagine them as overtones, or as loads on cars of a moving train, which can irritate the body in specific ways. Since every organ and every illness has its specific frequency patterns, irritations and illnesses can arise if irritating frequencies added to the field resonate with that illness.

Thus, there are places that cause or aggravate certain illnesses.

People developing cancer always have to check the places where they sleep to see whether there's an irritation that aggravates their illness. However, this basically applies to any illness.

 "Imagine lying in your bed for the whole night." Then test with your arms if there's stress.

Geopathic stress in the workplace

One of my patients always had a migraine around noon on one specific day of the week. Only on that day was she sitting in a certain place to work, directly on a spot with geopathic stress. She proceeded to move her chair by 20 inches and found that she no longer had migraines.

Harmful energetic interference in living and work spaces

Rooms or other spaces store energies. Fields stay stuck in them, and entities (beings) can be present there.

Nightmares are always a sure sign that entities are present. These can also be souls of people who already passed away that are attached to the intermediary world.

What matters is to identify the source of that interference—when it started and when it occurs. Was that interference already in these living or work spaces before you got there?

Do these energies come in through a human being who lives there?

And then, it's about finding a way to cleanse these spaces.

When energies are tied to objects, pictures or books, you can try to cleanse them or remove these objects. If energies are in a living or work space independent from objects, it's often possible to clear that space with music, crystals or through smudging. The most effective way is to treat the space using *innerwise*, as you would with a living being.

You can also successfully treat the entities themselves. Then, the healing symphony for the room or other space is saved to an *innerwise* disc and positioned in the optimal spot, as guided by the support of the arm-length test.

The optimal spot is the one where the healing energies are intensified the most and have the strongest impact—the place of resonance. This spot could also be outside the respective room or space.

"Is the room/space clean?" is not an ideal test question, because we all have different ideas of what "clean" means, thus obtaining contradictory results.

It's better to ask: "Is the room/space filled with pure white light?"

Not taking space for myself

How much freedom does a human being need?

And how much space for him- or herself?

Having space for yourself can mean having your own study, your own bedroom; being free to decide on the colors you wish to use in your room, on the floor covering and on the pictures on the wall. Or it can mean going to the movies or a café alone without any bad conscience vis-à-vis your partner, or going on a vacation alone.

Taking your own space always means no longer being considerate of how your partner, parents or friends feel or what they need.

It also always means looking at things in your own way, and being able to stop somewhere during a walk and observe something as long as you want.

Your own space is that which is sufficient for your own energy field.

Especially in families, this individual space and what belongs to each parent degenerates into "common property."

It's a good thing to have your own space that nobody—not even other family members—is allowed to enter without your permission. People can knock at the door and ask, and if they get a "no" for an answer, that's okay, too.

Test questions
- My partner/wife/girlfriend decides what I wear.
- I am worthy of having my own space.
- Nobody has the right to dominate me.
- I do what I want.
- My partner has to sleep next to me.
- I also grant others the freedom that I take for myself.

Being overwhelmed

Being overwhelmed always results from deep exhaustion creating an imbalance between one's ability to perform and one's challenges.

When your children are finally asleep and you're facing six hours of concentrated work almost every evening, then what's left is to dope yourself with coffee or chocolate, grit your teeth, treat yourself using *innerwise*, for example, and get to work.

There are only two major reasons for being overwhelmed:
- Not having enough energy, such as a level of life energy of 30 percent.
- Going in the wrong direction in life, thus losing even more energy.

Therefore, there's not too much work; there's only too little energy to take care of it.

Everyone knows how it is when you're exhausted and try to get something done which, the next morning, will go very smoothly and take little time.

What's essential is to keep your energy at an optimal level, not to do anything that's not part of your life plan and to always find the right moment to become active.

I always draw up a list of what I have to do, and then I test what to start with and the optimal moment to do those things.

Food toxins

As I'm writing this, a legal ruling is being passed stipulating that honey has to be free of genetically modified ingredients. And this has happened thanks to the courage of one beekeeper who sued an entire country.

But who sues the manufacturers who add toxic colorants to food? Or chicken farmers, because their chickens are being pumped full of antibiotics? Or restaurant owners who warm up chocolate in the microwave, thus rendering it unusable for the body?

For us, the only safe way out of this dilemma is the arm-length test.

So, test everything already at the supermarket before buying it in order to determine if you and your family can tolerate it.

It makes sense to divide food into groups and then test them in order to identify the source of the toxin as quickly as possible.

Test questions
- Everything I drink
- Everything I eat
- All the meat
- All the vegetables
- All the sweet food
- …

Test Card 12   Systems

The test card for issues specific to systems, projects, companies and organizations

For the greatest good

Which intention is behind a project? Does it serve to deceive others, sell a bad product at a high price, or is the product an expression of creativity and Creation, serving the "the big plan"? This rules out all manufacturers of weapons of war as *innerwise* customers. However, not just them … but anybody with dishonorable intentions.

Clarity

This refers to the inner clarity and structure of a project.

Goals and objectives

What is that project good for? What is the goal of the project? Which strategies are in place to reach that goal? Are all those participating in the project connected to its goal? Is it about the value of the products? Is it about happy product users? Is it about quality, and also about the joy and fun involved in creating something together?

Stability

Is the project like a tree—firmly rooted with a clear direction of growth? Can it move in the wind and adjust to the different seasons?

Nourishment

Is the project nourished on all levels: on the structural level; regarding the inner chemistry; in the processes; on the mental, emotional and energetic levels; and the soul of the project?

Toxins

These are the great poisons that can destroy all creation: fear, manipulation, guilt, greed, envy, sabotage, disappointment, consciousness of lack.

Identification

Can all those participating in the project identify with it? "I love my work, I'm glad to be able to participate and contribute, and I take an active role."
Or would it be better to take certain people out of the project and include others who really love it?
Personally, I no longer work with people who don't love their work.

Communication
Can everyone involved talk to one another openly, honestly, free of fear and projections, and across all structures?

Names and logo
Do they even fit into the project? Do they express the project's intention and values optimally?
If not, they have to be changed—in an unrelenting and honest way. A project is an artistic synthesis, and what doesn't fit needs to be modified. It's possible to test the name and logo with the arm-length test, but also tune in to them to feel what they trigger.

Products
Are these products of value? Are they products that stand for quality and love, or should they merely keep three days beyond their warranty period and continually require further purchase?

Balance
If the whole project was a scale, how would it look (in balance or out of balance)? This refers to the male and female energies of the system. (And I don't mean the number of men and women!) Also look at the levels of decision-making, inner workflows and more.

Competence
What are the competencies of those involved? Are they in the right position? Do they have the right qualifications for their area? Do they have the possibility to grow in their area?

Management
How is the project managed? What are the related qualifications? How about organizational and leadership skills, authenticity, honesty and truthfulness?

Processes
This topic has two sides: internal workflows and business processes on the one side, and growth processes on the other. Growth is process work, and it's necessary to let this happen, otherwise it turns into a dictatorship. This includes social and interactive process understanding, clarification and resolution, growth, and the ability to accept processes in gratitude. Anything that remains unresolved internally can be sensed in the products in the end.

Site/location

Has the right country been chosen for the project? Is the project located in the right region, with the right transport connections? And what about the company or organization itself: Is there environmental pollution or stress, electrosmog in the workplace, geopathic interference, or are there charges and energetic influences from previous users of this site or building?

Freedom

Are individuality, freedom of choice, creativity and freedom from manipulation desirable, and are they lived? Don't try to coach projects using *innerwise* that don't count freedom among their goals. This would be an abuse of *innerwise*.

Vertical integration

Are all the structures integrated that exist in a vertical line one on top of another—that is, the internal hierarchy? How are decision-making processes passed on and implemented from top to bottom? How is information transmitted from the "lower levels" to the management of the company or organization and integrated into the management's decision-making?

Horizontal integration

Are parallel structures, such as teams and areas, integrated? Are all working together with the bigger picture in mind and as part of one entity, or does every area try to reinvent the wheel?

Values

Is this company or organization based on inner values? Or is the price of shares the only value?
Owner-based companies (such as family-run businesses) have a clear advantage when it comes to living their values, because the people who created them are still the ones in the driver's seat.

Flow

Is the project in the flow?
In a flow of creativity, of money, of goods?
Are decisions also taken in the flow, or only based on directives and schedules?

Future

What does the project future look like? If everything continues as it is now, how does the project feel in two years?
Does the project invest in its future? Is research done with responsibility toward the environment, resources and people?
Is there a holistic view? Is there a measured approach?
Is this project carried by a vision?

Heart

Is the project considered a living and lovable being? When looking at the project only with one's heart, how does it feel? What is its aura like? What does it generate in the people who will be associated with the project, the company or organization, and the products?

Test Card 13   Integrity

Integrity is my way

From the Homo sapiens to the Homo integer—the integrated human

The meaning of *Homo sapiens* refers to the reasonable, wise, judicious and understanding, diplomatic human. Being reasonable doesn't necessarily mean being honest, being understanding isn't as broad as being circumspect, and diplomacy involves lying. Humans currently behave like they have been named. Reality follows the field, the sound and the energy. It's similar to being on a dance floor: the music determines how people move. If you want to change the moves, change the music. It's as simple as that. If we want to change the world, the easiest way to do so is to give people a new name, changing their sound: *Homo integer—the integrated human.*

Homo integer: the honest, pure, decent, intact, whole, sound, unblemished, unspoiled, pristine, authentic, unbroken, complete and incorruptible human.

What a world that would be! It's time for the Homo integer; and for an honest, whole, sound, lovable Earth worth living in! Let's live our dreams, break meaningless rules, think freely, be honest with ourselves and others, walk our own true path of life and thus have access to unlimited energy.

Integrity is my way

Be part of this movement of like-minded people who've made the conscious decision to live with more integrity. The *Integrity is my way* movement was initiated by Uwe Albrecht in order to share the opportunity to publicly commit to integrity and jointly create a field that supports the transition to a more livable world. This movement serves as a platform to jointly create reality and implement new projects together with inspiring individuals. *Integrity is my way* is a nonprofit movement. *www.integrity-is-my-way.com*

Integrity

These parameters and percentage levels provide you with a good overview on where you are in life at any given moment. They're not intended to create judgment; rather, they aim to offer understanding on how things are connected, as well as help you determine where you stand and set the next objectives on your life's journey.

Integrity in %
How high is your level of integrity right now?

Honesty in %

Your honesty toward yourself in all your thoughts, emotions and actions constitutes the basis for your ability to be honest with others. We can only give what we
have and live ourselves.

Authenticity in %

Do you live your life by your values and words? Do your thoughts, emotions and
actions match? If so, your authenticity can serve as an example, and you will be
able to inspire others with your Being.

Compromises in %

You recognize a compromise by virtue of the fact that it saps energy. With compromises, you lie to yourself and to life. They are the forces that prevent you from
experiencing the abundance of life, because you give too much power to your
fears.

Completeness in %

It's possible to experience the completeness of our soul, of our glow and Being.
Often we lose much of that over the course of our lives. Our eyes lose their shine,
our sound loses its beauty, our inner fire loses its strength, our time loses its slow
quality, and our amazement loses its greatness. It helps to know the current actual level of completeness in order to then be able to increase it again; in doing
so, there are no limits unless you set them yourself.

Self-responsibility in %

Have you created your life yourself, or are you a victim of life? Can you change
your life, or is someone supposed to save you? How much self-responsibility do
you live?

I am responsible for my life, as I alone have created it, and I am also the only one
who can change it. This phrase is the essence of being and acting like an adult. It's
not always easy to recognize that we've created our lives ourselves by attracting
issues and learning tasks through our resonance with them. We like to see ourselves as victims, yet in reality, we've done it 100 percent ourselves. Often simply,
because our individual life plan has foreseen these experiences to lead us to insight.

Charges

You may call it energetic charges, hatred, fear, aggression, self-destruction or negative focus—it's all the same: charges represent all that love is not. Many people have a charge level between 50 and 80 percent. Frequently, however, our optimal or feel-good range only sets in below 20 percent. Charges are *the* cause of aggression between people, ranging from energetic, emotional or physical aggression … all the way to war. Someone with a high charge level discharges him- or herself toward another individual with a lower level. Charges are also *the* cause of illness, as self-destruction manifests itself in this form.

Actual level in %
How high is your actual charge level currently in percents? This can change quickly, sometimes within minutes. It can rise when we take on charges, and fall when we've re-established our inner balance.

Fear-based decisions in %
How many of your decisions are based on fears? These include deep fears, such as the fear of pain, the fear of starving or the fear of not being loved, as well as more superficial fears that are part of daily life. The alternatives to fear-based decisions are decisions based on trust—that is, allowing life to happen.

Optimal level in %
How low should the level of charges that you carry be so that you feel good about yourself, experience peace and a sense of inner balance, and are able to trust yourself? This is your personal optimal or feel-good range regarding love. As your consciousness continues to evolve and grow, this level often keeps declining, residing between 20 and 0 percent—that is, 80 to 100 percent love. As you're leaving this range by taking on charges, you may feel restless inside, nervous and energetically dirty. Find ways to "be love" as much as possible, and on a long term basis; if you leave this feel-good range and your level of charges—that is, the opposite of love—is increasing, balance yourself in order to re-establish your optimal level.

Sources I am an instrument for

It's not the fields within us, but the forces, programs and sources that work through us; and for those, we made ourselves available, either voluntarily or not. These can include our own life purpose, but also other sources that aren't so pure. Independent of whether or not we know what works through us, we're still responsible for that which works through us and which has an effect.

Sources can have one of two qualities: pure or impure. Only our own life purpose is pure; it's the Divine within each individual, which stems directly from Oneness and wants to unfold through each of us. All those sources that have been tainted with duality on their path are impure, as they always include both light and dark aspects.

Sources connect to us via higher complex spaces—that is, through reality spaces that are beyond both the "plus space"—the light space, and the "minus space"—the dark space. These spaces are usually beyond our perception. This makes these sources hard to identify. Frequently, we have to find and connect to our individual life purpose, our soul passion, and we can also lose this connection again. Connections to impure sources come from initiations, drugs or manipulation. In this way, we become an instrument for these sources that can exert their effect through us on other people, thereby often weakening them energetically. In return, we receive a kind of energetic commission. We need to separate from and let go of these impure sources, and then find, or find again, our connection to our own pure source.

Number
Test the total number of sources that work through you.

Number of impure sources
How many of these sources are impure?

Presence of the pure source in %
If a pure source exists, it can be present to a varying extent; or how much you surrender to this source can vary—that is, how much you allow your connection to be. Measure the presence of the pure source in percents.

The need and the necessity

These are the words of the great writer Doris Lessing. In her book *The Sirian Experiments,* she describes three different civilizations: one that lives following the principle of maximum growth; another that lives on stolen energy, and yet another that makes all decisions according to the need and the necessity. The latter is the only stable and balanced civilization.

Living in accordance with the need and the necessity describes the ability to surrender to our individual life purpose, the big plan, and to let it guide us. Often we wish to create our lives based on our needs and wants. In most cases, this isn't very successful. Alternatively, we can allow our life plan to ensure that we can fulfill our soul purpose; then, we also receive all the support to make this possible. We can then experience a kind of flow and abundance that is unknown to most people.

Responsibility in %

In case of a burnout, you have too many responsibilities; with a boreout, it's too few. In my experience, the optimal range lies between 25 and 40 percent. Then your life is filled with meaning, but you're not overwhelmed. Of course, we can also handle a responsibility level of 95 percent for a short period, but not long term. Now you might ask: What is 100 percent responsibility? This is the point when you have exceeded the maximum level, the utmost limit of what you can perform, and collapse under the weight.

I live in accordance with the need and the necessity

This is not just about your individual needs, but *the* need and *the* necessity—that is, the goal is to live in accordance with my life plan *and* the overall all-encompassing plan. With this statement, you'll get only a "yes" or "no" response. To find out further details, you'll need to measure the exact percentage of the extent to which you live according to the need and the necessity.

Actual level in %

Currently, how high is your actual level of living according to the need and the necessity? In different situations this can vary largely. You can also test this percentage in regard to individual decisions.

Optimal level in %

What should be your minimum level of accordance with the need and the necessity so that your life plan can guide you and you can live life in flow, lightness and ease? These percentages can vary greatly. Some people already feel fine with a level of 60 percent, others only at 98 percent. The higher the value, the more radical and clear your decisions in life have to be in order to experience the abundance of Being—and the greater your life will be.

If you're still searching for your life purpose, your soul passion, let me share my experience: You can't find it. *It* finds you—when you clarify and put an end to all compromises in your life. Then, your life purpose is what remains. Life can be easy and beautiful if we surrender to our life purpose, thereby becoming an instrument of Creation. Then, our inner struggles and all other types of destruction are over.

"No, you can't always get what you want. But if you try sometimes, you just might find you get what you need."

From "You Can't Always Get What
You Want" by the Rolling Stones

Test Card 14   Make Me An Instrument

Make Me An Instrument

Creation reveals itself essentially through mathematics and numbers. Numbers serve as gateways to particular energetic and information patterns here. To activate a specific pattern, you can use a number code that you either create freely or with the help of the *innerwise* healing-code generator, which you will find at *www.innerwise.com*. If the question is clear and precise, the right number code will show. Number codes can be long—usually, up to 25-digit codes suffice.

Healing codes

These complex number codes have the power to activate certain functions in the hologram.

Visualize being in the hologram and letting the number code manifest its healing effects like a sound cloud in the hologram and thus also in you.

There is no need to learn the number codes by heart; simply look at them or put your hand on them, and take them with you *virtually* into the hologram.

Purification

Purification

5547632543852735-5547632543852748-5547632543852759-5746986
3707777325-64536952157426-74680535831-64795357425

We can experience irritations and poisonings on all levels—the physical, biochemical, rhythmic, mental, emotional, energetic, spiritual or unknown levels.

Pure sound

Code for pure sound

63840584634807413-63840695745918524-594843473-73652673-5937
63752541752-6737847737626

Sound emanates from people, animals, living and work spaces, and systems. It can be beautiful and harmonious, or unpleasant and disharmonious. Disharmonies hurt; they're ugly. They always reflect interrupted flow. They lead to struggle and loss. Disharmonious people squeak like unlubricated doors. We can harmonize our sound by cleaning up our lives, clearing charges and finding peace within ourselves. Nada Brahma—the world is sound.

Pure structure

Code for pure structure

53268342158336836-53379453269447947

The body of a newborn is so pure, so perfect. Forty years later it's a different story. The body starts to age and hurt here and there; old and foreign charges have accumulated. What is foreign—that is, not ours—and what is old, sound different to what is our own and what is clear. It is from this difference in sound that we can recognize it.

Healing energetic and spiritual trauma
Code for healing energetic and spiritual trauma
58484920757574935-529476158-54853-9627
Even after we forgive and forget, energetic scars or fissures often still remain in our field.

Getting back lost time
Code for getting back lost time
37236874752985941-37236874752196052-674931496317
Time is alive; it changes speed, direction and flow. Continuous and linear is the one thing that time is certainly *not*. Why does it appear to pass more and more quickly in the course of our lives? Is it really getting faster or only thinner?
Imagine time as a wide river when we incarnated—so wide that we had all the time in the world to feel amazed—but getting thinner and thinner during our lives. That's why it seems to go faster—just as water flows faster through a narrow tube than a wide one. And at some point, time is up. The time available has become thinner because some parts of it have been lost, frozen rigid as a result of shocks, gone backward in a nostalgic homage to the past, or disappeared into other dimensions as we fled from reality. Where is this lost time? It isn't gone, but exists somewhere in infinite space. The 12-dimensional image-layer structure of the *Make Me An Instrument* hologram represents this infinite space. It's all in the hologram, thus, lost time is in there, too. We simply have to get it back. As Michael Ende would say: "Let's crack the Timesaving Bank!"
Imagine standing in the most centrally located sphere of the hologram and sending out a lightwave that fills the whole hologram, the entire space—a wave that awakens your lost time and sends it a signal that you're ready to reintegrate it into your life. Once the entire hologram is activated, imagine this time flowing back to the center where you're standing. It can densify to white light, for example, which you then reincorporate, breathe in and integrate.
Be more careful with your time and never allow the men in gray from the Timesaving Bank to steal it from you again.

A whole and complete soul

Code for a whole and complete soul
9204042479214741581-9204153580325852692-920426469143696370
3-674594842488527-57487374168425825739124024247424734 1607
33825635147363683927

Having, being and living with a whole and complete soul is everybody's dream. Most people, however, are light years from that goal. As a result of the many traumatic experiences in life, most parts of the Self, the soul, have fragmented and disappeared—or so it seems. Being a complete soul, being in the now, feeling the divine flow through you and living as an instrument of peace is a high, and the only truly meaningful purpose in life.

Transforming charges into love

Code for transforming charges into love
5638270683254289-95257980642367346786325743210485274357964
-76141685346789 5326357-46534760263856934 1273682-3639582634

Love and charges are key to understanding and healing. We all harbor energetic charges within us. They're the opposite of love and are visible in fear, manipulation or many other ways. Charges and hatred lead to the destruction of oneself and others. Charges can be used to trigger and control a vicious circle of self-destruction. Many people have a charge level between 50 and 80 percent. The higher this level, the greater the negativity these people emanate. Some even have a charge level of 98 percent. Those used to living with a low charge level (below 20 percent) who experience a sudden dramatic increase due to an irritation of some sort, see themselves unconsciously as energetically unclean, even infectious, and begin to hide, to destroy themselves, to tear out what is ill, even if it's the soul itself. It's an attempt to prevent something worse. In the end, trying to counteract this with treatment even exacerbates the situation, since the self-destruction mechanism is not recognized as an ultimate form of protection. And a huge amount of energy is lost in the process. So, reduce your charge level as much as you can.

Better sleep

Code for better sleep
46848484-4164184379170-636735841738-135792468018

Sleep is more about *dis*charging all absorbed energies than recharging. The more that's discharged, the better your sleep. Good night!

Supporting spiritual growth

Code for supporting spiritual growth

3737373848595061627374 5-373737384859506162737 4548494041424
3444546474849404184248 2001168169527

The freedom to move within the 12 dimensions of Being and to be able to see from these dimensions is the gift of spiritual growth.

Resolving issues carried for others at their source

Code for resolving issues carried for others at their source

58946852749317537974752 5942595358537531695384 247003690744
69635842585374247526908 6000000053795380000000 00000000000001

On average, about one-third of our irritations and symptoms aren't based on our own issues; we only *carry* these issues, or we pay for them or pass them on. The most important source of the charges that cause these irritations and symptoms are our parents and ancestors. What hasn't been resolved will be passed on to the next generation. Other sources are all those people whose loads we want to ease. Such loads include traumas, secrets and charges we've taken on. However, we can only resolve issues where they come from: at their source.

With this code, we open up the connection to the source of the issues even if they go back generations, give back the unresolved charges and resolve them at their source.

Ending manipulation

Code for ending manipulation

642595026158-73925217-846428631753863-9190-4263773504273597
43-5761903456186158-55378538663910-764950852-586249-5385-637
6259742-536847935902673-63485205705074 2486375-5849731741693
83-85705269528458-4674642736346-74747368472749-274838493829
1038-483927166061626364 65666768696106047392666-73593279063
583836-7858428947939327 8392-53739536942593134-642794274831
95283840-584642441694273-63748074603738538417 4804273-64948
392

Many people are hungry for energy because they aren't nourished by life through being connected to their soul purpose. They steal energy from others.

Cutting the links to impure sources

Code for cutting the links to impure sources

A Purifying my own field
   76264848536

B Bidding adieu to impure energy sources by focusing the code on their energetic center
   58382827362826379826-636248362-713627579237904735262-83838
   3818181-463790705060403020109 08222

C Letting go of impure energy sources
   49367284952-99723707317-9999963652941-65248426384-852368637
   63-65337484276

D Activating my own pure source
   281605637350483429419536096952642584839418489600407586858
   59093

We are often energetic servants of unknown masters, using energy sources or allowing them to use us. All initiations, for example, open gateways to energy
sources. If these are pure, it's a gift. If they're impure, however, the energy we radiate as an instrument of these sources becomes ever darker and more manipulative
with time. You *can* separate from impure sources.

But this also means giving up on the power potential that you were able to tap
into by being connected to these sources. Follow the steps in order: A, B, C, D.

Test Card 15   The Seeing Space

I see what you don't see.
The Earth is flat, says the hiker.
The Earth is huge and round, says the Moon.
The Earth is small and revolves around me, says the Sun.
From their own perspectives, they are all correct.

The Seeing Space

The field

What is foreign

Parts, fields, energies or sources left in the individual that were taken in on a voluntary basis, or left through manipulation, or implanted.

What is lost

Parts, fields, energies or sources of the individual that were given away by him- or herself on a voluntary basis, left somewhere, or taken away by others on an involuntary basis.

Gateways

Gateways into or out of individuals, enabling influencing. They can be created or used in two ways.
1. by something foreign left in the individual, or
2. by a part or parts of the individual that separated from him- or herself or were removed, and are located outside of that individual.

Intelligent fields

Fields that are independent of matter and have their own intelligence. Depending on their degree of purity, they can offer positive support or manipulate in negative ways. Manipulating fields, in particular, are hard to discern and identify as the cause of irritations due to their complexity, changeability, diversity and polymorph nature.

The cause

1. Interactive

Originating in the interaction between individuals, related issues need to be resolved there.

2. Intrapersonal
Originating within an individual, related issues need to be resolved there. Personal life issues.

3. Family-related
Originating in the family and the ancestors' field, related issues need to be resolved there.

4. Local
Originating in places where people lived or live, related issues need to be resolved there.

5. Regional
Originating in the region, related issues need to be resolved there.

6. Cultural
Originating in the cultural history and identification, related issues need to be resolved there.

7. National
Originating in the nation or tribe, related issues need to be resolved there.

8. Religious
Originating in religious influences and imprints, related issues need to be resolved there.

9. Related to evolutionary biology
Originating in evolutionary processes throughout time, related issues need to be resolved there.

10. Species-specific
Originating in the species, related issues need to be resolved there.

11. Cosmic
Anchored in the cosmic field, related issues need to be resolved there.

Seeing

I see

This offers the lowest quality of seeing things—from our individual perspective, tainted by personal inner judgment, expectations and experiences. Our vision is always limited, and we look at things subjectively, which often leads to biased results.

It sees

Be an instrument of seeing—*it* sees through us. Moving from a subjective to an objective way of seeing things. Freeing our vision from what's individual, as well as time and space, it becomes possible to see things objectively. Our vision is broadened as we look at things from the higher dimensions of Being according to Burkhard Heim, which further improves the quality of seeing. In the end, only those who look at something from the same dimension will also obtain the same results as they test and look at things. You can test from which of the 12 dimensions you are looking at something, or whether *it* is looking through you.

With the *Make Me An Instrument* hologram and the number code "Supporting spiritual growth" (37373738485950616273745-37373738485950616273745 48494041424344454647484940418424482001168169527), you can gain access to vision involving the higher dimensions according to Heim.

Inner wisdom

We never experience the same quality in our vision, whether *we* see, or *it* sees—that is, when we are an instrument of seeing; neither is our ability to see things and the quality independent from us. Rather, they always depend on the next steps that we are meant to take in our evolution and growth. For many things, we need to go through the actual experience, which will allow us to grow. The goal of our growth is always greater clarity and purity. Thus, what we are given the opportunity, and are able to see, becomes ever more clear.

The following may serve as an image to illustrate the above: Imagine a lake; you are able to see everything that is above the surface of the water. If the water level drops as a result of our experiences in life and growing inner wisdom, things and issues will become visible that, so far, remained under the surface. The lower the water level, the more issues will be visible that we weren't able to see before. And only once all the water is gone, we will have reached our full inner wisdom. You can also test in percents how high the water level is right now, giving you an idea of what is not yet visible to you at this very time.

The space

Multiple reality spaces

Besides the "light" side, the "plus space," which we like to display in public, and which we utilize when resolving issues on the surface, there is also the dark side, the "minus space." Only few people want to enter it in order to look at issues and their roots there, and resolve them. These two spaces make up duality. But this doesn't suffice to describe life. We still need the third space. This space represents all possible further reality spaces—that is, an infinite number of them. In these spaces, we will find the cause of many complex issues, such as the connection to impure sources. By consciously involving these complex reality spaces that are also described in quantum physics, we can target healing energies and let them manifest their effects precisely and successfully there.

Individual space

This refers to our usual way of looking at an individual with his or her structure, field, energies, rhythms and space.

Space equivalents

These refer to spaces surrounding an individual; spaces that don't seem to be related to the individual but that create the space within which the individual exists, and through which he or she is connected to other individuals. Those spaces are as important as the direct space—that is, the individual space, when it comes to creating reality. With space equivalents, we are leaving the causal relation between an individual's issues and his or her life, experiences, energies and fields, and allow other spaces that are not related to the individual to influence him or her as an expression of Creation's systemic complexity.

System Test Cards

Tools for your professional work with systems, companies and organizations, projects and teams. 30 test cards offering around 400 specific topics to analyze systems and guide you with confidence throughout your coaching, in ways you are already familiar with from the other testing systems.

Here you can find an overview of the test cards, each covering 10 to 20 thematic complexes.

System test card topics

Parameters
Staff
System management
Products & services
Heart & soul
Creativity
Workflow
Growth & transformation
Graphics & design
Inner world & environment
System structure
Sources of energy
Perspective
Manipulation & influencing
Energetic charges
Integrity
Identity
Finances
Communication/integration
Flow regulation
History
Marketing/PR

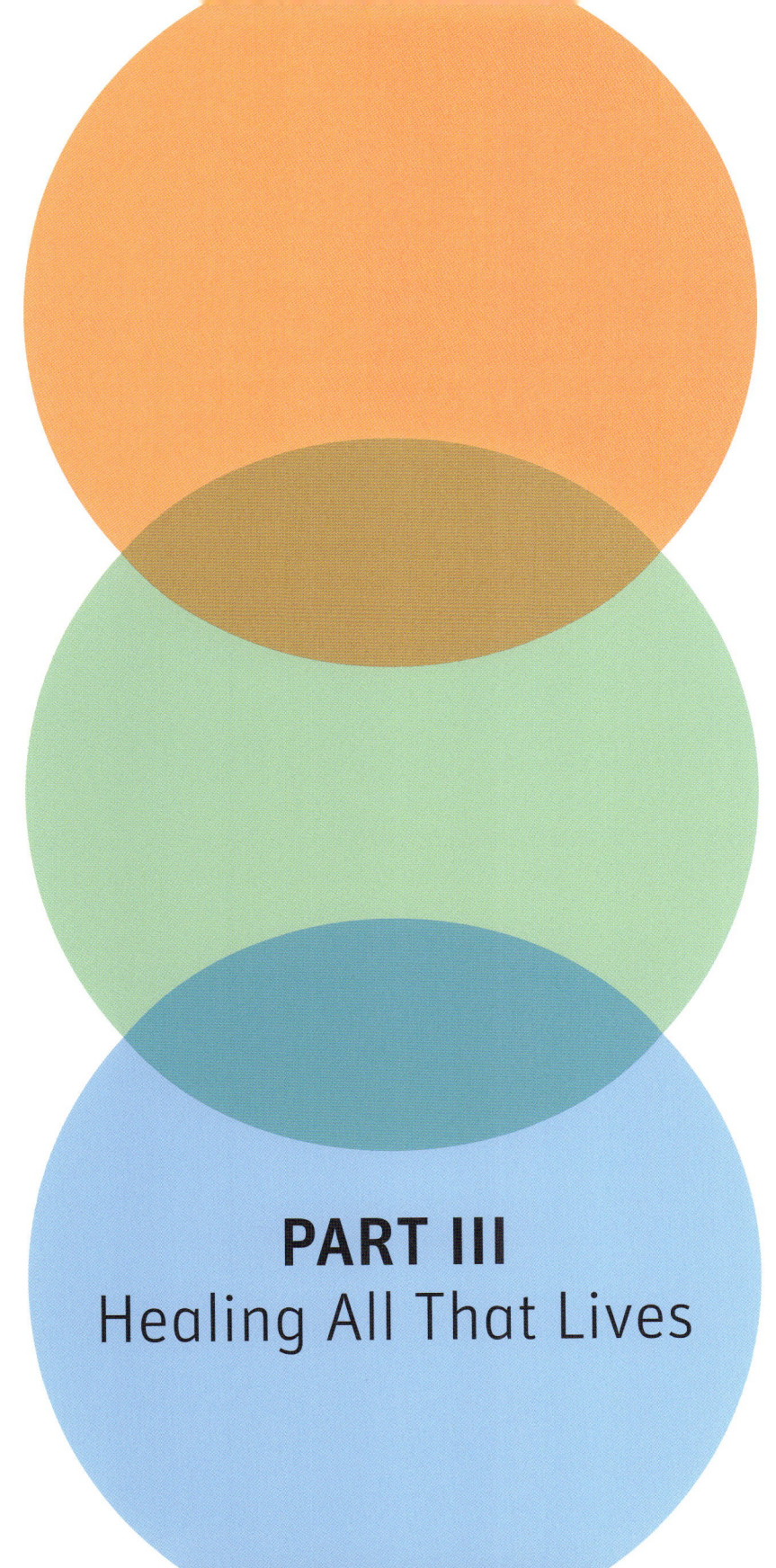

PART III
Healing All That Lives

Overview

The third part includes using *innerwise*

- to heal people, animals, plants, buildings and landscapes,
- for learning, creativity and relationships
- and in the work with companies and organizations, projects and systems.

1. How to Use *innerwise*

Step by Step

Feeling, sensing, tuning in, experiencing a true encounter and developing empathy

At first, it's about feeling and sensing oneself—and then the person or system we're working with—in order to gain an overview and be able to empathize, as well as to have the option to compare the current state with the initial situation during the treatment.

Diagnostics using the arm-length test

We "grasp" the initial state with the arm-length test. This includes testing the basic parameters, such as identity, life energy and integrity; performing a diagnosis on the organic, structural and rhythmic level; and clarifying the client's treatment goals.

Letting ourselves be guided by the testing system

The testing system guides us toward healing in the most effective way. We intuitively select the first test card and place it on the client. If it causes stress in the client, this will show up in the arm-length test. However, only one of the 10 to 20 topics included in the test card is active. It can be sensed intuitively (active topics feel different from others) or identified with the arm-length test. At any given moment, only one topic of the entire testing system is active; it's precisely the one that shows the most effective way through the healing process.

Composing the healing symphony

With the help of the healing cards, we compose a healing symphony by drawing cards intuitively. This can be one or several healing cards for each issue. We can always refer to the arm-length test to double-check the result: "Does this suffice for this issue?" "Do I need another card?" Some issues can be resolved with one healing card; others need more. Then, the healing cards are placed on the client.

If the client is lying down, simply put it on his or her belly or chest. When treating yourself or when working with someone who's standing up, put the healing cards in a pocket of the clothes. At this point, clients can often sense changes in their body themselves, and the therapist can observe what has changed in the client's body compared to the status diagnosed initially. Double-checking the testing topic with the arm-length test using the client's arms will show if the issue is already resolved.

Process: Identify the issue through testing, resolve the issue with healing cards and observe the changes resulting from that process until the testing topic no longer creates stress. This can take from five minutes to one and a half hours.

In between, the therapist leads the communication in order to explain the connections and guide the client through the therapeutic process.

Perceiving the changes

This is about feeling and sensing the changes. Even if no test cards cause stress anymore and all symptoms are stress-free in the arm-length test, this doesn't mean that they're necessarily all gone. The ground has been prepared so that they can disappear. Now the therapist lets the client tune in to him- or herself again and describe the changes. Oftentimes, it's also a good idea to ask clients to tune in to how they'll feel in two, four or six days, because some changes need time.

Checking symptoms and completing the treatment

To complete the treatment, a final check with the arm-length test serves to once more test all parameters that revealed stress in the initial diagnosis. If clients still need healing cards, they're added at this point. Only then are all symptoms checked with the arm-length test to determine if they still create stress. If they do, add additional healing cards, as required.

Now clients can once more visualize all wishes regarding their treatment goals.

With the arm-length test, we double-check once more whether any of the topics create stress that can be balanced using healing cards. The question "Is the treatment complete for the client?" should yield a "yes" response. However, it can still be the case that the treatment is complete for the client but not for his or her environment.

Yet we want the changes to be integrated. Therefore, it's better to ask, "Is the treatment complete for all involved?"

This is followed by the two mandatory final questions: "Is there something else I can do? Is there something else I'm allowed to do?" If we get a "no" to both questions, the treatment is finished even if the client would like more, or if the therapist likes to play the hero and wants to "make it all nice." Making it all nice for clients, taking away their self-responsibility, is detrimental to them in the long run and only builds dependency on the therapist. "Can you recharge my batteries?" "Can you make my pain go away again?" It's not our responsibility as therapists to "make it all nice." Rather, it's about giving again clients the possibility to change their lives and to no longer "need" their symptoms.

The easiest way to determine whether the treatment is complete is by testing the following statement: "I have done everything that I was allowed to do for all involved." If this statement yields a "yes" response, the treatment is complete.

Copying the healing symphony to the amulet

Copying the healing symphony to the amulet is really easy: Place the amulet or Balance Card in one palm, lay the copy card on top of it, put the healing cards on top of the copy card, and hold your other hand over the top. An energy field is created below the upper hand. Meanwhile, the therapist once more feels the healing symphony that was composed, and in doing so, completely separates from the connection he or she had built with the client for the duration of the treatment. An energy wave goes through the healing cards into the amulet or Balance Card and expands from there into the space around you. Thus, the healing symphony is available to the client via the amulet or Balance Card. Sensitive people will notice that the copy card isn't needed to transfer the energies. This is correct, but not usually a common scenario. If therapists resonate with an issue raised during the treatment, and as a result, lose some of their clarity and concentration, the copy card always ensures a reliable transfer of the healing symphony.

Instructing clients how to use the arm-length test

I show all clients how they can do the arm-length test themselves. In this way, we help them to live and make decisions with greater self-responsibility.

Using the amulet

Wearing the amulet. Now clients may wear the amulet, and a few times a day, take a moment to visualize their wishes and listen to the sounds of the healing symphony with their heart. This can also be called *meditation.*

Changing your life

Everyone may do this alone.

Follow-up treatments

They take place according to the client's needs. Here, it's important to give the client time to integrate the results. Therefore, there can be several months between individual treatments. Applying the arm-length test is the best way to determine the interval, or we leave it up to the client when he or she wants to contact us again.

In follow-up treatments, new healing symphonies are transferred to the existing amulets, Balance Cards or discs.

Is it necessary to erase the amulets?

Since *innerwise* is based on the principle of resonance, we only sense those energies that we still resonate with; no memory has to be erased. In fact, the energies only come through the system; they're not directly stored in something.

When asked the question as to whether amulets or discs need to be erased, I like to respond, "You didn't kill every former lover either, did you?" When the resonance is gone, it's gone.

2. The Art of Healing

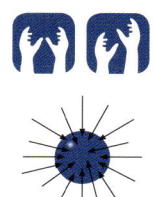

> ## Testing topics
>
> - Use the arm-length test to determine if there's stress in your liver.
>
> - Test how freely the energy flows in your solar plexus.
>
> - Feel your breath.
>
> - If a sick child comes to see you for a treatment, do you treat the child, or do you first treat the parents?
>
> - What is the percentage of couples who hope to conceive but who haven't been successful thus far, and who don't show stress in the arm-length test when asked to imagine being pregnant or becoming a father?
>
> - Do you also feel confident working with animals and buildings?

No matter who uses *innerwise*—**whether physicians, dentists, psychologists, alternative health practitioners, energy practitioners or anybody treating themselves—they all use the same basic tools, and give a treatment based on their competencies and experience.**

For 20 years I've been working solely with *innerwise* in my medical practice. I no longer write prescriptions for conventional medical drugs, and hardly ever need lab or imaging diagnostics. This is possible.

In treatments, the key is that we no longer try to treat symptoms, but instead, search for the causes, find them and resolve them. Then, symptoms can disappear by themselves because they're no longer needed.

If I treat symptoms, I don't change anything about the basic charges behind them, which will make their presence felt again with irritations at the surface. If they aren't allowed to surface in one place, they'll show up again in another.

Intuitive diagnostics

Consultation
"What can I do for you today?" instead of the usual "How are we doing today?"

At the beginning, clients have the opportunity to explain why they came and what they expect from the therapist—a "classic" start, if you like. At this point, the therapist's interest is awakened. Then, I show patients who've come to see me for the first time how the arm-length test works.

It's important that therapists don't engage in "victim" or "poor-me" talks. Neither is it about offering solace, but rather, bringing the conversation back to the client's self-responsibility while keeping an open and loving heart.

The arm-length test
The arm-length test is the best way to convince even skeptical clients, or at least provide food for thought. It's a bridge that builds trust. In the case of skeptical husbands, you can also pull their arms a bit more vigorously when they're standing up to get them to think about it.

Then, I ask my patients to lie down on their back on the massage table, and I have a close look at them—at the length of their legs, pelvic position, how they're lying there and how they're breathing.

With the help of the arm-length test, I check the initial state of their ground regulation:

• Are both arms equally long when the patient says "yes," or aren't they?
• Do the arms differ in length when the patient says "no," and if so, how big is the difference?

This clearly reveals whether patients have an open ground regulation, experience initial stress, are in a panic or are in a state of rigidity.

If the client's state is irritated, it always makes sense to go back in time to determine how long this irritation has been present:
"Imagine that it's yesterday (one year ago, five years ago)." Or, "Now we're going back in time. How was your state four days ago (six months ago, two years ago)?"

In this way, you can identify the cause very quickly, especially in the case of a rigidity.

Once, a patient came to see me in my practice after a motorcycle accident. He was in a state of rigidity, which had started five days prior to the accident. Therefore, we had to clear this rigidity first before working on the accident and its consequences.

Feeling, sensing, perceiving

"May I tune in to you in order to sense you?"

With this question, I ask permission for a very deep contact with the patient. This occurs when we sense someone as if we *were* this person. Apart from a few exceptions where I don't want to tune in to the energy or prefer to feel it by virtually placing it on my hand and sensing it there because the energies involved are so unpleasant and manipulative, I identify with the patient for a few seconds, which enables me to feel their pain, blockages or emotions within myself. To do so, I close my eyes in order to be able to concentrate better.

This moment offers a great opportunity to be able to gain a better understanding of that person, and also move freely in time. Within seconds, I can move through this person's life as if I were in an elevator, and determine when certain patterns and irritations originated.

When sensing people, it's important to pay attention to their stance, how the load is distributed between their right and left leg, their breathing, their rhythms, and their ability to move through life. Sometimes one has the feeling that people can't get going, that their feet are stuck solid in cement, that one half of their body feels different from the other, or many other things.

Basic topics and symptoms

Then, I sit down on the massage table next to the patient's legs, and I start testing the wishes that the patient came to see me for, using the arm-length test.

However, in the event that in the arm-length test, patients showed initial stress or were in a state of rigidity, I first pick healing cards to resolve this. Guided by your intention to find the right cards, you can draw them intuitively from the set of cards and test their effectiveness by placing them on the patient and repeating the arm-length test.

After that, I ask the patient to participate actively:

"Imagine being healthy again and having a zest for life!"

"Imagine still being alive in ten years!" (with cancer patients)

"Imagine having a partner; being pregnant; having a job that you enjoy; being able to breathe freely again; singing the musical note *A* loud and clear!"

The result often comes like a shock to the patients—the arms reveal a stress response in all cases of such statements and imaginations.

"How is something supposed to happen that you can't even imagine?"

This reveals the unconscious programs that create reality with a manifestation power of 95 percent (compared to the 5 percent of the conscious mind). It's important to show the patients what their unconscious wants, and also does.

Testing organs

Now it's time for you to gain an overview of the organs.

For this purpose, you can either touch the skin above the organ—as if you intended to exercise light pressure on that organ—or you can touch the organ energetically with your hand at a distance of a couple of inches, and then check the reaction to this stimulus with the arm-length test.

"Hi liver, how are you doing today?" Such a witty question feels good, and in treatments, people should always laugh as well.

Always keep in mind that you want to see and test organs on all levels. If the arm-length test reveals stress in the client's liver, this stress can reside on the organic, biochemical, mental, emotional, energetic, spiritual or an unknown level; or, it can involve more than one of those.

For a more precise understanding, test the liver on all levels individually:

"Liver on the organic level."

"Liver on the biochemical level," and so on.

Naturally, the liver's most commonly affected level is the emotional one. This stems from swallowing so much and being angry at oneself for having denied one's own Self once again.

As you can see in the checklist, it makes sense to start with the upper abdomen and then continue with the kidneys, lower abdomen, chest, head, rhythms and then stance and structure. In this way, you can perform a complete diagnosis within one to five minutes.

For therapists, it's important to keep practicing their sensing skills, such as by sensing the body's rhythms with their hands, or the energy fields of irritated organs.

Or, the client is asked to take a deep breath and then exhale so that the therapist can check the respiratory function using the arm-length test. Alternatively, therapists can also imagine that their hands are the lungs of the client. With their hands, they carry out the client's breathing cycle and are able to precisely determine that "during a deep inhale, there's a blockage in the left lung," for example.

Rhythms

It's important to sense the fine rhythms—the freedom and proper functioning of the nerve plexuses, craniosacral rhythm and cranial breath.

If you hold your hand above the solar plexus (stomach area) with the palm facing up, and imagine that your hand *is* the solar plexus, and you try out how freely it moves by moving your hand up and down, you can check the nerve plexus. If it's free, your hand can move as if there is zero gravity. If it's blocked, your hand can only move with difficulty, the feeling may be heavy and/or viscous; or your hand won't be able to move at all, depending on the extent of the blockage.

The nerve plexuses carry out the fine-tuning of all organs. If they're blocked, the organs are thrown out of kilter.

Now check the pelvic plexus, which regulates the entire lower abdomen (sexual function, a woman's cycle, etc.); the navel plexus—an important remnant from the time of the umbilical cord connecting us to the source that was nourishing us; the solar plexus, regulating all organs of the upper abdomen; and the left and right cervical plexuses, which regulate the left or right upper-body quadrants respectively, with the brain, heart and lungs.

To sense the cranial breath, virtually place your hands on both sides of your client's head—that is, your hands don't touch the head itself. Now imagine that your hands *are* the cranium, and try to gently press them together. Then do the same from the front and back, and from above and below the cranium.

A free cranium can be pressed together slightly, as if it's a fully inflated air balloon. When the cranium is blocked, it feels more like a concrete block. In that case, people often have a headache as well, or they feel at least slight pressure in the head.

To feel the craniosacral rhythm—that is, the rhythm that transcends the spine and connects everything—virtually place one hand underneath the cranium, and the other underneath the sacrum. Now imagine that your hands are the ligaments and tissues, which can move freely in the structures, and try to move both of your hands simultaneously, like a swing.

If the rhythm is free, it has a beautiful sound, and you can feel that person's way of life and the sound of his or her soul.

However, the rhythm is often blocked in one or both directions (in the direction of the pelvis or cranium). Sometimes it also feels mechanic; it has lost all its aliveness. Instead of the original rhythm, there's a foreign substitute rhythm, similar to artificial respiration replacing someone's natural breathing.

Structure

Always remember that 99 percent of all differences in leg length are functional in nature. That means that they can also go away again. This applies to all structural imbalances. We just have to find the key causes, remedy them, and then our structure and stance often realign by themselves.

The length of our legs is a simple parameter, and it's really impressive to see a difference disappear with a few healing cards.

Then, the therapist moves the upper and lower ankle joint to test their state. Therapists can immediately determine irritations in the joints by applying the arm-length test with their own arms.

In doing so, they keep the following question in mind: **"Is the joint free of irritations?"**

Regarding the knees, it's important to check the collateral ligaments by testing the legs in a bow-leg or knock-knee position. The meniscus on each side can be tested by virtually twisting thigh and lower leg against one another. The cruciate ligaments can be tested by virtually pushing down the thigh while pushing up the lower leg, and vice versa. This test can also be performed by moving the joint's structures directly in the way medical doctors are trained to do, and combining this with the arm-length test.

When I say *virtually,* it means that therapists carry out the movement only with their hands while imagining that their hands *are* the respective body parts.

Next, the hip joints are tested by visualizing how the legs move in all directions. If there's any uncertainty regarding the test result, the therapist can also move the leg physically anytime and repeat the testing.

Now the therapist's hand "becomes" the client's tailbone, and the therapist tries to move it in all directions. In doing so, therapists will feel any limitation in movement. If they now go on a journey through time and imagine doing the test 5, 10, 20 or 30 years earlier, they will feel the tailbone's ability to move at the respective age. The field has stored everything; we only need to access it. Often the tailbone is irritated if the person fell at some point, or through giving birth in women. As the pelvic plexus of the autonomic nervous system is located above the tailbone, this plexus also gets irritated, which, in turn, can lead to irritations or disorders in the lower abdomen.

The sacrum is tested next. Once again, the hand "becomes" the sacrum and moves in all directions.

It's important to stay aware of the fact that clients can feel everything; for them, it feels real—as if their bones are moving. Therefore, it's essential to tell them what we're doing as therapists: our hand turns into a kind of cyberhand that moves through the body.

All bones enjoy the freedom to move in all directions. Thus, freedom means being able to move freely in all directions even if these movements aren't big—they don't have to be.

As for the spine, therapists can sense the ability to move every single vertebra individually. And they can double-check the results with the arm-length test at any time, using either their own or the client's arms.

About 80 percent of the body's muscle chains go via the hyoid bone. Virtually, this bone can be moved in all directions, which enables the therapist to detect any tension.

Regarding the lower jaw, clients can move it in all directions themselves, and the therapist tests every direction using the client's arms. Teeth can also turn and move in all directions—forward, backward, upward, downward or sideward.

Even if their movements are minimal, they're still extremely important for the body's overall structure and stance—this is demonstrated by cases of scoliosis developing due to dental braces, and by the reduced blood supply to the brain as a result of tension in the neck.

The therapist's hand "becomes" every individual tooth, and can thus try out its ability to move.

As you can see, therapists develop what could be called "piano-player hands," which are extremely sensitive, yet have the advantage that heavy-duty gardening work doesn't adversely affect their abilities.

Clients can also push their individual teeth themselves into a certain position using their tongue, and the therapist tests. This matters in particular when it comes to misaligned teeth: pushing them with dental braces into a certain direction where they don't want to go means forcing movement onto them, and is quite questionable from a therapeutic point of view.

There are orthodontists who've integrated *innerwise* into their practice and first treat their patients with this system. If the patients are children, they also work with their parents, if need be (that is, if the child carries issues for his or her parents), and only then apply braces. This often reduces the overall time required for the orthodontic treatment by half, because the blockages that created the misalignments are resolved first; only then are mechanics used to support the body in correcting the teeth's alignment toward their normal position. In the case of my oldest son, I could correct his misaligned incisors exclusively with *innerwise*.

To conclude the testing of structure and stance, we test the cranial breath and the cranial bones' ability to move. Once more, the cyberhand comes into play, which is applied together with the arm-length test.

Also, cranial bones remain movable, to a minimum degree, in all directions throughout our entire life.

The precise examination of structure and stance helps therapists learn.
While working on serious issues originating in childhood, for example, structure and stance of the client will change, and the therapist can observe which issues have manifested in what form in the body.
An exact statement of the testing results is not relevant for the client, as after half an hour of working with *innerwise*, everything will be different again; and in an optimal scenario, everything will be free again.

Testing medications

All medical drugs and food supplements should be checked using the arm-length test. Here, it's necessary to sort them as to whether they're needed and helpful, or useless but can be tolerated; whether they can't be tolerated, or whether there's an allergic reaction to them.
It's possible that patients show an allergic reaction to a medication that they need nevertheless. At that point, it's necessary to find another medicine to replace it.
Then, the dosage has to be double-checked to see if it's optimal. "Do you need 75 (100, 125) micrograms of thyroid hormones per day?"
Any medication to which the patient reveals an allergic reaction has to be stopped as soon as possible, or replaced. The safest way is to test this with the arm-length test:

- "Can the patient stop taking this medication immediately?"
- "Does the patient have to reduce it gradually?"
- "Over how many weeks (days, months) does it need to be gradually tapered off?"
- "What should the dosage be in one (two, three, four) weeks?"
- "Should the withdrawal of a medical drug be supported with another remedy?"

This sounds like a lot of diagnostic work and time spent. And if you prefer, this can take you a long time. But it may also only take five minutes, because you just need to identify the parameters that are important and interesting to observe.

Note for all self-users: Please adjust any medication only after consulting a qualified physician.

Checkup—overview of basic parameters

The checkup serves to quickly get an overview and gain clarity on key parameters. It serves as an inspiration, and I use it intuitively, too, testing which parameters should be tested.

I recommend that anyone starting to use *innerwise* always determine all parameters of the checkup during the first few months in order to be able to recognize how everything is connected. Those who are able to juggle freely with all tools will only work selectively then.

Now, the moment of truth has arrived. Who is actually lying there in front of you?

- *"Please say: I am I."*
- *"Okay, now repeat this using your first name: I am …"*
  In 50 percent of the cases, you'll have someone in front of you who isn't him- or herself.

Now you can follow up with the provocative question:
- *"If you're not yourself, who are you? And whose life are you living, because you're not living yours!"*

Next, you want to find out how many energy fields the client has—that is, how many clients are really lying there in front of you.
- *"You have 1 (2, 5, 10, 100, 1,000) energy fields in you!"*

Then you want to find out how high the client's level of life energy is.
- *"Your life energy in percents is 50 percent!"*
  (Next, you can ask whether it is 60, 70, 80 or 40, 30, 20 percent.)

What age corresponds to the client's behavior?
- *"Your social maturity is … years!"*

And how old are your cells?
- *"Your biological age is … years."*

"How much integrity does the person have?
- *Integrity in percents: …*

And here you can find a complete overview of diagnostic parameters:

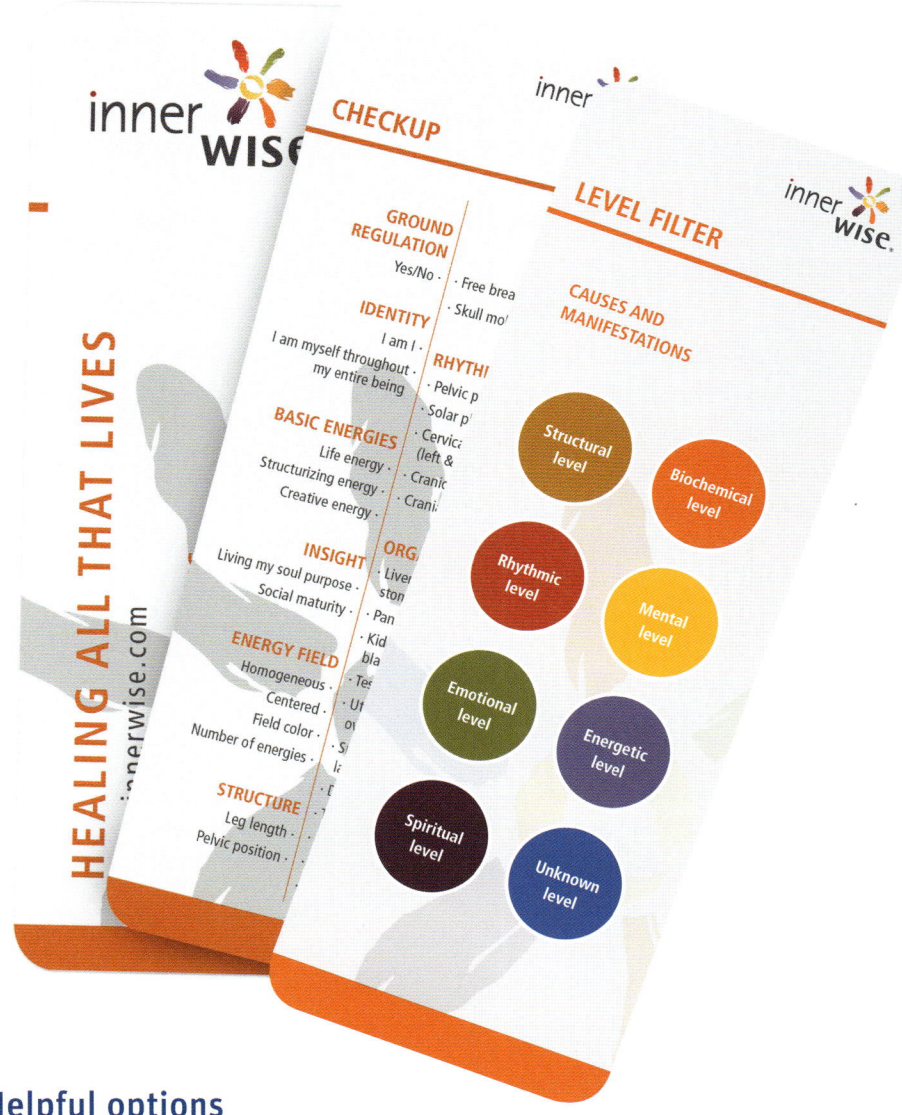

Helpful options

Finding out when a trauma occurred

Identify the point in time when certain issues originated by using the arm-length test. Was it at the age of 50 to 40 years? Was it at the age of 40 to 30 years? And so on.

The Level Filter

With the Level Filter, you can intuitively identify the level where a specific issue originated, and you can also identify the levels where it has manifested at this point in time.

These can be the structural, biochemical, mental, emotional, energetic, spiritual or unknown levels.

With the symbols used on the Level Filter, each level has its own specific energy. You can touch it intuitively with your finger and double-check the result with the arm-length test.

Treating people

Individual treatments

In individual treatments, *innerwise* is applied following the steps described in the section *Step-by-step*.

When patients come to see me in my practice, they lie down on their back on a massage table with their clothes on.

Treatments for couples hoping to conceive

Here, it's not about doing what's possible, but what the therapist is *allowed* to do. Therapists have to abide by and serve the big plan. We can't play God and force something to happen.

"Am I allowed to do this?" is the most critical question in this kind of treatment.

Part 1: Individual treatments

This treatment should always be done with both partners. In exceptional cases, it's also possible to just work with the woman.

Both partners come with a desire to have a child.

"Imagine that you're pregnant and have a baby."

The arm-length test will reveal that this causes stress to both partners. Not being pregnant doesn't create stress, but the fulfillment of what has been their great wish for years does.

Now both partners receive a complete individual treatment. Here, therapists have to focus in particular on previous abortions, miscarriages, energetic sexual manipulation, and tailbone traumas with a subsequent blockage of the pelvic plexus. Often an *innerwise* Imago of the uterus proves very effective.

Then part 2 of the couple's treatment follows.

An Imago is particularly suitable to see the energetic constellation of both partners. How do they stand with regard to one another? Do they look at each other? Are they equally tall in this visualization? (Their height, and thus, level of responsibility should be equal.) The next question is: Do they both even have soul contracts with children with each other?

Part 3: Looking at the soul

Once parts 1 and 2 are complete, it's time to look for the child's soul. Is it far away? Is it one or two souls? When twins are coming, you can already perceive them before the conception as two points of light.

"Is it also okay for you to have twins?"

"I've always wanted to have two children anyway; then they're both here at once," one patient replied who gave birth to twins a bit more than nine months later.

Sometimes it's necessary, and the therapist is also allowed, to send healing cards to that soul. Then, this can also be done by the future parents themselves. Give them the cards and ask them to pass them to the child's soul.

Now comes the control test for both parents:

"Imagine that you're pregnant and have a baby."

To be sure, all steps are now tested individually with both partners: conception, pregnancy, changes in the woman's body, birth, cutting of the umbilical cord, breast-feeding, not sleeping through the night for a year and a half, being fully in the service of the child for the first two years, possibly years without sex, a flabby belly, changes in the woman's breasts and a certain mental "hormonal drunkenness" during the time of breast-feeding.

If individual topics still cause stress as revealed by the arm-length test, you can balance them with healing cards as needed.

If both partners can now say "yes" to all of the topics listed above, you only need to wait for their happy call during the next two to four weeks. The success rate is about 80 percent.

These are the most beautiful treatments I've experienced with *innerwise*.

Treating unborn children

Souls are so perfect and complete at the beginning of the pregnancy, and so vulnerable.

It's one of the greatest gifts that you can give to a child—that he or she is born as whole and complete as possible.

If you ask adults to imagine their own conception and the time in their mother's womb, they almost all show stress.

About 80 percent react negatively when testing conception with the arm-length test, and almost with delight when it comes to the pregnancy. It's easy to identify the main stressful events by testing the individual pregnancy months:

- not being wanted at the time of conception;
- doubts of the parents during the pregnancy as to whether they want the child and will be able to handle this;
- relationship stress;
- medical interventions such as ultrasound or amniocentesis;
- accidents and events in the lives of the parents.

Unborn children absorb almost everything and have little protection.

During the treatment, I touch the belly and ask the child: "How are you doing today?"

It's the mother's or my own arms that give the answer.

If there's stress, I use the testing system and work with healing cards in a targeted manner on the child.

It's also possible to feel the rhythms of the child with our hands as our hands, are moving freely in space and expressing the movements.

At the end of the treatment, it's the mother who receives the symphony of healing cards.

What's important with pregnant women is that the treatment stops at the point where it's enough for the child. It's not the mother who decides what she needs, but the child.

Some issues can only be resolved with the mother after she has given birth.

Treating children

Children love their parents, and they're ready and willing to "help" share their burden even if they break down under the weight. When parents come for a treatment of their child, I always work with the parents first. Often the child needs less or no treatment anymore afterward, as it was just the parents' issues.

Treating children although the issues aren't theirs is a form of child abuse. Because when the children are cleansed from the charges, they can take on even more from their parents, leaving their role of being children more and more—they become little adults.

Couples' treatments

Husband and wife are lying on two massage tables next to each another. He has problems with the liver, and she has heart problems, both of which reveal themselves in the arm-length test. Now you're treating an issue on his side (such as the lover and lies in life), and on her side, the heart problems disappear.

Then you treat the causes of her manipulative behavior *(I need you, I can't live without you),* and his liver is stress-free again.

Couples often give up their own Self and have a mixed "we/you/myself" field. Often it's no longer clear on whose side an issue originated.

Therefore, it's particularly important here to make clear which projections and manipulations are present, whether one of the partners suffers along voluntarily, and what parts of all this a couple even *wants* to resolve.

If love no longer carries them and they're honest with themselves again, this can also result in a separation.

Or, they may prefer staying with the "You're killing me!"

After all, they're grown up and free to suffer as long as they want.

Coma patients

With coma patients, treatments work really well. The arm-length test shows big differences between "yes" and "no" responses, revealing results very clearly and distinctly, and is well suited to guide the therapist through the treatment.

Here, it's important that the therapist test at the very beginning whether the patient even wants to wake up again. Otherwise, it could be that the therapist has to live with the words: "It's your fault that I continue living. I wanted to die."

If the arm-length test reveals that they want to wake up again, you can test directly, asking: "What is needed to wake up again?"

Trauma patients

I work regularly with patients of the *Weißer Ring,* an organization that helps victims of violence. These patients suffered a severe trauma two to four weeks before. They were assaulted or raped, or experienced attempted murder. All of them are in a state of total rigidity—that is, it's not possible for them to deal with the trauma. It's a state of total shock.

After dissolving this rigidity with the help of *innerwise* frequencies, it's possible to work on the deep roots and charges, and then to address the manifestation in the current trauma and resolve it. *Resolving* means that being reminded of a trauma causes no more reactions whatsoever in the arm-length test. Since this test is a direct response from our unconscious that determines our lives at a rate of roughly 95 percent, this approach offers an opportunity to effectively transform fundamental issues without having to reactivate traumas.

Treating animals

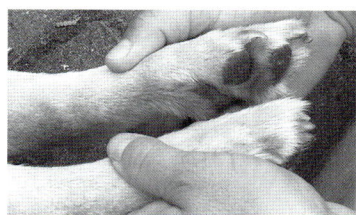 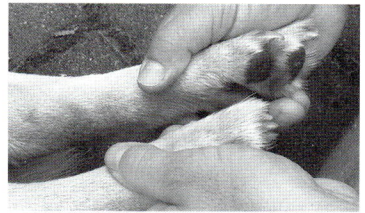

Polly's arms say "yes"   ... and "no"

Treating animals isn't substantially different from working with humans. Animals like to take over issues and illnesses from their owners. Cats are known to do that, but they're not the only ones. Dogs, horses and other animals do that as well. Thus, it's often necessary to work with the owner first. "Is the animal carrying a burden for people?" "Should the person be treated first?"

When working with animals, therapists test on behalf of the animal using their own arms.

The testing systems are used in the same way as when working with people.

The finished healing symphony can be copied to an amulet that is attached to the animal, or the symphony is copied to an *innerwise* disc that is used to energize the animal's food or water, or it is copied directly to water that you can keep in bottles and give to the animal.

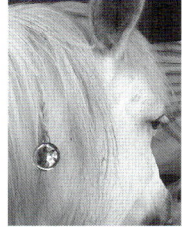

Treating buildings

Buildings are also alive and can be treated. Often they even have to be treated, if irritations in humans are caused by them. Memories are stored as energy fields in buildings, or there can be beings or entities that can irritate the people there. These can be souls of people who already passed away who are stuck in the intermediary world, such as victims of a murder or war victims.

Completing a treatment

When is a treatment complete?

- When no test card causes stress anymore in the arm-length test.
- And when both of the following questions get a "yes" response:
    1. Have we done everything that we were allowed to do today?
    2. Is the treatment complete for all involved?

Copying the healing symphony to amulets, discs or cards

With the help of our hands, the energies of the healing cards are copied to an amulet, disc or card.

- **For people,** they're copied to an amulet or Balance Card.
- **For animals,** they're copied to an amulet that is then attached to the animal, or to a disc that is used to energize the animal's food or water. For that purpose, the disc is placed underneath the feeding dish.
- **For living and work spaces, systems or projects,** the energies are copied to a disc that is then placed in a spot where they can unfold their maximum effect, and attached there. This spot can be identified with the arm-length test.

Using amulets, discs or cards

- **For people:** Wear the amulet or Balance Card. To reinforce the effect, hold it in your hand a few times a day and meditate with it, visualizing your visions and wishes.
- **For animals:** They can wear an amulet, or eat food or drink water that has been energized with the healing symphony.
- **For living and work spaces, systems or projects:** Position the disc in the spot where the energies can unfold their maximum effect.

Homework

What matters is to let people be self-responsible. For that purpose, homework is often needed as support.

When patients call after some time, my first question is: "Have you done your homework?"

If they reply with a "no," they won't get another appointment for a treatment until they can respond honestly with a "yes."

Patients expect us to do the best possible job, and we can demand their cooperation.

Emergency help in case of a blockage

Easy steps to treat yourself:

- **You're caught in a state of rigidity.** Draw healing cards intuitively until the rigidity is dissolved again. It will be a maximum of eight cards.
- **When saying "yes," your arms differ in length—you're experiencing initial stress:** Draw healing cards intuitively until your arms are equally long again. It will be a maximum of five cards.
- **You have a problem or symptom:** Think of the problem or the symptom that bothers you. Your arms will differ in length. Draw healing cards intuitively until the difference in length has disappeared. It will be a maximum of ten cards.

3. The Art of Living

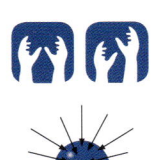

> ### Testing topics
>
> - How much of your creativity do you express?
>
> - Can you be in a bad mood when you're in the flow?
>
> - Do children really need education?
>
> - Isn't it finally time to reinvent school?
>
> - How many politicians have integrity?
>
> - Have you ever had energetic group sex with your partner's ex-partners?
>
> - Say all letters and test them individually to identify those that cause stress to you.

Sing like no one's listening,
love like you've never been hurt,
dance like nobody's watching,
and live like it's heaven on earth.

Mark Twain

What is life without creativity? Who am I, and what do I live when there is a problem with my identity? How do I get happy? How can I avoid having love turn into a dependent relationship? How can we bring our relationship back to love? Can learning really be that simple? How do I attract success? How can I design living and work spaces to support their purpose in an optimal way? How do I manage to live up to my potential? How do I succeed in living with integrity in all areas of life? How do I find the strength to change my life and live my dreams? What is my life purpose? How can we keep up the zest for learning in children although they have to go to school? How can really good schools be created? How can I connect heart and mind?

Bad mood

You're looking at your child, wondering whether this moody being is really yours. In the morning, the child was still radiant, happy and open.

Coming home from kindergarten, your child is grouchy and screaming, the face looks different, the voice sounds different, and she/he is hurting her-/himself.

Yes, deep inside, it's your child; but on the surface she/he probably has the identity of another kid—breathing differently; and feeling heavy, sad and angry.

After two hours of intense attention, your child is rising back to the surface. And at night, after your child has finally fallen asleep, you're asking yourself once more whether you should really bring your son/daughter back to that place the next day because this alienation recurs on almost a daily basis.

On the other hand, your child quickly learns the difference between being oneself and "being beside oneself." We can't save our children from that. It's important, however, that we support them in re-establishing their balance quickly and easily. Children learn very fast to treat themselves using *The Complete Healing System,* or at least, to ask us for help. We then take a few healing cards, and a couple of minutes later, sunshine returns to the face of your little loved ones. A sigh of relief follows, and a hug occurs between you so you can feel each other really intensely again. It's like a miracle.

Give your children the gift of feeling how it is to be in the flow as often as you can, because this state is addictive, and later on, they will keep striving to experience it again. Children who don't know this state of Being—and unfortunately, there are many—won't know what they're looking for in life, yet they'll still be searching.

Education? No, thank you!

My experience of having eight children confirmed my conviction that children don't need education. What they need, however, is an inner structure, and this results from living with integrity.

The higher people's integrity, the fewer external rules they need. Therefore, it's our primary task to support our children in raising the level of their integrity and to then find suitable schools, or set them up if they don't exist. And for that purpose, we have to live with integrity ourselves and serve as living examples, since this is the only way that we, as parents, can impart values. **Integrity? Yes, please!**

Behavior and inner balance

My large family keeps giving me the opportunity to experience interactions first hand.

My two little girls had talked to their mother on the phone (she lives in a spiritual community). Subsequently, the girls (then three and six years old) were really out of sorts for a couple of days; they were more restless and unhappy, had little accidents, and being with them was very exhausting. Then, I'd enough. I asked them to lie down on the massage table, and both of them were caught in a state of rigidity.

After their rigidity was dissolved, I tested their identity—both had the identity of their mother. Five minutes later, they had their own identity back and were in balance again. And I once again had two happy girls who could play together wonderfully. The tangible disharmony was gone.

Our behavior is directly linked to our energy field. Each irritation in our field has an impact. False identities, states of rigidity or foreign energies can be sensed directly as disharmony, heard in our voice and seen in our face.

The artist

Being crazy, looking at things in crazy ways, creating crazy things—each artist needs another perspective to *create* art. In fact, he or she doesn't create art, it's the art that is created through him or her. This makes it clear that blockages prevent this flow of creativity.

Neither could this book be written under pressure or in every situation. On the one hand, I have to keep bringing myself back in the flow; on the other, I have to find the inspiration that lets the words bubble out of me. There were weeks when I wasn't able to work on it. Then, there were other times. In such times, I'm living only in the text, I'm part of the book, and the text keeps flowing out of me.

I compose a book like a painting, with an inner flow like in a musical piece. I paint the energy of the book in the air and keep changing the text until I'm absolutely satisfied with the energetic image of the book. For me, it's a living being, and any perceptible disharmony reveals a lack of clarity that still exists.

Being crazy simply means having another perspective. And if you recall the *Dimensions of Being* on test card 9, none of these perspectives is wrong; they're just different.

Schools

I had a wonderful experience with a school that I was given the opportunity to be involved with for years—from energetically cleansing the building and site; to supporting the staff in their selection of materials; to coaching the team, designing the garden, facilitating processes and showing students the arm-length test so that they could balance themselves with colors in the morning in order to feel good, and be able to learn and study in optimal ways. I even served as the school physician. In the summer, I set up my massage table in the school courtyard and worked individually with parents and children. It was a great time!

What fascinated me about this school was the trust it was built on. In the first year, there were 5 kids; in the second, 30, and in the third, 65 children attended this school. These are huge growth processes. A project born out of flow that keeps blossoming.

One of my next projects is to create a completely new school system that does justice to the children of these new times—a school where the zest for learning never dies, but keeps growing.

Science

Creation is logical, but can also be experienced and understood intuitively.

Even mathematical formulas come as intuitions. Suddenly, they appear, similar to crop circles. No one knows how they're created, yet they're often perfect from a mathematical and geometric point of view. The discovery of the benzene ring structure is a known example. The solution appeared as an intuition to chemist August Kekulé in a dream.

innerwise itself has been a research institution for 18 years, aiming to understand energetic and systemic principles and to create solutions that can be applied immediately.

For all these years, independence has been of paramount importance to me—not accepting how something is supposed to be, not attempting to publish results scientifically, and no sponsors. What has always mattered to me is inner work—

clearing blockages that arise and seeing myself in the service of the being of *innerwise*—and in return, being carried by divine providence. If something was meant to happen, it always came at the right time.

innerwise is applied science in the flow. Results have proven the success of this path of combining science and its application in practice.

Politics and policymaking

Integrity, authenticity and *honesty* are foreign words in this métier.

Since these are precisely the values that we want to achieve in our *innerwise* work, people working in the areas of politics and policymaking don't yet figure among the most frequent clients for *innerwise* coaches.

Yet, this is precisely our strength—a quick systemic analysis and the possibility to clear even complex energy fields rapidly and efficiently, thereby achieving flow. But this contradicts the manipulative power struggles found in political circles.

We've had wonderful experiences accompanying political reform projects with *innerwise*, increasing the effectiveness of political meetings and supporting many regional projects.

In essence, this work corresponds to the coaching of complex structures; however, finely sensing the limits of what is permitted, and what kind of energetic influence is allowed and optimally effective, and when, is critical.

Design

Designers have already been using *innerwise* for a long time, since their work is to convey information, values, energies and atmosphere in their products. This is something that's not feasible using only one's rational mind or logic. A logo and all that it projects has to match a company's vision; as do the corporate name, the company's marketing and advertisement, its website, etc. Only if everything is considered as an artistic synthesis can all elements and aspects support one another, and is it possible to achieve an optimal result.

Research and development

I've developed many products myself and have supported companies in optimizing their existing products. We can virtually sense the effectiveness of vitamin pills in any tissue of our body. With the help of the arm-length test, we can test the ingredients in cosmetics and determine if they can be tolerated. If the test reveals irritations, alternatives can be found. We can even attain remarkable results in technical processes, as shown by the following text:

Electrolysis research

With *innerwise*, technical processes including the structural and surface properties of gold and palladium can be modified. Read about the experimental results found by Dr. Jan Marwan, a leading researcher in the field of cold fusion:

> My experiments led to the following findings: Generally, treatment of the electrochemical cell with the *innerwise* crystal placed underneath the cell for five minutes prior to each experiment significantly changed the catalytic reactivity and physical and chemical properties of the analyzed metals, gold and palladium. During the experiment, the electrodes in the solution were protected from any kind of contamination.
>
> Here, two important distinctions have to be made: On the one hand, the reactivity in oxygen generation was strongly reduced as a result of the *innerwise* procedure, suggesting passivation of the metal surface. On the other, kinetic processes in hydrogen generation and the diffusion of hydrogen into the palladium grid were accelerated considerably due to the IW (*innerwise*) procedure.
>
> This can only lead to the general conclusion that the effect of the crystal significantly alters the structural and surface characteristics of the examined metal.

In principle, we don't do anything different here than when we sense and treat people.

"Happiness comes to the happy."

So says Connor Mayfield, and he's right. People who can't imagine being happy on all levels—the conscious and the unconscious ones—will never reach it.

Relationships

If this is supposed to refer to one's ability to compromise, I prefer to do without. "But we need to meet in the middle!" my then-partner said during a conflict we had.

I replied, "We don't have to meet in any middle, but in truth, or nowhere."

In partnerships, it often helps to look at or draw a situation as an Imago. This serves to quickly gain a clear overview of that situation.

What's important is to keep testing whether there's an involuntary exchange of energy between both partners. Who gives away voluntarily, or loses against his or her will, how much of his or her energy in percents to the other? Frequently, it also happens that one of the partners takes on the other's identity.

Couples' treatments are very beautiful and rewarding work. When working with both partners individually and together, patterns become clear quickly, and major changes are easily possible. Of course, it can also happen that a treatment considerably accelerates a separation that has been postponed.

Sex

Suddenly, I can't stand my partner anymore.

You may relate to this: You're lying next to your partner, feeling almost disgusted at the idea of touching him or her. Nothing drives you to melt with each other erotically, and the bed can't be large enough to be as far away as possible. You're starting to wonder whether he or she is the right partner, or whether you aren't worth going for a fling. Yet, a little while ago, your love and mutual attraction was still so wonderful, and the sexual energy was exhilarating.

Now you're testing—and your partner has the identity of his or her ex-partner. Old, unresolved aspects concerning the two were reactivated through a contact. But you don't want to be with that other person. If your partner radiates another energy, you can't recognize him or her on the love level.

After an *innerwise* treatment, you will once again feel the resonance and desire within just a few minutes.

Energetic waste dumps and ties

Sexuality creates the strongest energetic ties between people, which often don't detach by themselves. These links are often used or abused energetically, involving a continuous flow of energy via these ties, which often goes in one direction only. In order to be free for your current partner, it's important to cut all old sexual energetic ties.

For women, they're mostly in the uterus.

This must be related to men's fundamental desire that Woody Allen described as follows: "I have an intense desire to return to the womb. Anybody's." And from there, men don't want to leave anymore.

However, these ties can also be attached to the clitoris, the vagina, the tubes, the ovaries or the pelvic plexus. These energy fields can be perceived when sensing the energy flow in the vagina, uterus or the tubes, or when the woman does an Imago of her uterus.

For that purpose, she closes her eyes and imagines her uterus as a room, a space, which she then describes.

Ideally, this space is bright and beautiful; and feels light, free, sound and whole. Instead, women often see darkness, a black space. These are the manipulative and possessive energies of their past and current sexual partners.

As if many former partners had left an unpleasant sound there, and all of them together sound horrible.

How can an organ stay healthy under such circumstances?

How is it supposed to be open and experience sexual ecstasy?

Sometimes a new partner can also sense these old energies as if they downright bit his penis. "This is our space—go away!"

For men, the old energies of former partners are often in the prostate or pelvic plexus.

Interestingly enough, these are precisely the places in women or men respectively, where cancer frequently arises.

When entering a new partnership, I urgently recommend the following: first, cleanse yourselves if you want to spare yourselves the experience of energetic group sex with your predecessors.

Take into account that sexual energetic links can also be activated remotely. Suddenly, you're having erotic dreams with your ex-partner. For that to happen, it's enough if your former partner masturbates and thinks of you when having an orgasm.

This constitutes a particular problem for celebrities who are used for sexual stimulation. Officially, these stars have recurring bladder infections, problems with their voice or energetic irritations within themselves; in reality, there are many energy fields at their genitals, sapping their energy.

Consequences of abuse

When people have experienced abuse, their ability to enjoy their sexuality is often impaired. This is not only caused by that memory, but also by the related energetic and spiritual trauma. Frequently, a part of the soul is torn out when that happens. Sometimes the aggressor can use this as an energetic fountain of youth for years.

I've often experienced that deep healing can set in once these parts of the soul have been retrieved. That person becomes whole again. It's like with *any* severe trauma in life: Forgiveness is only one part of the healing. The other, even more important, part is healing the wounded soul.

From my experience, combining the card system and the healing breath works best.

In the event that a part or parts of the soul are still in the aggressor: By visualizing the eyes of the aggressor, it's always possible to access him or her deep inside, with the opportunity to find and retrieve the stolen soul fragments. It's similar to dragons in the fairy tales: Through their eyes, you can look into their soul.

From my experience, combining the card system and the healing breath works best.

In the event that a part or parts of the soul are still in the aggressor: By visualizing the eyes of the aggressor, it's always possible to access him or her deep inside, with the opportunity to find and retrieve the stolen soul fragments. It's similar to dragons in the fairy tales: through their eyes, you can look into their soul.

Creativity

Our goal in life is to be an instrument of creative energy, to have the strength and clarity to manifest it, and to experience the joy of creating something meaningful in life.

Yet, how is this supposed to work if the creative energy has the water level of a dried-up river?

Test anxiety

Tests or exams are stressful, and this stress often blocks one's access to knowledge. If testees or examinees aren't even able to imagine passing the test or exam beforehand, how are they supposed to manage?

This can be determined easily using the arm-length test.

Once the person has been balanced with *innerwise*, it becomes possible, and success can happen.

Why make life difficult if it can also be easy?

Talking, writing and singing

The body is the temple of the soul, and ideally, it is also its "organ of resonance."

Let's start with spoken language

Test all letters from A to Z as to whether they cause you stress when you imagine saying them out loud. Make a note if the answer is "yes." Once you've tested all letters and also the numbers 0 to 9, treat yourself regarding those that created stress.

You can also feel this, because a free letter resonates in your entire body, while a blocked one will resonate only in certain areas.

Letters and numbers are often blocked as a result of negative experiences connected to words that start with that letter.

Once you've successfully treated all blocked letters and numbers, imagine visiting your parents, and partly return to the children's role.

Then, check all letters and numbers once more and balance those with *innerwise* that still cause stress.

You'll be amazed by how your voice will change, as well as how your environment will react to it.

Writing

With your eyes closed, write one letter after the other in the air using one hand (make your letter as large as possible), and sense which one is blocked. Then, treat these letters and the underlying issues.

Singing

Sing the individual tones and treat yourself regarding those that don't sound good, that don't come from within your whole body, or that cause stress in the arm-length test.

Energetic design of living and work spaces

Design and create living and work spaces in harmony with their purpose. Clear them from any source of interference and energy loss. Become the energy architect of your living and work environments. Redesign your home, your garden, your life!

Let go of everything that you don't love. Clear up the spaces—they're neither waste dumps nor museums of your life.

Energetic cleansing of your living and work spaces

Energies don't create dust and can't be removed with a vacuum cleaner, but they pollute the space differently.

If the souls of people who have passed away are present in buildings, these buildings smell stale and musty, like a humid basement, and this odor can't be eliminated.

Energetic pollutions can recur, depending on who's coming to your home or workplace, or which objects you bring in.

A secondhand chest of drawers brings along its entire history as it moves into your house.

"Nice" visitors might not only leave a pile in the toilet, but often something energetically similar in your living spaces as well.

Frequently, however, we already have a feeling beforehand that there's something unclear about certain people and that they don't have a pleasant aura. If you still decide to welcome such visitors, you might just have to cleanse your space afterward.

Especially when you move, it's important not only to repaint the walls, but also to cleanse your new home energetically so that you don't have to pay for the issues of the previous tenants or owners.

In addition, treat the new apartment or house in the same way that works for humans: using the testing system and healing cards, saving the healing symphony to a disc and positioning the latter in its optimal place.

4. The Art of Business

innerwise for systems, teams, products, companies and organizations, projects, regions and situations.

Change the field and reality follows.
Successfully applying creative lateral thinking and action to interconnected systems.

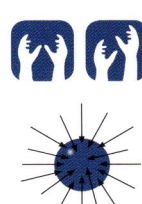

Testing topics

- Does your team squeak, or is it well-oiled?

- Are projects delayed?

- Have your employees resigned all but their job titles?

- Is the budget exceeded on a regular basis?

- Do good employees or partners leave?

- Is there a lack of innovation?

- Do processes take longer than average?

- Are you no longer fulfilled by what you do?

- Are results only suboptimal?

- Are you ready for unconventional solutions?

"There are no formal design reviews, so there are no huge decision points. **Instead, we can make the decisions fluid.** Since we iterate every day and never have dumb-ass presentations, we don't run into major disagreements."

Jonathan Ive about Apple[2]

Let the person who's in charge of the project, company, organization or system—or the person whose idea it is—draw it intuitively on a sheet of paper.

Draw it!

What counts is *what* is drawn *where* in the picture—as it applies to an inner Imago. How are the elements connected to one another? How big or small are the individual elements that are drawn in that picture? What's the basic structure of the whole system?

It helps to first draw a frame that represents the project, idea, company or organization. This makes it possible to also identify elements outside the frame and draw them there—that is, elements that aren't integrated, for example.

In the case of one manufacturer, for instance, it was the products that were outside the frame. How are sales supposed to work under such circumstances?

Everything that's important is drawn within the frame: the people involved; the goals and objectives; the values, names, products, clients, investors (or even money itself), the building, etc.

Intuitively, everything finds its place, and thus, is an image representing reality.

The *innerwise* consultant can apply the arm-length test at any time to verify if an element is drawn in the right location or if something has been forgotten ("Two components are still missing").

This is how a real image of reality, an Imago drawing, is created.

Now, both the client and the *innerwise* consultant see and test whether the elements have stress with one another, whether they're placed in their optimal position, and how the structure created in this way represents an image of the blockage that is supposed to be cleared with the *innerwise* treatment.

Next comes the *innerwise* treatment:

* Guided by the testing system, the *innerwise* consultant (and/or client) picks healing cards and places them directly on the drawing.
* The drawing represents the actual client.
* It's the art of the consultant to find out where to start the treatment. He or she has to identify the points that guide the work most effectively.

---

2 Translator's note: Walter Isaacson, *Steve Jobs* (New York: Simon & Schuster, 2013), p. 346

- If one's inspiration doesn't suffice, there's always the arm-length test. "Where should I start? Here … ?"
- Applying healing cards, the work on the image continues until one feels that much has changed and that a new drawing will show the changes and re-establish clarity.
- The work continues with this new drawing until it's time for another new drawing.
- This process can be repeated a few more times until there's a structure and degree of clarity that optimally supports the goal of the project, company, organization or system.
- Often, this requires two to four drawings.
- Then, these healing cards are copied to a Flowmaker disc, *Make Me An Instrument* hologram, or a Homo Integer when it's about large systems, which is available in the dimensions 35.4 x 35.4 inches, 58.9 x 58.9 inches and 81.9 x 81.9 inches. The copying process is the same as it is when copying healing cards to an amulet. Place the healing cards in the middle, hold your hand on top of them and let them be copied.

Working with *innerwise* changes the fields so that reality can follow easily.

Apart from this basic application, as described above, all consultants will work in their unique ways according to their qualifications.
This may involve:
- including the strategic planning of the company or organization;
- reworking the logo and names;
- facilitating team processes;
- checking the products and suggesting changes;
- verifying whether the energy of the premises of the company or organization optimally supports its function;
- directly supporting decision-making processes.

All of the above involves the basic inner tool—one's ability to feel, sense and perceive. That is, to tune in to a building or imagine how an employee feels who works there. Or to sense products and feel their effects on the user.
A consultant acquires all these abilities in working with people and can then apply them to other things as well.

Often, it might be necessary to have individual sessions with key people in the system (the boss, his lover, wife and secretary, if the latter hasn't been mentioned yet).

I would like to emphasize the high degree of responsibility of the consultant, since changes in a system's energy field impact all and everything involved.

Therefore, it's often a good idea and even necessary for two consultants to work together, and thus, be able to take turns and check each other's work.

To sum it up in a structured way, it involves the following steps:
- Analysis and fine-tuning
- Treatment
- Integration
- Aftercare

In addition, a prevention program has to be set up for the future to recognize and clear serious blockages at an early stage.

Aftercare and prevention also involve becoming aware of the need that those in charge have to maintain the flow and ensure the use of the essential tools in order to recognize irritations themselves at an early stage and clear them.

Of course, it's also possible to create—together with the flow coach—a new occupational profile for reviewing and assessing the system and its systemic fields on a continuous or regular basis.

We also offer an educational program to become an *innerwise* Consultant at the *innerwise* Business School. This program focuses on
- System Diagnostics
- System Development
- Systemic Therapy
- Systems in a Network

We will be examining the following types of systems:
- Ideas & projects
- Companies or organizations & teams
- Buildings, sites & landscapes
- Regions & regional developments
- Processes & crises
- Political structures

5. The Developer

My life

Anybody can learn and use *innerwise*. My daughter Gaia was able to use it by herself when she was only two years old. One day she stood before me and said: "Daddy, you need something." Then she ordered me to lie down on the couch, crawled on top of me and tested with my arms. She chose the appropriate healing frequencies, and when everything was done, and especially when she was happy with the result, she proceeded to copy it all to an amulet so I could use it whenever necessary. I was so happy that I was given the opportunity to have this experience that it left me speechless!

I studied medicine at Humboldt University in Berlin, and became a medical doctor in 1994.

In my third academic year, I found a book on neural therapy in my mother's bookcase which she had received as a gift from a pharmaceutical representative. This book described how pain in different areas of the body had disappeared by merely injecting a local anesthetic in the gums around a particular tooth. "**HEALING** really does exist after all … ," I thought. After three years of studying medicine, I'd already given up hope.

So my search began. In addition to my medical studies at the university, I started studying Traditional Chinese Medicine for several years—or to be more precise, its philosophy, pathology and medicinal herbs. I trained in neural therapy under Dr. Horst Becke, and was given the opportunity to work with Dr. Johann Abele, one of the last medical doctors who still mastered detoxifying treatments based on methods by Hufeland.

The *Karl and Veronica Carstens Foundation* sponsored two clinical studies that I conducted to examine the correlations between focal infections, chronic inflammations and the reflex zones in the throat and neck area; I also worked to prove the effectiveness of cupping therapy in the treatment of carpal tunnel syndrome, which otherwise often results in surgery. The studies were published internationally.

All of this was great fun, and it allowed me to meet wonderful people such as Dr. G. Draczynski, who had worked with Professors Alfred Pischinger and Felix Perger in the 70s and who gave me precious information and texts on the ground regulation system. Through the *Deutsche Arbeitsgemeinschaft für Herdforschung* (German Working Group on Focal Infection Research), I learned more about the implications of focal infections and their correlations within the body.

From there, my journey of discovery took me to Walter Kunnen and his son Konrad in Belgium, who became my teachers on electrosmog and geopathology. In the field of conventional medicine, I worked in different hospitals at the time. In Berlin, for example, Professor Friedrich Luft taught me to always base my therapies on the most recent studies. This became so deeply engrained in me that since then I no longer read studies and have instead set out on a journey of discovery myself. My experiences in a rheumatic clinic focusing on autoimmune diseases (self-destructive diseases), matched exactly what I discovered later using the arm-length test: people who are ill, unconsciously want to be ill.

My last stint in the field of conventional medicine was my experience working at a pain therapy clinic. There, the credo was: those who can provide healing are right. My ward physician Dr. Michael Fischer granted me every therapeutic freedom one could possibly dream of. Since I had started to learn about a kinesiological system known as physioenergetics from Raphael van Assche on the side, I began using it at the clinic. And was kicked out. Testing with the arms went too far for the head of the clinical department.

Additional training followed, including profound experiences using osteopathic techniques, homeopathy, systemic constellation work and emotional therapies. For a number of years, Professor Bernd Senf worked with me using bioenergetic bodywork based on Wilhelm Reich's methods, and during one weekend I lost 1.5 diopters, thus getting rid of my glasses. Another miracle!

Originally, I was supposed to take over my mother's general practice. Yet, with the knowledge I had already gained at the time, 60 patients a day with only five to ten minutes for each of them was no longer conceivable to me.

This meant that I now had to stand on my own two feet and also manage to feed my family with my small private practice. If you're good and able to help, people come to you. If you aren't, they don't.

This also meant I needed a healing system that really worked … and so I developed one myself. This system is known as *innerwise*: healing by accessing one's inner wisdom. With this, I had found a way to combine everything I had learned so far and to use this power to continue my research and to discover something even greater.

For me, *innerwise* is a living healing system that unites the best from all cultures and times. It's an open system, and any technique or method can be integrated. It enables us to discover the individual correlations, thereby developing a new understanding of what illness is. It's both the essence and the abundance that can be applied intuitively.

Every aspect of this system is something we have experienced ourselves. As a result, together some friends and I went through hell a few times and back, but also found ourselves back on cloud nine time and again.
Authenticity can't be gained any other way. I'm grateful for all experiences.

If I had to describe my path in just a few words, they would be:

- From chaos to my own identity: I am myself again, I am I.
- Clearing old charges
- Putting an end to compromise and being honest with myself
- Trusting myself
- Finally growing up and taking responsibility for myself and my life
- Reintegrating lost soul fragments
- Learning to be happy with myself
- Loving myself

At the age of 45, I could already look back at my lifework with joy, let it go and look forward to all that life still has in store for me.

6. Learning How to Use *innerwise*

Books

To date, the following books on *innerwise* have been published:

- *Yes/No: Using the Arm-Length Test for Instant Answers and Wellbeing*
- *Der Heilatem: Atme dich frei. Atme dich gesund. Atme dich glücklich* (The Healing Breath: Breathe Yourself Free. Breathe Yourself Healthy. Breathe Yourself Happy) (in German)
- *A Course in Healing*
- *Heilung für alles Lebendige* (new edition in 2016: *Intuitive Heilung/Intuitive Healing*) (in German, English, Spanish and Portuguese)
- The audio book *innerwise Meditationen: Der Heilatem* (*innerwise* Meditations: The Healing Breath) (in German)
- The audio book *innerwise Meditationen: Mutter Erde* (*innerwise* Meditations: Mother Earth) (in German)
- *Besser schlafen, besser leben* (Sleep Better, Live Better) (in German)
- *Integrity is my way* (in German)
- The audio book *innerwise Meditationen: Der Fluss des Lebens* (*innerwise* Meditations: The River of Life) (in German)
- The audio book *innerwise Meditationen: innerYoga* (*innerwise* Meditations: *innerYoga*) (in German)
- *Heilmeditationen/Healing Meditations* (in German and English)
- *Intuitive Diagnostik* (Intuitive Diagnostics) (in German; English coming soon)

Treatment sets and other products

- *innerwise: The Complete Healing System*
- *innerwise Cardsystem*
- *Unconscious Mind Coach*
- *innerwise Quintessence*
- *innerwise IMAGO Game*
- *Live! The Healing Game of Life* by *innerwise*
- Please visit *www.innerwise.com/en/shop* for all other products, such as amulets, posters, discs, energizers or the E-Cover.

Videos

You can watch numerous videos on how to use *innerwise* at *www.youtube.com* and *www.innerwise.com*.

Mentors

Experienced *innerwise* mentors in a number of countries are glad to offer you guidance. You can find their contact information at *www.innerwise.com.*

Workshops and online courses

The following workshops are offered in different countries:
- *Yes/No: How to Use the Arm-Length Test*
- *Basic Workshop*
- *Intensive Workshop*
- *Intuitive Diagnostics*
- *Integrity—Success through Truthfulness*
- *Various Practice Workshops*

All workshops and online courses offer the opportunity to work with mentors directly so that everyone can find the support he or she needs.
Visit *www.innerwise.com* to find the dates of workshops and online courses.

Treatments and coachings

There's a growing number of experienced professional *innerwise* therapists and coaches worldwide.
Under **Coaches** at *www.innerwise.com,* you can find *innerwise* coaches and practitioners who have successfully completed the full educational program, have extensive experience working with *innerwise*, and participate in *innerwise* refresher programs on a regular basis.

Learn more on our website at www.innerwise.com.

Index

Checklists

These checklists comprise the basic parameters that should be checked on a regular basis and balanced as needed.

Permanent check

Your identity, "I am I," should always be clear. Don't let yourself be "off," that is, "beside yourself," if you want to enjoy life to the fullest!

Daily checkup:

	Optimal value	
Initial state	Arms equally long; balance	
Reaction to stress or "no"	Arms differ in length	
I am I	Yes	
Number of energy fields	1	

Weekly checkup

	Optimal value	
Life energy	100%	
Biological age	Younger than your actual age	
Actual creative potential	At least 30%	
Social maturity (alone, with your partner, at work, with your children)	Age-appropriate	
Heart	Stress-free	
Breathing	Stress-free	
Kidneys	Stress-free	
Liver, gallbladder	Stress-free	
Pancreas	Stress-free	
Nervous system: brain, spinal cord, nerves	Stress-free	
Autonomic nervous system: pelvic plexus, solar plexus, cervical plexus	Stress-free	
Yes to change	Stress-free	
Yes to love	Stress-free	
Yes to the body	Stress-free	
Yes to life	Stress-free	
Yes to honesty	Stress-free	

	Optimal value	
Yes to happiness	Stress-free	
Yes to health	Stress-free	

Monthly checkup

Organ tested	Balance or stress	Balancing healing cards or remedies
Liver		
Gallbladder		
Stomach		
Pancreas		
Spleen		
Blood		
Lymph		
Adrenal glands		
Kidneys		
Ureters, bladder		
Small intestine		
Large intestine		
Testicles, prostate		
Vagina, uterus, Fallopian tubes, ovaries		
Parasympathetic nervous system: pelvic plexus, cranial nerves		
Sympathetic nervous system: cervical plexus, solar plexus		
Diaphragm		
Breasts		
Heart		
Lungs		
Thyroid		
Teeth		
Sinuses		
Tonsils		
Ears		
Eyes		
Brain		
Nerves		
Skin		

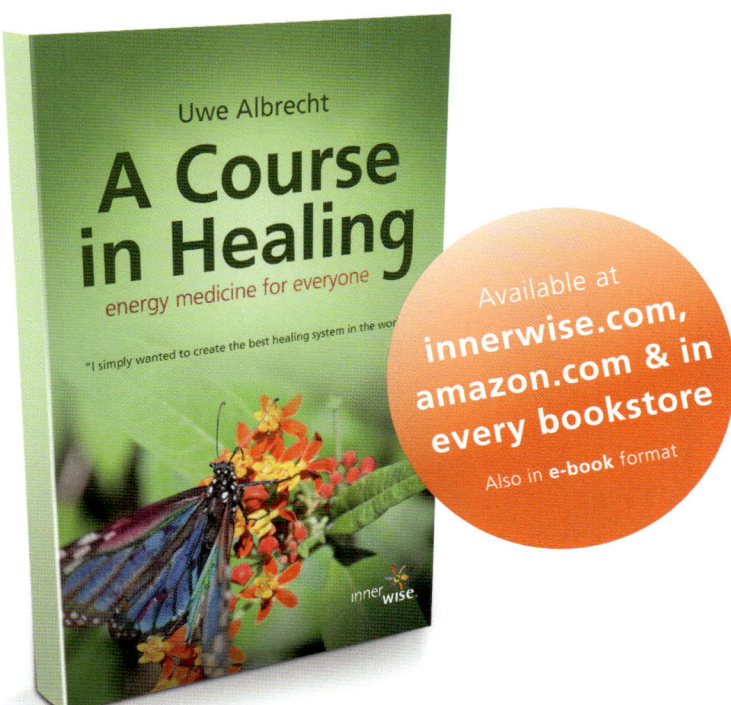
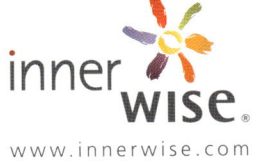

All about

inner**wise**

AND UWE ALBRECHT

• Story • Background • Videos • Coaches • Courses

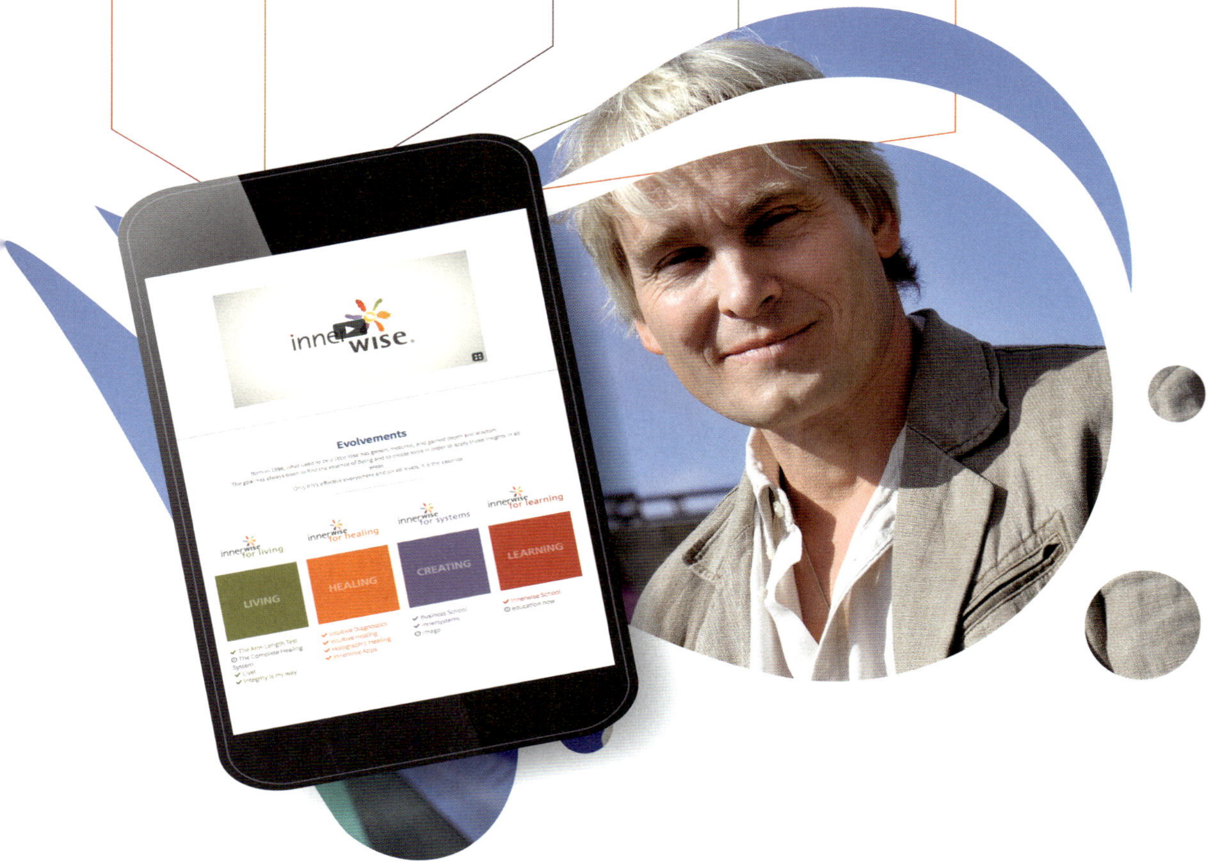

www.innerwise.com

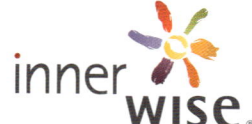

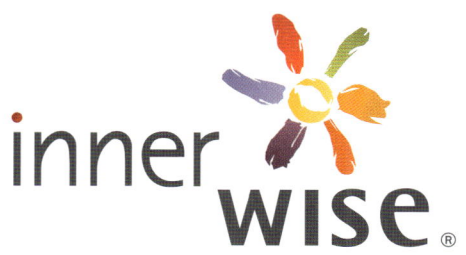

app.innerwise.com

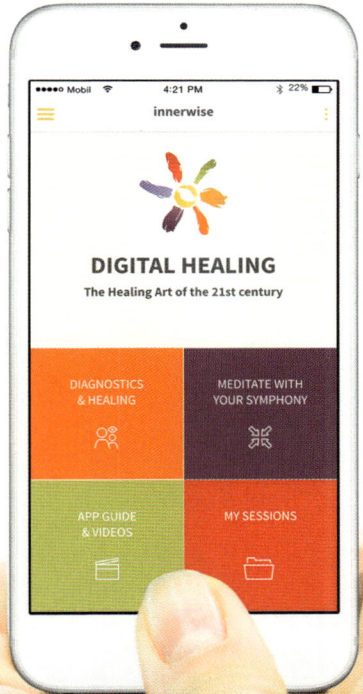

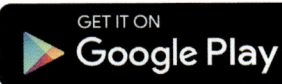

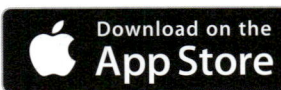

inner**wise**

Live
WORKSHOPS

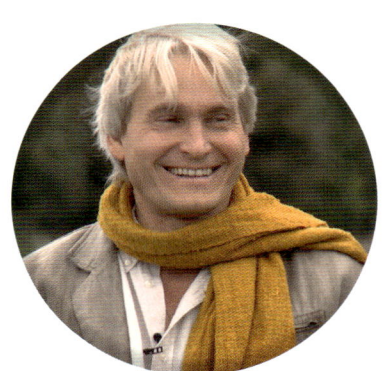

Learn _inner**wise** live_
from Uwe Albrecht
or a certified mentor.

▶ Small groups
▶ Lots of practical experience

Once you have completed the workshop, you will be ready to apply _inner**wise**_ and integrate it into your daily life and profession.

HEALING

YOURSELF

FAMILY

PETS

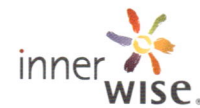

*inner*wise

Online
ACADEMY

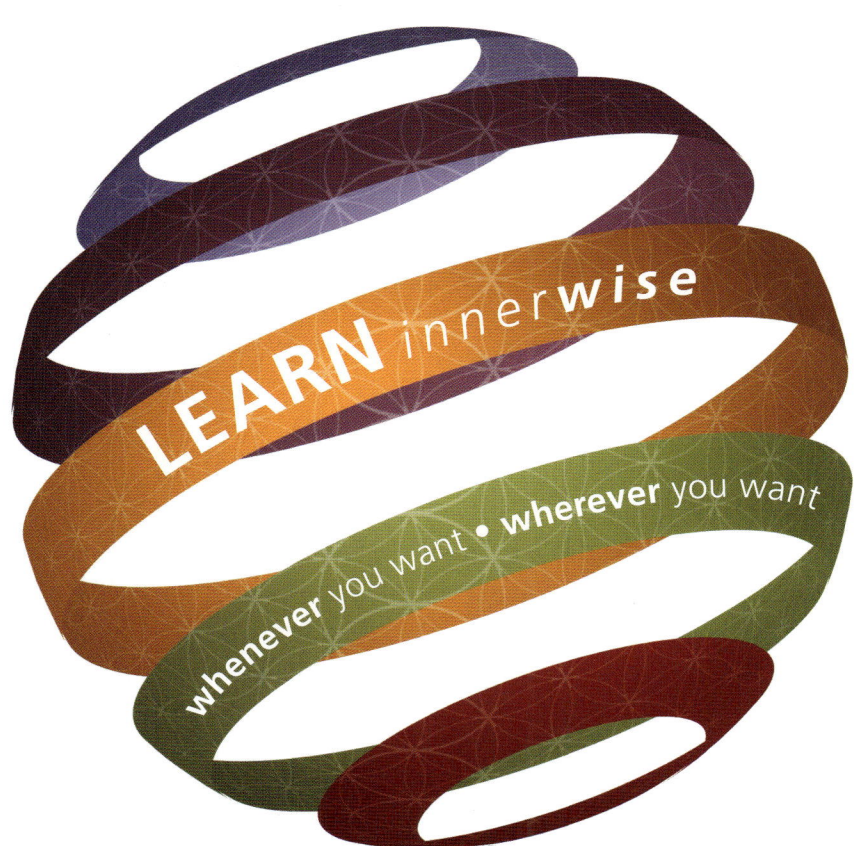

LEARN *inner*wise

whenever you want • **wherever** you want

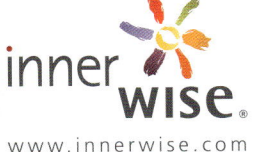

inner
wise®

www.innerwise.com

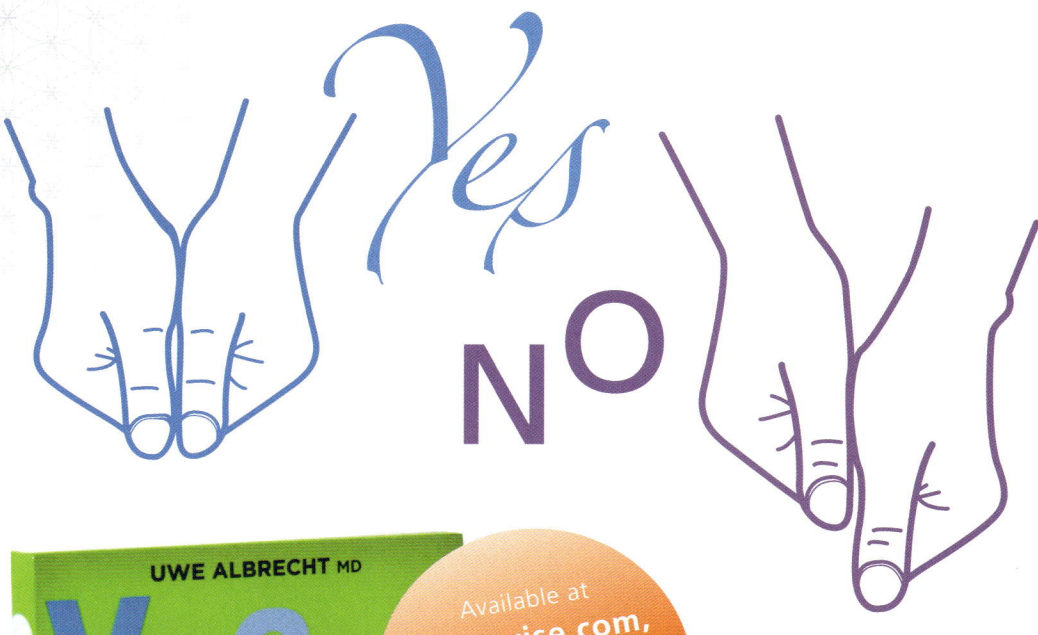
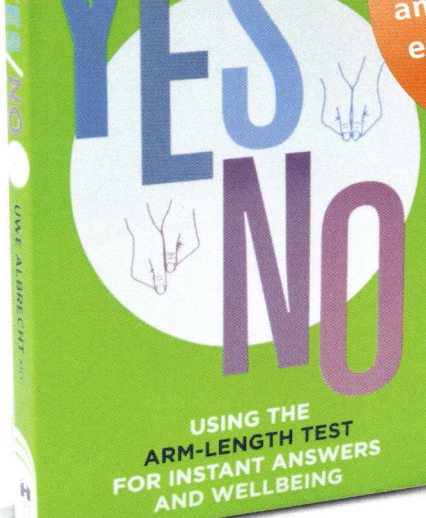
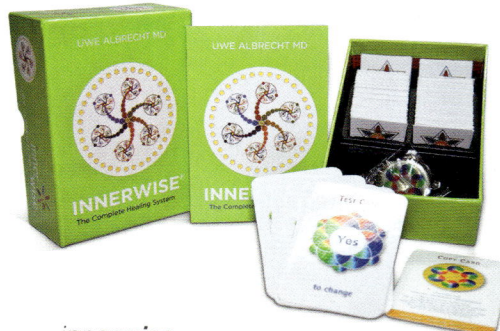
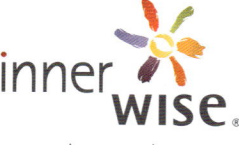